Robin Fisher
W9-AMQ-062

Multivariate Analysis
Part 1
Distributions, ordination and inference

KENDALL'S ADVANCED THEORY OF STATISTICS
and
KENDALL'S LIBRARY OF STATISTICS

Advisory Editorial Board: P J Green, University of Bristol; R J Little, University of Michigan; J K Ord, Pennsylvania State University, A J Scott, University of Auckland; S Weisberg, University of Minnesota

The development of statistical theory in the past fifty years is faithfully reflected in the history of the late Sir Maurice Kendall's volumes THE ADVANCED THEORY OF STATISTICS. The ADVANCED THEORY began life as a two volume work (Volume 1, 1943; Volume 2, 1946) and grew steadily, as a single authored work, until the late fifties. At that point, Alan Stuart became co-author and the ADVANCED THEORY was rewritten in three volumes. When Keith Ord joined in the early eighties, Volume 3 became the largest and plans were developed to expand, yet again, to a four-volume work. Even so, it became evident that there were gaps in the coverage and that it was becoming increasingly difficult to provide timely updates to all volumes, so a new strategy was devised.

In future, the ADVANCED THEORY will be in the form of three core volumes together with a series of related monographs. The three volumes will be:

1 Distribution Theory
2A Classical Inference and Relationships
2B Bayesian Inference (a new companion volume by Anthony O'Hagan)

The series of KENDALL'S LIBRARY OF STATISTICS monographs will encompass the areas previously appearing in the old Volume 3, such as sample surveys, design of experiments, multivariate analysis and time series as well as non-parametrics and log-linear models, previously covered to some extent in Volume 2. In the preface to the first edition of THE ADVANCED THEORY Kendall declared that his aim was "to develop a systematic treatment of [statistical] theory as it exists at the present time" while ensuring that the work remained "a book on statistics, not on statistical mathematics". These aims continue to hold true for KENDALL'S LIBRARY OF STATISTICS and the flexibility of the monograph format will enable the series to maintain comprehensive coverage over the whole of modern statistics.

Available: MULTIVARIATE ANALYSIS Part 1 Distributions, Ordination and Inference, W J Krzanowski (University of Exeter) and F H C Marriott (University of Oxford)
1994 300pp 0 340 59326 1

Forthcoming: MULTIVARIATE ANALYSIS Part 2 Classification, Covariance Structures and Repeated Measurements, W J Krzanowski (University of Exeter) and F H C Marriott (University of Oxford)
DESIGN OF COMPARATIVE EXPERIMENTS, R A Bailey (University of London)
STATISTICAL LOGIC, A P Dawid and M Stone (University of London)
ROBUST INFERENCE, T Hettmansperger (Pennsylvania State University) and J McKean (Western Michigan University)
TIME SERIES ANALYSIS, M Priestley (University of Manchester)
GENERALISED LINEAR MODELS, R Gilchrist (University of North London)

MULTIVARIATE ANALYSIS
Part 1
Distributions, ordination and inference

W J Krzanowski

Professor of Statistics, Department of Mathematical Statistics and Operational Research, University of Exeter, Exeter, UK

and

F H C Marriott

Department of Statistics, University of Oxford, Oxford, UK

Edward Arnold

A member of the Hodder Headline Group

LONDON MELBOURNE AUCKLAND

Copublished in the Americas by Halsted Press
an imprint of John Wiley & Sons Inc.
New York – Toronto

© 1994 Edward Arnold

First published in Great Britain 1994

Copublished in the Americas by Halsted Press, an imprint of John Wiley & Sons Inc., 605 Third Avenue, New York, NY 10158

British Library Cataloguing in Publication Data
Available upon request

ISBN 0 340 59326 1

Library of Congress Cataloguing in Publication Data
Available upon request

ISBN 0470 233826

All rights reserved. No part of this publication may be reproduced or transmitted in any form or by any means, electronically or mechanically, including photocopying, recording or any information storage or retrieval system, without either prior permission in writing from the publisher or a licence permitting restricted copying. In the United Kingdom such licences are issued by the Copyright Licensing Agency: 90 Tottenham Court Road, London W1P 9HE.

Every effort has been made to trace copyright holders of material reproduced in this book. Any rights not acknowledged here will be acknowledged in subsequent printings if notice is given to the publisher.

Printed and bound in Great Britain for Edward Arnold, a division of Hodder Headline PLC, 338 Euston Road, London NW1 3BH by the University Press, Cambridge

Preface

In late 1991 Edward Arnold approached us with an invitation to participate in what seemed an exciting venture: a radical updating of 'KENDALL'S ADVANCED THEORY OF STATISTICS', which would reflect the enormous growth of the subject since the first appearance of this classic work and provide a worthy successor to it for the start of the new century. The idea – of which Alan Stuart and J Keith Ord were the principal authors – was to have two central volumes containing all the core material which every statistician needs to know before he or she specialises, accompanied by a volume presenting the same objectives from a Bayesian viewpoint, and then to augment these central volumes with a library of advanced monographs covering all the various specialisations. Our task was to provide coverage of multivariate methodology for this library.

Mindful of Sir Maurice Kendall's special interest in multivariate analysis and multidimensional geometry, and remembering with affection his two early Griffin monographs on these topics, we felt honoured by the invitation. Our initial enthusiasm was somewhat tempered, however, when the full extent of our task became apparent. The breadth of the present-day subject surely demanded not just one, but two monographs! Also, how should the material be divided? Not without a certain amount of heartsearching, the split we finally agreed upon was that Part 1 should contain all the 'basic' material (such as data description, data visualisation and projection techniques, basic inference, general linear models, and nonlinear generalisations of the foregoing) while Part 2 would concentrate on 'specialised' techniques (such as discriminant analysis, cluster analysis, latent variable techniques, graphical modelling and path analysis, and repeated measure analysis). This book is the resulting Part 1; we are now wrestling with Part 2, and hope to have it ready for publication before too long.

Our philosophy for both volumes, broadly speaking, has been to adhere as far as possible to Kendall's original aims: to provide a comprehensive account of the subject as it currently stands, in as readable and 'user friendly' a fashion as possible. We have realised only too clearly as we have progressed that a full coverage of every topic of interest would result in an impossibly long and totally indigestible work, so we have not gone into unnecessary detail in the text but have either consigned it to the exercises at the end of each chapter or provided sufficient references for the reader to be able to fill it in for himself or herself. In addition, the exercises cover some rather more specialised algebraic extensions of the central ideas. Our hope is that the two volumes together will give a good overall picture of the subject as we reach the mid 1990s.

Since the first approach by James Griffin, we have been encouraged and guided by various other people at Edward Arnold, among whom we would particularly like to mention David Mackin, Richard Stileman and Diane Leadbetter-Conway. We are grateful to an anonymous reader who provided some useful comments on the first draft of the manuscript. As always, however, we accept full responsibility for any errors or infelicities (to echo Sir Maurice Kendall), and would be grateful to have them pointed out by readers. Last, but certainly not least, we must thank our long-suffering wives and families for their patience and support throughout the whole endeavour.

W J Krzanowski
Exeter

F H C Marriott
Oxford

Contents

	Preface	**v**
1	**Introduction**	**1**
	Multivariate data	1
	Populations and samples	6
	Multivariate description	7
	Models and inference	13
	Computer-intensive methods	15
	Missing values	16
	Scope of this book	17
2	**Multivariate Distributions**	**19**
	Distribution theory	19
	Marginal and conditional distributions	20
	Transformations	21
	Second order analysis	21
	The multivariate normal distribution	24
	Spherical and elliptical distributions	25
	The Dirichlet distribution	28
	Distributions for compositional data	29
	Generalisations of the Gamma distribution	31
	Multivariate discrete distributions	32
	The multinomial distribution	32
	The multivariate hypergeometric distribution	33
	The multivariate Poisson distribution	34
	Mixed binary and continuous data	35
	Multivariate stable distributions	36
	Matrix-valued distributions	39
	Exercises	40

3	**Initial Data Analysis**	**43**
	Graphical displays of multivariate data	43
	The detection of outliers	50
	Tests of normality	55
	Transformations of data	59
	Descriptive statistics for multivariate data	64
	Similarity, dissimilarity and distance	69
	Exercises	71
4	**Projections and Linear Transformations**	**75**
	Principal components	75
	Scaling	78
	Size and shape	79
	Population principal components	80
	Common principal components	81
	Choosing subsets of variables	82
	Three-mode component analysis	85
	Comparison with other techniques	85
	Biplots	86
	Canonical variables	88
	Canonical variables in classification	91
	Projection pursuit	92
	Criteria for projection pursuit	94
	Projection pursuit and significance testing	97
	Projection pursuit regression	97
	Projection pursuit density estimation	99
	Function optimisation	100
	Exercises	104
5	**Distance Methods and Ordination**	**105**
	Ordination	105
	Proximity matrices	105
	Geometrical objectives and fundamentals	106
	Metric scaling	108
	Non-metric scaling	115
	Individual differences	120
	Contingency tables	127
	Correspondence analysis	131
	Indicator matrices and higher-order tables	133
	Procrustes analysis	134
	Generalised Procrustes analysis	141
	Exercises	145
6	**Inference: Estimation and Hypothesis Testing**	**147**
	Point estimation	148
	Interval and region estimation	156
	Hypothesis testing	161
	Single-sample normal data: tests of the mean	163
	Single-sample normal data: tests of dispersion	166

	Multi-sample normal data	169
	Non-normality	172
	Exercises	174
7	**Multivariate Linear Models**	**177**
	The univariate linear model	177
	The multivariate linear model	179
	Multivariate calibration	180
	Inference in the multivariate linear model	181
	Multivariate analysis of variance	182
	Multivariate analysis of covariance	187
	Simultaneous inference	187
	Presentation of means	190
	Selection of variables	191
	Redundancy indices and redundancy analysis	192
	Exercise	194
8	**Nonlinear Methods**	**195**
	Nonlinear principal components	195
	Nonlinear biplots	200
	General nonlinear systems	203
	The Gifi system	204
	Distance approach	214
	Exercises	219
A	**Appendix A. Normal Theory Sampling Distributions**	**221**
	Multivariate generalisation of Student's t	221
	Further properties of the Mahalanobis distance	223
	The Wishart distribution	224
	Related distributions	225
	Likelihood ratio tests	226
	Union-intersection tests	228
	Testing linear models	229
	Choice of test statistic	232
	A test of dimensionality	233
	Eigenvalue distributions	235
	References	**237**
	Author Index	**267**
	Subject Index	**275**

1

Introduction

Multivariate data

1.1 Statistical data arise whenever any responses or attributes are either measured or observed on a set of individuals. Each particular response or attribute is referred to generally as a *variable* or *variate*; if just a single observation or measurement is made on each individual then the data are said to be *univariate*, whereas if more than one observation or measurement is made on each individual then the data are said to be *multivariate*. The values of any given variable can be taken at any of the recognised levels of measurement (i.e. nominal, ordinal, interval or ratio), but a more useful classification is probably into one of *quantitative* (i.e. numerical) or *qualitative* (i.e. categorical). A special case of a qualitative variable is one that has just two possible categories (e.g. presence or absence of a particular attribute), and such a variable is said to be *binary*.

A standard method of displaying a multivariate set of data is in the form of a *data matrix* in which rows correspond to sample individuals and columns to variables, so that the entry in the ith row and jth column gives the value of the jth variate as measured or observed on the ith individual. When presenting data in this form, it is customary to assign a numerical code to the categories of a qualitative variable and to label the variables by an algebraic symbol and subscript. For example, Table 1.1 gives a portion of a larger set of data obtained during an investigation into psycho-social influences on breast cancer in women. Here x_1 is a binary variable giving the menopausal status of the subject (0=pre-, 1=post-menopausal), x_2 is the age of the subject in years, x_3 is the age at menarche of the subject in years, x_4 and x_5 are both binary variables denoting presence (1) or absence (0) of allergy and thyroid disorder respectively, while x_6 is the subject's weight in kilograms.

An alternative tabulation when the variables are all categorical is in the form of a *contingency table*, which gives the incidences in the data set for all combinations of categories of each variable. Variables x_1, x_4 and x_5 from Table 1.1 are tabulated in this manner in Table 1.2.

Table 1.1 Data concerning psycho-social influences on breast cancer. Reproduced with permission from Krzanowski (1988a)

Unit	x_1	x_2	x_3	x_4	x_5	x_6
1	1	49	15	1	1	52.46
2	0	59	17	1	1	60.83
3	0	49	11	1	0	48.70
4	0	58	14	1	1	57.33
5	1	49	13	0	1	64.26
6	1	43	11	1	0	53.90
7	0	46	16	1	1	52.45
8	0	59	14	1	1	66.18
9	0	53	14	1	0	49.54
10	0	51	11	1	1	53.88
11	0	50	21	0	0	58.46
12	1	50	16	1	1	50.22

Table 1.2 Contingency table showing the incidences for the three binary variables of Table 1.1

		Thyroid Disorder Present	Thyroid Disorder Absent
Pre-menopause	Allergy Present	5	2
	Allergy Absent	0	1
Post-menopause	Allergy Present	2	1
	Allergy Absent	1	0

1.2 The popularity of multivariate analysis has spread rapidly over the past twenty years, fuelled in the main by the dramatic advances in computing power, by the easy accessibility of increasingly sophisticated software, and by the pervading culture in research that demands a firm quantitative basis for any conclusions reached. The upshot is that multivariate data sets can now be found in almost every branch of study, including some in which quantitative work would have been almost unthinkable at one time. The following brief list gives some examples of typical multivariate data sets, as well as demonstrating the range of possible applications.

- Agriculture: Fenlon and Beever (1976) give the net flows of sixteen amino acids in grams/day across the rumen of 96 wether sheep that had been distributed among 33 different diets.
- Archaeology: Brothwell and Krzanowski (1974) describe the analysis of a data set comprising eleven cranial vault measurements taken on a large number of skulls from various different burial sites in Great Britain.
- Biometry: Corbet *et al* (1970) consider the differences between British and European water voles, using thirteen epigenetic characters observed on each vole.

- Chemistry: McReynolds (1970) gives the gas chromatography retention indices of ten representative test compounds on 226 different liquid phases.
- Education: Yule *et al* (1969) give the results of ten cognitive tests from the Wechler series as applied to 150 children graded according to reading ability.
- Geology: Chernoff (1973) analyses data on twelve variables representing mineral contents from a 4500-foot core drilled from a Colorado mountain-side.
- History/Classics: Boneva (1971) lists the incidences of thirty-two different sentence endings in the 45 works of Plato.
- Medicine: Armitage *et al*, (1969) consider the problem of distinguishing between success and failure of ablation on a sample of women suffering from breast cancer, using a variety of diagnostic indicators.
- Psychiatry: Everitt and Dunn (1991, p230) present a subset of the data obtained in a large psychiatric study in which normal people and people diagnosed by the psychiatrist as ill were asked a series of questions relating to feelings of tension, inadequacy etc.
- Psychology: Fleishman and Hempel (1954) report the results of administering eighteen tests concerned with such matters as mechanical aptitude, rate of movement, comprehension of spatial relations, and so on to 197 airmen.
- Sociology: Hartigan (1975a) gives the number of crimes of different types per 100 000 population in various American cities.
- Soil Science: Webster and McBratney (1981) consider methods for the analysis of measurements on soil profiles sampled along a transect. A typical soil science set of data, taken from Kendall (1980, p20), is given in Table 1.3 showing percentages of sand content (x_1), silt content (x_2), clay content (x_3) and organic matter (x_4) along with pH (x_5) of 20 soil samples.

1.3 The above examples contain multivariate data sets of modest size and exhibiting a traditional structure, in that the number of individuals exceeds (sometimes greatly) the number of measured variables. These are perhaps the typical sorts of data set that classical multivariate techniques were designed to handle. More recently, however, various electronic and other automatic data recording devices have been developed which enable data to be gathered much more easily than before. This has led to the collection of much larger data sets. Moreover, these data sets are often ones in which the number of variables greatly exceeds the number of sample members. Thus modern multivariate data sets incur a number of new problems, and give rise to additional questions. We give here a few examples; it is convenient to classify such data sets into several distinct categories.

The first such category contains all those data sets in which the observations on each individual (or sample member) comprise a *function* rather than a few discrete values. One common application is that of spectroscopic data, as found in the modern area of chemometrics. Here a chemical sample is exposed to an energy source, and the resulting absorbance is recorded as a continuous trace over a range of wavelengths. Mark and Tunnell (1985) give a number of examples, including the one shown in Fig. 1.1 for two samples. Such a trace is

Table 1.3 Five variables observed on each of 20 soil samples; see text for description of variables. Reproduced with permission from Kendall (1980).

Soil sample	x_1	x_2	x_3	x_4	x_5
1	77.3	13.0	9.7	1.5	6.4
2	82.5	10.0	7.5	1.5	6.5
3	66.9	20.6	12.5	2.3	7.0
4	47.2	33.8	19.0	2.8	5.8
5	65.3	20.5	14.2	1.9	6.9
6	83.3	10.0	6.7	2.2	7.0
7	81.6	12.7	5.7	2.9	6.7
8	47.8	36.5	15.7	2.3	7.2
9	48.6	37.1	14.3	2.1	7.2
10	61.6	25.5	12.9	1.9	7.3
11	58.6	26.5	14.9	2.4	6.7
12	69.3	22.3	8.4	4.0	7.0
13	61.8	30.8	7.4	2.7	6.4
14	67.7	25.3	7.0	4.8	7.3
15	57.2	31.2	11.6	2.4	6.5
16	67.2	22.7	10.1	3.3	6.2
17	59.2	31.2	9.6	2.4	6.0
18	80.2	13.2	6.6	2.0	5.8
19	82.2	11.1	6.7	2.2	7.2
20	69.7	20.7	9.6	3.1	5.9

then digitised by reading off the absorbances at suitably chosen (usually, closely spaced) wavelengths, and the latter form the variables of the data set. Pyrolysis mass spectroscopy yields about 200 such variables for each chemical sample, near infrared spectroscopy yields about 700, while infrared spectroscopy yields around 1700. Other related molecular activity techniques can yield up to 4000 variables. In all of these cases the number of chemical samples is usually severely restricted, often to fewer than 100, so a very unbalanced data set is the end product. Brown *et al* (1991) discuss statistical matters associated with such data sets.

Spectroscopic data result from measurement of absorbance arising from an energy source; similar continuous traces, and hence similar statistical problems, are encountered by measurement of sound (e.g. in speech recognition problems – see Juang and Rabiner, 1991) or by monitoring electrical impulses (e.g in electroencephalogram or in electrocardiogram analyses – see van Bemmel, 1982), or by taking continuous measurements off a motion picture. An interesting example of the last-named is that of gait analysis (Olshen *et al*, 1989), in which the angular rotations of various joints in the body are recorded continuously while a subject walks a given distance. Fig. 1.2 shows the traces obtained from the hips of 39 normal 5-year-old children, over a gait cycle consisting of one (double) step taken by each child.

It may be that the measurements do not form a continuous trace which has to be digitised, but are already discrete values that can be treated as the individual variables. Such situations arise when a single quantity is measured repeatedly over a certain period of time. The inevitable correlations between successive values of the observation suggest that a good way of treating the

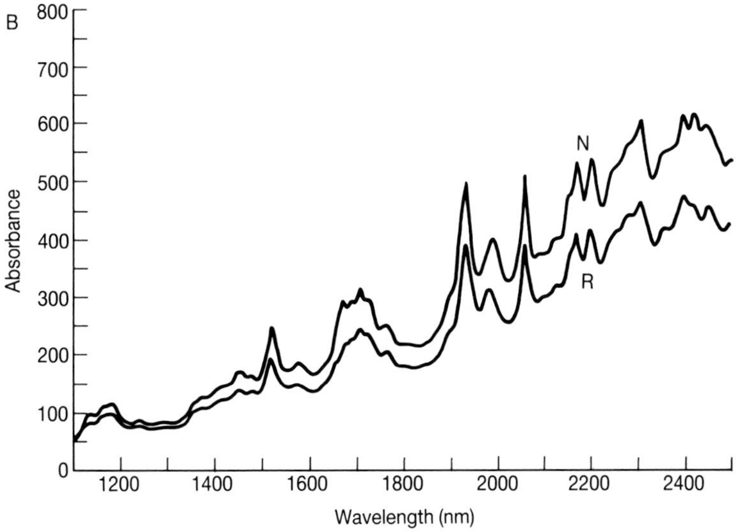

Figure 1.1 Spectroscopic traces of two chemical samples. Reproduced with permission from Mark and Tunnell (1985).

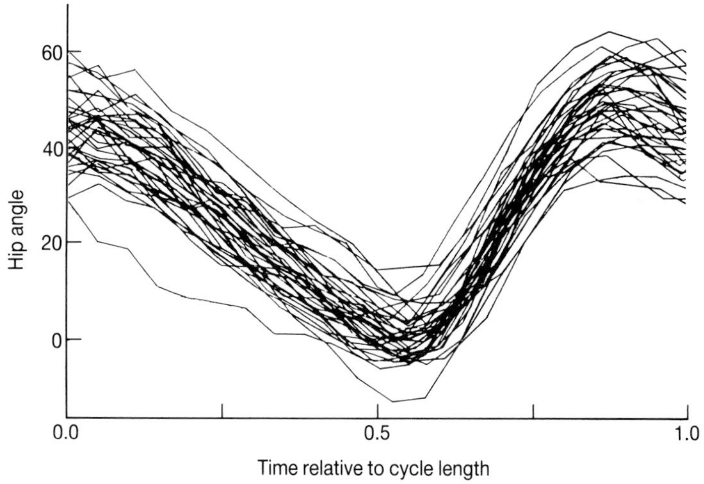

Figure 1.2 Observed records of angular rotation of the hip in the saggital plane over one gait cycle in each of 39 subjects. Reproduced with permission from Rice and Silverman (1991).

measurements is to view each time point as a separate variable, and then a particular time sequence of values can be treated as a single multivariate observation. For example, the blood haemoglobin might be measured at weekly intervals for a period of three months after calving for a number of cows, or seismic readings might be taken every hour for several days after a shock is experienced in a particular geographic region. A common objective is to distinguish between two or more groups on the basis of such readings (for example between cows on several different feed regimes, or between earthquakes and shocks experienced after an underground nuclear test). If the number of time points is large, then these problems can be classed as discrimination between time series (Shumway, 1982).

The second category of modern multivariate data sets comprises all those sets that involve the reconstruction and classification of *images* from observed measurements that are subject to various forms of degradation, such as blurring, noise or geometrical distortion. Typical instances of such data arise in geography (remote sensing of an area of the earth's surface from a satellite by means of a multispectral scanner – Swain, 1982), medicine (photon emission tomography – Aykroyd and Green, 1991) and astronomy (Ripley and Sutherland, 1990). In all these applications, multivariate observations (typically from a set of spectral components) are available for each point (*pixel*) of a rectangular area of material (ground, bodily organ, or portion of sky respectively in the examples above). The area in question usually contains very many such pixels (typical numbers being 64×64, 128×128 or 512×512) and the pixels are themselves spatially correlated (thereby introducing further complications into any analysis). The usual objectives of the analysis are to identify specific patterns in the data or to classify the pixels into one of a given number of types.

A third category of data set associated with digitised readings is one concerned with *shapes* of individuals. Such data sets arise commonly in biology, archaeology, astronomy and cartography, but have also been increasingly evident in medicine, geology, geophysics and other sciences. The data usually consist of the coordinates of p labelled points (or *landmarks*) for each individual. For example, Moss *et al* (1987) give such data from radiographs of the lateral (sagittal) sections of close-bred, pre-weaned male rats 21 days old; here there were $p = 20$ landmarks digitised for each of 10 rats in each of 4 dietary regimes imposed on the mother, and the substantive question to be investigated was whether differences in shapes of the rats' skulls could be associated with differences in dietary regime. The special feature of such data is that the shapes of all individuals are invariant under translation, rotation and reflection so that any analysis must take this feature into account.

Having surveyed the most common types of multivariate data encountered in practice, we now turn to an overview of the methods that have been developed for analysing such data.

Populations and samples

1.4 Statistical investigations generally concern some form of description of a *population* of individuals, typically by attaching numerical values to a *parameter* (or parameters) of interest. These parameters are usually simple descriptors of location (e.g. mean, median, mode, etc.), dispersion (e.g. variance, standard deviation, range, etc.) or association (e.g. covariance, correlation, etc.). Sometimes it may be possible to observe the values of any variables of interest on *all* the individuals in a population; for example, the heights could be measured for all students in a particular city, or the number of syllables could be counted for all the sentences in the works of Plato. In this case the relevant descriptors for each variable or pair of variables are the appropriate summary statistics (mean, variance, correlation, etc) calculated from all the population values. However, more commonly, it is not possible to observe all individuals in a population (either because the population is very large or because it consists of an infinite number of hypothetical values) and it is necessary to take a *sample.* By following well-established statistical procedures (see, e.g. Barnett, 1974) it is possible to ensure that the sampling preserves independence among individuals and is as efficient as possible. Nevertheless, any summary values computed from these individuals pertain only to the sample, and *statistical inference* is required if statements are to be made about the population. Probability models form the cornerstone of statistical inference, and statements about populations then involve such techniques as point and interval estimates or hypothesis tests which have such models as their basis. Volume 1 of Kendall's *Advanced Theory of Statistics* (Stuart and Ord, 1987) is devoted to probability models and Volume 2 (Stuart and Ord, 1991) to inferential aspects for the univariate case.

The general principles remain the same in the multivariate case, but description of a population now involves more measurements and hence more parameters. Each individual has a number, p say, of variables observed on it. These variables can be denoted by the vector $\boldsymbol{x}' = (x_1, \ldots, x_p)$, while the actual values observed for the ith individual can then be written as the vector $\boldsymbol{x}'_i = (x_{i1}, \ldots, x_{ip})$. If n individuals have been observed then the data matrix has size $(n \times p)$, and $\boldsymbol{x}'_i$ forms the ith row of the matrix. Description of the data thus requires a summary in some sense of the patterns existing among this set of numbers.

To assist in such description, it is convenient to adopt a geometric approach. We can associate an orthogonal axis in p-dimensional Euclidean space with each observed variable x_j, and treat the values $(x_{i1}, \ldots, x_{ip})$ of these variables for an individual as coordinates of a point in this space. In this way the data matrix can be represented as n points in space, and a description of the data can be effected by describing the structure of these points. If the data comprise the whole population, or a non-random subset that can equivalently be treated as a population, then such description is all that is required and any relevant technique can be termed *descriptive multivariate analysis.* If the data are a random sample, however, then we are really after a description of the parent population and we first need to formulate a probability model for this population. This model specifies the likely distribution of all possible individuals from the population throughout the p-dimensional space; a description of the structure of this distribution is the province of *inferential multivariate analysis.*

We now give an informal overview of the problems that are tackled in each of these areas, and a brief introduction to some of the multivariate techniques that have been developed for this purpose.

Multivariate description

1.5 If the multivariate data set does not have any probabilistic aspect, either because it is the complete population of study or because it is a non-random subset of a population (e.g. all patients arriving for treatment at a doctor's

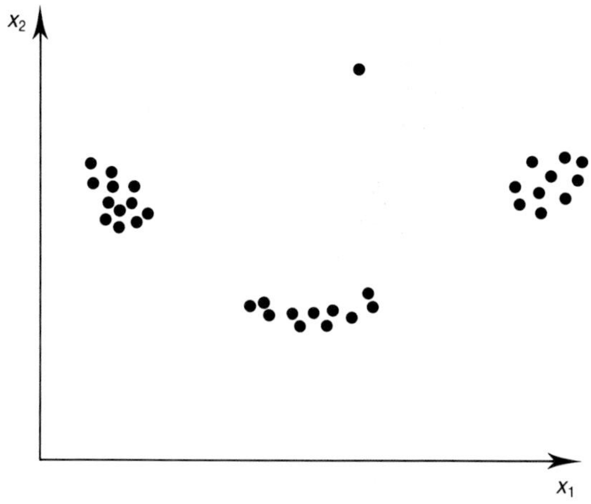

Figure 1.3 Pictorial representation of a bivariate sample

surgery), then our primary objective is to simplify the data and uncover any patterns or structure that may be present. For example, it is of interest to determine whether there are any relationships, either linear or nonlinear, among the variables; whether the individuals fall into more or less distinct groups as opposed to constituting a single homogeneous mass; whether there are any outliers, unusual features or influential observations present, and so on. Such features will show up readily in the geometrical representation described above, but the question is how to visualise this representation. There is no problem in depicting a bivariate sample, as n points in 2 dimensions can be plotted easily; Fig. 1.3 shows such a bivariate sample in which the individuals exhibit three distinct groups, there is a moderately strong nonlinear relationship between the two variables, and there is also one very clear outlier.

Suppose now, however, that the number of variables is substantially more than two. Then the visual presentation of the scatter of points can only be handled by projecting it on to planes. This visual presentation can be thought of as viewing the points in (p-dimensional) space through suitable (two-dimensional) 'windows'. The problem is that, just as different windows will provide different views of the outside world so will different planes highlight different features of the data; the best plane for showing up a nonlinear relationship will not generally be the same plane that identifies the outliers in the data or highlights the separation into several groups. Consequently, much effort has been invested in the multivariate area into finding the most useful projections of a data set for highlighting specific features of interest. Moreover, if it is known *a priori* that some structure exists, then this knowledge can be built into the multivariate technique. For example, if the data matrix is known to consist of individuals from a given number of distinct groups, then we might seek the projection of the data that maximally emphasises this particular grouping.

There is a further matter associated with such descriptive techniques, namely that of interpreting the resulting projections. Any plane in p-dimensional space

Table 1.4 Coefficients in linear combinations of white leghorn fowl data

Original variable	Coefficients a_i y_1	y_2	y_3	y_4	y_5	y_6
x_1	0.35	0.53	0.76	-0.04	0.02	0.00
x_2	0.33	0.70	-0.64	0.00	0.00	0.03
x_3	0.44	-0.19	-0.05	0.53	0.18	0.67
x_4	0.44	-0.25	0.02	0.48	-0.15	-0.71
x_5	0.44	-0.28	-0.06	-0.50	0.65	-0.13
x_6	0.44	-0.22	-0.05	-0.48	-0.69	0.17

can be defined by specifying two lines at right angles within it. Moreover, if the axes of the space are associated with the variables x_i as described above, then any line in this space is defined by an appropriate linear combination $a_1x_1 + \ldots + a_px_p$ of the variables. Given the physical interpretation of each x_i, it is often possible to interpret a linear combination of the x_i in terms of a physically meaningful quantity. Hence it may be possible to associate a simple meaning with each axis of any obtained projection, and gain further insight into the data under study. Such a process of interpretation is known as *reification.* Although it has long been used by multivariate analysts, it is still a topic of current interest and research (see Arnold and Collins, 1993). Another current application of multivariate projections is in the context of dynamic and interactive graphics, where a series of appropriate two-dimensional projections are sought either as scatterplot matrices or in such a way as to provide a continuously varying three-dimensional 'view' of the data. Linking successive projections gives the possibility of 'spinning' the views and 'brushing out' particular observations from the picture. Weihs and Schmidli (1990) describe a computational strategy for such online multivariate exploratory graphical analysis.

Example 1.1

Table 1.4 presents the coefficients in six linear combinations $y_1, \ldots, y_6$ obtained from a principal component analysis (see Chapter 4) of six bone measurements $x_1, \ldots, x_6$ made on each of 275 white leghorn fowl (Wright, 1954). The six original measurements were: skull length (x_1), skull breadth (x_2), humerus (x_3), ulna (x_4), femur (x_5) and tibia (x_6). Thus the first two were skull measurements, the third and fourth were wing measurements, and the last two were leg measurements. In interpreting derived variables, we can ignore any coefficients 'close to' zero (as the corresponding variables will hardly contribute to the derived quantity) and we can round values fairly liberally in order to simplify matters.

We can now interpret each of the derived variables y_i of Table 1.4 quite easily. For y_1, all coefficients are approximately equal (to 0.4). Thus y_1 is approximately equal to $0.4(x_1 + x_2 + x_3 + x_4 + x_5 + x_6)$. Now large fowl will tend to have large values for all x_i and hence for y_1, while small fowl will tend to have small values for all x_i and hence for y_1. Thus y_1 can be interpreted as a measure of 'size' of the fowl. For y_2, we note that the coefficients of x_1 and x_2 are not very different (and positive) while the other four coefficients are negative and approximately equal. Thus y_2 is approximately of the form $a(x_1 + x_2) - b(x_3 + x_4 + x_5 + x_6)$. Fowl with large x_1, x_2 (i.e large heads) but small x_3, x_4, x_5, x_6 (i.e small wings and legs) will have the most extreme values on the positive side of y_2, and conversely those with small heads but large wings and legs will have the most extreme values on the negative side of y_2. Consequently, y_2 measures 'body shape' of the fowl.

The remaining derived variables follow a similar reasoning to that of y_2 for their interpretation, but with the additional feature that coefficients near to zero imply that the corresponding x_i can be ignored. Thus we have approximately (for constants c, d, e, f):

- $y_3 = c(x_1 - x_2)$ ('head shape');
- $y_4 = d(x_3 + x_4 - x_5 - x_6)$ (again a 'body shape', but this time contrasting just wings and legs);
- $y_5 = e(x_5 - x_6)$ ('leg shape');
- $y_6 = f(x_3 - x_4)$ ('wing shape').

1.6 Projection techniques, as described in the previous section, are based on the notion that there exists a configuration of points in a higher dimensional space, and this in turn requires the multivariate data to be quantitative so that data values can be used as coordinates of points. This feature seems to exclude multivariate qualitative data from this body of descriptive techniques. However, all such projections can be viewed as methods of obtaining two-dimensional approximations to a p-dimensional scatter of points, and alternative ways of achieving this objective are possible. One such way is to construct *directly* a two-dimensional configuration which optimises some goodness-of-fit function based on the p-dimensional scatter, and a possible such function is one that matches all inter-point distances in the two-dimensional configuration with their counterparts in the full space. For example, if D_{ij} is the distance between points i and j in p dimensions and d_{ij} is the distance between the corresponding points in two dimensions, then we might seek the two-dimensional representation that minimises the discrepancy $V_1 = \sum_i \sum_j (D_{ij}^2 - d_{ij}^2)$, or perhaps the one that minimises $V_2 = \sum_i \sum_j (D_{ij} - d_{ij})^2$, or even the one that minimises $V_3 = \sum_i \sum_j w_{ij}(D_{ij} - d_{ij})^2$ for selected weights w_{ij}.

It turns out that constructing a two-dimensional configuration to minimise V_1 subject to the constraint that $d_{ij} \leqslant D_{ij}$ for all i, j produces exactly the same configuration that is obtained on projecting the data into the plane that maximises the scatter of the points. Thus we can derive this projection in effect *without* starting from a p-dimensional configuration of points; all we need are the computed inter-point distances. Now the idea of distance between two points in space can be linked readily to the concept of 'dissimilarity' between the two sample individuals that the points represent, and there are many possible ways of measuring this dissimilarity. Moreover, dissimilarity can be measured from qualitative variables just as well as from quantitative ones, so that we can readily find all inter-object dissimilarities for such data. Thus we can obtain a configuration of points that represent the objects and for which

Table 1.5 Data on mean mandible measurements for groups of canines. Taken from Manly (1986).

Group	x_1	x_2	x_3	x_4	x_5	x_6
Modern Thai dog	9.7	21.0	19.4	7.7	32.0	36.5
Golden jackal	8.1	16.7	18.3	7.0	30.3	32.9
Chinese wolf	13.5	27.3	26.8	10.6	41.9	48.1
Indian wolf	11.5	24.3	24.5	9.3	40.0	44.6
Cuon	10.7	23.5	21.4	8.5	28.8	37.6
Dingo	9.6	22.6	21.1	8.3	34.4	43.1
Prehistoric dog	10.3	22.1	19.1	8.1	32.3	35.0

the inter-point distances approximate the inter-object dissimilarities, in the sense of minimising one of the above functions. This means that descriptive geometrical techniques exist for multivariate qualitative as well as quantitative data. Techniques that produce such configurations are grouped under the general title of *multidimensional scaling*.

1.7 All the above descriptive techniques work by providing a geometrical picture representing the data, and then allowing the analyst to inspect this picture and determine whether there are any patterns in the data. The main problem with them is that the pictures on which the deductions are based are usually low-dimensional *approximations* to the true pictures, so that some distortion is almost inevitable. Consequently, false deductions are always a possibility.

An alternative approach is to use the *full* set of data, but to seek some other compression of information for descriptive purposes. One way of doing this is to attempt a partition of the data into subgroups, in such a way that individuals within a subgroup are 'similar', while individuals in different subgroups are 'dissimilar'. This type of data summary had its origins in biology (more precisely in numerical taxonomy), but is nowadays applied in very many different disciplines. It is generally termed *cluster analysis*, and it has a number of variants. *Optimisation* methods of cluster analysis produce the partition of the data into a specified number of groups by optimising some suitable objective function similar in spirit to the functions V_1, V_2 or V_3 above (Marriott, 1982). *Hierarchical* cluster analysis, on the other hand, provides a complete 'family tree' (*dendrogram*) of partitions, in which the g-group solution is obtained by splitting one of the groups in the $(g-1)$-group solution (or the $(g-1)$-group solution is obtained by fusing two of the groups in the g-group solution). Such a tree provides an overview of the data structure, and allows the analyst to choose the most appropriate number of groups for summarisation. A review of the methodology is given by Cormack (1971).

Hierarchical clustering has traditionally been the most popular approach, partly because of its relative ease of computation and partly because it reproduces the sort of structures familiar in biology (i.e. divisions of organisms into genera, species, families etc). However, recent increases in availability of computing power has produced an upsurge of interest in optimisation methods.

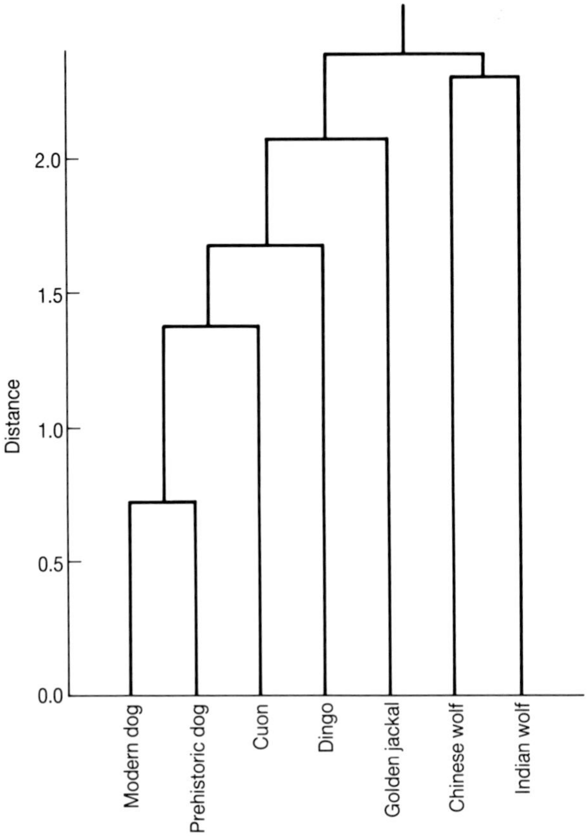

Figure 1.4 Dendrogram from nearest-neighbour cluster analysis of canine data. Reproduced with permission from Manly (1986).

Example 1.2

Table 1.5 shows some data on mean mandible measurements (mm) of different groups of canines, extracted by Manly (1986, p10) from Higham *et al* (1980). The variables are breadth of mandible (x_1), height of mandible below first molar (x_2), length of first molar (x_3), breadth of first molar (x_4), length from first to third molars inclusive (x_5), and length from first to fourth premolars inclusive (x_6). Manly summarises this table by a dendrogram (Fig. 1.4) computed from a nearest-neighbour cluster analysis of the canine groups, and concludes from this dendrogram that the prehistoric dog is closely related to the modern Thai dog, with both of these being somewhat related to the cuon and dingo and less closely to the golden jackal. The Indian and Chinese wolves are closest to each other, but the difference between them is relatively large.

Models and inference

1.8 If the data are a random sample from some population or populations and the objective is to describe these populations, then the first step is to choose an appropriate probability model for them. There are many different multivariate distributions that can be used for this purpose, including generalisations of most of the familiar univariate distributions. However, by reason of tractability on the mathematical side and the central limit theorem on the statistical side, the overwhelming majority of cases of inferential multivariate analysis of quantitative data use the multivariate normal distribution as the underlying model. This distribution is governed by two parameters, the vector $\boldsymbol{\mu}$ (location) and the matrix $\boldsymbol{\Sigma}$ (dispersion). The former fixes the position of the centre of the population in the p-dimensional data space, while the latter quantifies the scatter of potential points in this space and characterises the associations between the variables. Multivariate inference mainly centres upon these parameters.

1.9 All the familiar techniques of univariate inference extend to the multivariate case in an obvious way, but with some additional features induced by the higher dimensionality of the data. *Point* estimation of $\boldsymbol{\mu}$ and $\boldsymbol{\Sigma}$ provides a single sample quantity for each parameter, these quantities estimating respectively the centre and spread of the population in the data space. In place of univariate confidence intervals for the mean, however, we now need to find a confidence *region* for $\boldsymbol{\mu}$ in view of the higher dimensionality, while region estimates for $\boldsymbol{\Sigma}$ are not in general a practical proposition. Derivation of *hypothesis tests* about either parameter is founded on similar principles to those of the univariate case, but for many of the standard multivariate tests there now exist a number of competing test statistics. This is because most null hypotheses specify a unique point in data space, but the corresponding alternative hypotheses can be satisfied in various ways and each competing statistic will be geared to detecting departures from the null hypothesis in one of these ways.

For example, suppose that there are k populations and the null hypothesis is that all their means are equal. In both univariate and multivariate cases the general alternative hypothesis of 'nonequal' means can be satisfied if the means all differ from each other, or if one differs from the rest which are all equal, or if there are two different groups of coincident means, and so on. However, in the multivariate case there are additional possibilities: a set of nonequal means could lie on a line in space, or on a smooth curve, or at the corners of a simplex, or they could have some less regular arrangement. Different test statistics will in general be best for different structures. Finally, imposition of a *linear model* structure on the means of a set of populations can be done exactly as in univariate analysis, and the associated regression and analysis of variance techniques then find direct multivariate counterparts.

1.10 In addition to these direct univariate generalisations, multivariate inference exhibits a number of special features. Consider first inferences about means. Suppose again that the sample observations comprise values from k populations and that a test of hypothesis has established that the means of the populations differ in some way. The experimenter will often wish to investigate the nature of these differences further. In the univariate case there is not much trouble in doing this, because the k sample means can be ranked along a single dimension and then either individual tests of selected pairs of means, or multiple comparisons among the means, can be conducted to determine the structure among the groups. While multivariate generalisations of such tests do exist, the more important aspect is the descriptive one of inspecting differences among the sample means, but the data are now in a higher dimensionality and can no longer be ranked uniquely. This problem can be overcome if we are able to link a projection of the data into a small dimensionality with the testing of mean differences, and the most appropriate projection will be one which maximises group separations in some sense. A multivariate technique for achieving this objective is *canonical variate analysis*.

A second, allied, problem arises in the same context if we envisage receiving future observations that are known to come from one of the k populations but not which one, and we would like to use the available variable values to identify the population from which a particular observation has come. Intuitively, one believes that the more variables that are measured, the more information we have about each individual and hence the more likely we are to allocate the individual to the correct population. For example, in a medical context, we may have a collection of signs, symptoms and laboratory measurements for a set of patients suffering from jaundice. Jaundice has a number, say k, of possible causes. Moreover, some of these can be treated by administration of drugs while others need surgery for successful cure, and the latter is both expensive and potentially dangerous for the patient. Thus when a new patient presents for treatment we would like to decide as accurately as possible the cause of the jaundice and whether surgery or medication is needed for treatment. If we only wish to use the signs, symptoms and laboratory measurements as a basis for this decision then we are in the province of multivariate *discriminant analysis*; a *discriminant function* can be constructed from the records of those previous patients whose 'true' diagnosis is known (either from previously successful treatment or from post-mortem examination!) and then this function can be used to *classify* each new patient to one of the salient populations. Statistical problems associated with this technique include the estimation of likely success rates with it, and the incorporation of external information into the allocation rule.

1.11 Turning next to inferences about the dispersion matrix, a particular facet that is specific to multivariate situations is the explanation of associations that exist between the variables. Typically, there is an association between two variables if they have some feature in common. Of course, in some cases the mere fact that two variables are measured on the same individuals is enough to account for the observed association. For example, Table 1.6 gives the correlation matrix between the six variables measured on the fowl of Example 1.1. Most entries in this matrix are moderately large and positive because the variables are bone measurements so will tend to be large or small together, depending on the size of an individual fowl.

However, in some cases it is plausible to postulate that there exists some deeper reason for a set of observed associations. For example, consider the

Table 1.6 Correlation matrix for white leghorn fowl data

x_1	1.000					
x_2	0.505	1.000				
x_3	0.569	0.422	1.000			
x_4	0.602	0.467	0.926	1.000		
x_5	0.621	0.482	0.877	0.874	1.000	
x_6	0.603	0.450	0.878	0.894	0.937	1.000
	x_1	x_2	x_3	x_4	x_5	x_6

data presented by Yule *et al* (1969). Here, the following subtests from the Wechsler Preschool and Primary Scale of Intelligence were measured on 150 children aged between $4\frac{1}{2}$ and $6\frac{1}{2}$ years: Information, Vocabulary, Arithmetic, Similarities, Comprehension, Animal house, Picture completion, Mazes, Geometric design and Block design. A correlation matrix computed from this sample again yields positive and moderately large associations among all pairs of variables. In this case it would be reasonable to suppose that there exists a small set of skills that are not directly measurable, such as 'general intelligence', 'verbal facility', 'spatial awareness', 'arithmetic ability', and so on. Each child possesses a particular level of each skill, and a child's score on each subtest is made up of some mixture of these levels plus a random component. Such a model might reproduce the observed correlations to within acceptable accuracy. Any variables which are not directly measurable, such as the skills described above, are termed *latent variables*, and models built from them are *latent variable models.* Multivariate techniques such as *factor analysis* and *latent structure analysis* have such models as their basis.

Computer-intensive methods

1.12 All the above methods of analysis may be termed *classical* multivariate methods. Many of them now have a long history, for instance principal component analysis and factor analysis originated late in the nineteenth century, and they are best geared to answering questions about the sort of data sets described in **1.2**. Many of the descriptive methods are *linear*, in that they rely on derivation of linear combinations of measured variables, and the inferential techniques are built exclusively round the *multivariate normal* distribution as model. In recent years, prompted in part by the problems encountered with the sort of data sets described in **1.3**, interest has turned increasingly away from multivariate normality and towards *nonlinear* and *computer-intensive* methods of analysis.

Such methods hinge on extensive use of the computer to provide empirical, data-based and non-parametric estimates of quantities of interest. Rather than assuming a distributional form such as the normal for the data, the most appropriate density is *empirically* estimated from the sample values using a technique such as kernel density estimation (Silverman, 1986) and this estimated density is then used as the basis for, say, discriminant analysis (Hand, 1982) or projection pursuit (Jones and Sibson, 1987). Instead of relying on approximate justifications such as the central limit theorem for basing inferential techniques on the multivariate normal distribution, hypothesis tests and confidence region calculations are conducted by intensive resampling from the available sample data using ideas such as the *bootstrap*, the *jackknife*, *Monte Carlo* methodology, *permutational* distributions and *cross-validation*. All these techniques operate by generating (artificial) replication from the underlying population and then using this replication to obtain estimated variances and covariances, confidence regions and hypothesis tests. Only Monte Carlo methodology requires specific distributional assumptions, the other techniques operating purely empirically on the given data sets. However, all the methods require much repeated sampling and hence extensive involvement of the computer. Similarly, instead of just a few parametric curve-fitting procedures for summarising a complex set of data there now exists a plethora of variants of nonparametric regression, spline and other smoothing procedures. Again, these techniques do not assume any functional form for underlying distributions but are built around many iterations of relatively simple arithmetic operations conducted empirically on the given data sets. Finally, various rule-induction methods such as genetic algorithms and neural networks have appeared in specialised applications. The revolution in computer power that has taken place since the late 1970s has made such methods not only feasible but indeed commonplace in multivariate data analysis.

Note that the most extreme deviation from multivariate normality comes when the data are qualitative or categorical. While some multivariate methods have been developed exclusively for such data, a general framework for their analysis is the log-linear model and this is covered in a separate book in this series.

Missing values

1.13 It can often happen that a (small) number of entries in the data matrix are missing, for example because some children were ill on the day that one of the Wechsler subtests was administered or because some laboratory test results on a jaundice patient were lost. While some multivariate techniques can be specially modified in the presence of such missing values, many will only work if the data matrix is complete. One possible approach in such situations (automatically adopted by some computer packages) is to exclude from the analysis any individuals that have missing values. This will enable the analysis to be performed, but may be a very draconian solution to the problem: if just one or two values are missing on each of a number of individuals, then the sample size may be drastically reduced and at the same time a lot of useful information could be discarded. A more satisfactory approach might be to estimate any missing values and then to fill out the data matrix with these estimates, a process known as *imputation*. The multivariate technique is then applied to the completed data matrix.

Various imputation techniques have been proposed over the years. The simplest, and historically oldest, is simply to replace each missing value by the mean of all values present on the corresponding variate (within a given group if necessary). Buck (1960) introduced a second step, following this crude imputation of means with a series of multiple regressions in which each variate containing any missing values is treated as the dependent variable, and all other variables are the explanatory variables. Each missing value is then predicted from the relevant equation. Beale and Little (1975) iterated on this procedure, and showed that the iterative procedure converged rapidly to give maximum likelihood estimates of the missing entries assuming that the parent population is multivariate normal. Dempster *et al* (1977) demonstrated that this iterative procedure is a special case of their general E-M algorithm for handling incomplete data. Krzanowski (1988b) suggested a method of imputation based on the singular value decomposition of the data matrix, which makes no distributional assumptions about the data.

Whichever method of imputation is employed, there is a danger that variances and covariances will be underestimated from the completed matrix, as the imputed values do not allow for natural sampling variation. One way of overcoming this is to add a small random value to each imputed one, another is to reduce the degrees of freedom when calculating the variances and covariances. For a full discussion of missing values and how to handle them, see the book by Little and Rubin (1987).

Scope of this book

1.14 The above is an informal introduction to the principal concepts of multivariate analysis, and to some of the problems which concern workers in the area. Our aim is to provide a comprehensive survey of the whole subject in its present state, including more formal and detailed coverage of all these ideas and problems. In view of the extensive developments that have accompanied the dramatic increases in computing power of recent years, it was felt that the material would be more manageably presented in two parts. These are being written and published sequentially, so there will be an inevitable delay before appearance of the second part. It therefore seems appropriate to conclude this introductory chapter by outlining the division of topics between the two parts and sketching our plans for the future one.

This first part concentrates on what might be termed the basic methods of multivariate analysis, including the fundamental distribution theory, the various descriptive techniques, and all those inferential techniques that generalise familiar univariate methods to the multivariate case. We start in Chapter 2 by surveying the necessary distribution theory that forms a basis for multivariate methods, and briefly consider all those multivariate distributions that have any practical applicability. Chapters 3, 4 and 5 are then devoted to descriptive methods of analysis, including all the techniques that go under the general umbrella of ordination and multidimensional scaling. Chapters 6 and 7 focus on formal models for inference, and the techniques that arise from them, while Chapter 8 is concerned with more recent developments in nonlinear methodology. The Appendix contains a number of technical results relating to sampling distributions, mainly of relevance for inferential applications.

This leaves various specialised multivariate models and techniques to be considered in the forthcoming Part 2. This volume will start with a survey of classification, encompassing both discriminant and cluster analysis and including such recent topics and application areas as neural networks, image analysis and temporal data. The next main section will be devoted to the extensive set of techniques that arise from modelling the dependence among observations. These range from path analysis through factor analysis and latent variable models to such recent developments as covariance structure modelling and graphical modelling, as exemplified for example in the texts by Bollen (1989) and Whittaker (1990). An allied technique that links covariance modelling with more traditional linear models is repeated measures analysis, and this will also be considered. Finally, we will give attention to a number of special forms of data that are of topical interest and relevance, in particular those stemming from modern developments in instrumentation that give rise to measurement of very many variables or attributes and hence to very large data sets. We aim to conclude the whole work with a discussion of various general strategic aspects of multivariate analysis.

2

Multivariate Distributions

Distribution theory

2.1 A multivariate distribution of the p random variables $\boldsymbol{x} = (x_1, \ldots, x_p)'$ can be defined in terms of the frequency function $f(\boldsymbol{x})$. This satisfies

$$\Pr(\boldsymbol{x} \epsilon A) = \int_A f(\boldsymbol{x}) d\boldsymbol{x} \tag{2.1}$$

where A is any region of R^p. The definition, with integration understood in the Stieltjes sense, covers continuous variates, for which $f(\boldsymbol{x})$ is a probability density, and discrete variables with a specified probability of taking certain values.

Multivariate distribution theory is fully covered in Stuart and Ord (1987), and many of the definitions and results are simple extensions of the univariate theory. They are briefly summarised in the following sections.

For simplicity, we shall adhere to the following conventions regarding notation: upper case bold to denote matrices, lower case bold for vectors, and lower case to denote *either* random variables (vectors) *or* particular values. The former will predominate in this chapter and the latter throughout the rest of the book. It will generally be evident from the context which interpretation is appropriate, but where necessary the distinction will be stressed.

2.2 The distribution function is defined as

$$F(\boldsymbol{x}) = \int_{-\infty}^{x_1} \cdots \int_{-\infty}^{x_p} f(\boldsymbol{x}) d\boldsymbol{x}. \tag{2.2}$$

This is not a very useful function, because it depends on the specific variables. Often it is useful to change the axes, ȧnd the region of integration has no easy interpretation in terms of the new variables.

2.3 Expectation is defined in the obvious way

$$E(g(\boldsymbol{x})) = \int_{R^p} g(\boldsymbol{x})f(\boldsymbol{x})d\boldsymbol{x} \tag{2.3}$$

and this leads to definitions of moments and generating functions,

$$\boldsymbol{\mu} = E\boldsymbol{x} \tag{2.4}$$

$$\mu_{ijk,\dots} = Ex_1^i x_2^j x_3^k, \dots \tag{2.5}$$

$$M_{\boldsymbol{x}}(\boldsymbol{t}) = Ee^{\boldsymbol{x}'\boldsymbol{t}} \tag{2.6}$$

$$\phi_{\boldsymbol{x}}(\boldsymbol{t}) = Ee^{i\boldsymbol{x}'\boldsymbol{t}} \tag{2.7}$$

$$K_{\boldsymbol{x}}(\boldsymbol{t}) = \log(M_{\boldsymbol{x}}(\boldsymbol{t})). \tag{2.8}$$

Here, $\boldsymbol{t} = (t_1, \dots, t_p)'$ is a vector of p terms, and the coefficient of $t_1^i t_2^j t_3^k, \dots$ in the expansion of $M_{\boldsymbol{x}}(\boldsymbol{t})$ is $\mu_{ijk,\dots}/i!j!k!, \dots$. The cumulants are similarly generated by $K_{\boldsymbol{x}}(\boldsymbol{t})$.

The properties of these generating functions are analogous to those of the corresponding univariate functions. In particular, the convolution of independent variates $\boldsymbol{x}, \boldsymbol{y}$ satisfies

$$M_{\boldsymbol{x}+\boldsymbol{y}}(\boldsymbol{t}) = M_{\boldsymbol{x}}(\boldsymbol{t})M_{\boldsymbol{y}}(\boldsymbol{t}). \tag{2.9}$$

Also, the characteristic function uniquely defines the corresponding frequency function.

Marginal and conditional distributions

2.4 Suppose $\boldsymbol{x}'$ is partitioned into

$$\boldsymbol{x}' = (\boldsymbol{x}'_A, \boldsymbol{x}'_B) = (x_1, \dots, x_q, x_{q+1}, \dots, x_p). \tag{2.10}$$

The marginal distribution of $\boldsymbol{x}_A$ is the distribution of $\boldsymbol{x}_A$ when $\boldsymbol{x}_B$ is unobserved, or has the distribution it has in the population.

$$f(\boldsymbol{x}_A) = \int_{R^{p-q}} f(\boldsymbol{x})d\boldsymbol{x}_B. \tag{2.11}$$

The conditional distribution of $\boldsymbol{x}_A$, given $\boldsymbol{x}_B = \boldsymbol{x}^*{}_B$, is obtained by replacing $\boldsymbol{x}_B$ in $f(\boldsymbol{x})$ by $\boldsymbol{x}^*{}_B$. The resulting expression is proportional to the conditional distribution, so has to be normalised.

$$f(\boldsymbol{x}_A|\boldsymbol{x}^*{}_B) = f\begin{pmatrix}\boldsymbol{x}_A \\ \boldsymbol{x}^*{}_B\end{pmatrix} \Big/ \int_{R^q} f\begin{pmatrix}\boldsymbol{x}_A \\ \boldsymbol{x}^*{}_B\end{pmatrix} d\boldsymbol{x}_A. \tag{2.12}$$

The expectation of $\boldsymbol{x}_A$ conditional on $\boldsymbol{x}_B$ is the regression (in general, the multiple regression) of $\boldsymbol{x}_A$ on $\boldsymbol{x}_B$. It is given by

$$E(\boldsymbol{x}_A|\boldsymbol{x}_B) = \int_{R^q} \boldsymbol{x}_A f(\boldsymbol{x}_A|\boldsymbol{x}_B)d\boldsymbol{x}_A \tag{2.13}$$

and is a function of the random variable $\boldsymbol{x}_B$.

Example 2.1
In an adult population, suppose x_1 represents height, and x_2 is a binary variable, $x_2 = 0$ for men, $x_2 = 1$ for women. The marginal distribution of x_1 is the height distribution for the complete (mixed) population. The distributions of x_1 conditional on $x_2 = 0, x_2 = 1$ are the height distributions for men and women respectively.

Transformations

2.5 The individual variables of $\boldsymbol{x}$ may be transformed to stabilise their variances, give approximately symmetrical (marginal) distributions, and so on using ordinary univariate transformations. They may also be standardised by linear transformations to have the same location and dispersion, given by the mean and standard deviation or some other parameters considered appropriate. Multivariate transformations of the Box–Cox type (Andrews *et al*, 1971) are discussed in Chapter 3.

If $\boldsymbol{y} = (y_1, \ldots, y_p)$ represents a smooth 1–1 transformation of the continuous variate $\boldsymbol{x}$, the frequency function of $\boldsymbol{y}$ is given by

$$g(\boldsymbol{y}) = f(\boldsymbol{x}(\boldsymbol{y}))|\frac{\partial \boldsymbol{x}}{\partial \boldsymbol{y}}| \tag{2.14}$$

where $\boldsymbol{x}(\boldsymbol{y})$ is $\boldsymbol{x}$ expressed in terms of the elements of $\boldsymbol{y}$, and $J = |\frac{\partial \boldsymbol{x}}{\partial \boldsymbol{y}}|$ is the Jacobian, the determinant of partial derivatives $\partial x_i(\boldsymbol{y})/\partial y_j$. One caution is necessary. Transformations based on the relationship among variables in the whole data set may not work well when the underlying distribution is a mixture. For example, cluster analysis may be intended to identify components of distribution mixtures. Many of the techniques work best when the components have roughly spherical contours. Standardising on the basis of the variances in the mixture will not achieve this.

Second order analysis

2.6 If $\boldsymbol{x}$ has a multivariate normal distribution, the distribution is completely specified by the mean and the second moments about the mean. Most of the classical methods of multivariate analysis are based on the corresponding statistics. The theory of correlation and regression is useful when regressions are roughly linear, and conditional variances are roughly the same for different values of the conditioning variables.

The covariance matrix $\boldsymbol{V}$ has elements of the form $v_{ij} = E(x_i - \mu_i)(x_j - \mu_j)$. It is positive semi-definite—positive definite unless there are exact linear relationships among the variates. The least squares linear regression of x_1 on $x_2, \ldots, x_p$ minimises

$$E(x_1 - \alpha - \beta_2 x_2 - \ldots - \beta_p x_p)^2.$$

This minimisation leads to a plane that is the best approximation, in the least squares sense, to the true regression surface. Minimising this expression gives equations for the parameters in terms of the means, variances and covariances, and they are exactly the same as the equations relating the least squares estimates to moment estimates. The whole theory of linear regression and correlation (Stuart and Ord, 1991, Chapters 26–27) then relates to estimates of parameters derived from the second order moments. Partial regression equations and correlation parameters may be approximations to conditional regressions and correlations, but they are also parameters in their own right.

Yule (1907) introduced the notation now standard for these parameters and the corresponding statistics. The general rule is that suffices following a dot indicate variables that have been taken into account, or eliminated. Thus $x_{i.j}$ is the component of x_i orthogonal to x_j, or the residual in the (linear) regression of x_i on x_j. Similarly:

$v_{ij.kl,\dots}$ is the covariance between $x_{i.kl,\dots}$ and $x_{j.kl,\dots}$.

$\beta_{ij.kl,\dots}$ is the coefficient of x_j in the regression equation of x_i on $x_j, x_k, x_l, \dots$ (note that the order of the first two subscripts is important).

$\rho_{ij.kl,\dots}$ is the correlation between $x_{i.kl,\dots}$ and $x_{j.kl,\dots}$, the 'partial correlation' with the effect of x_k, $x_l, \dots$ eliminated.

$R_{i(jk,\dots)}$ is the multiple correlation, the correlation of x_i with the best fitting linear combination of $x_j, x_k, \dots$. $R^2_{i(jk,\dots)}$ is known as the 'coefficient of determination', and is given by $1 - v_{ii.jk,\dots}/v_{ii}$, that is, it is the proportion of the variance of x_i accounted for by the regression.

There are relationships among these coefficients; for a full discussion see Stuart and Ord (1991), Chapter 27. The most important are given below; (l) in parentheses stands for one or more further subscripts.

$$v_{ij.k(l)} = v_{ij.(l)} - v_{ik.(l)} v_{jk.(l)} / v_{kk.(l)} \tag{2.15}$$

(by 'Gauss elimination', or pivotal condensation of the matrix $\boldsymbol{V}$).

$$\rho_{ij.k(l)} = \frac{\rho_{ij.(l)} - \rho_{ik.(l)}\rho_{jk.(l)}}{\{(1-\rho^2_{ij.(l)})(1-\rho^2_{jk.(l)})\}^{\frac{1}{2}}} \tag{2.16}$$

$$\beta_{ij.k(l)} = \frac{\beta_{ij.(l)} - \beta_{ik.(l)}\beta_{jk.(l)}}{1 - \beta_{jk.(l)}\beta_{kj.(l)}} \tag{2.17}$$

$$R^2_{i(jk,\dots)} = (1-\rho^2_{ij})(1-\rho^2_{ik.j})\dots \tag{2.18}$$

The inverse of the covariance matrix may be expressed in terms of partial variances and correlations. Consider the matrix equation $\boldsymbol{VA} = \boldsymbol{I}$.

This set of equations may be solved by elimination. After eliminating $x_3, \dots, x_p$, the equations for a_{11}, a_{12}, a_{22} are

$$\begin{pmatrix} v_{11.3,\dots,p} & v_{12.3,\dots,p} \\ v_{12.3,\dots,p} & v_{22.3,\dots,p} \end{pmatrix} \begin{pmatrix} a_{11} & a_{12} \\ a_{12} & a_{22} \end{pmatrix} = \begin{pmatrix} 1 & 0 \\ 0 & 1 \end{pmatrix} \tag{2.19}$$

giving

$$a_{11} = v^{-1}_{11.23,\dots,p} \tag{2.20}$$

$$a_{22} = v^{-1}_{22.13,\dots,p} \tag{2.21}$$

$$a_{12} = -\frac{a_{11}v_{12.3,\dots,p}}{v_{22.3,\dots,p}} \tag{2.22}$$

$$= -\frac{a_{22}v_{12.3,\dots,p}}{v_{11.3,\dots,p}} \tag{2.23}$$

$$= -\rho_{12.3,\dots,p}\sqrt{a_{11}a_{22}}. \tag{2.24}$$

The diagonal elements of V^{-1} are the reciprocals of the partial variances of $x_1, \dots, x_p$, each partial for all the other variables. When the matrix is standardised to unit diagonal, by dividing rows and columns by the square roots of the diagonal elements, the off-diagonal elements are the partial correlations, with sign changed, each partial for all the other variables.

In the multivariate normal distribution (see **2.7**) a zero element in this matrix implies the *conditional independence* of the corresponding variables, conditional on all the other variables. This concept is important, because it leads to simplified models of data structure in which conditional independence may make the relationships among variables more easily understood. The independence graphs introduced by Speed (1978) are based on tests of conditional independence in normal or log-linear models; for a detailed account of graph-theoretic models, see Whittaker (1990).

Example 2.2

Pearson (1898) calculated the correlation matrix of data published by Rollet (1889) on the stature (S) of 50 men, later dissected at Lyons to give measurements of the length of femur (F), humerus (H), tibia (T), and radius (R):

	F	H	T	R	S
F	1	0.8421	0.8058	0.7439	0.8105
H	0.8421	1	0.8601	0.8451	0.8091
T	0.8058	0.8601	1	0.7804	0.7769
R	0.7439	0.8451	0.7804	1	0.6956
S	0.8105	0.8091	0.7769	0.6956	1

Eliminating F gives the partial correlations:

	H	T	R	S
H	1	0.5682	0.6068	0.4007
T	0.5682	1	0.4574	0.3569
R	0.6068	0.4574	1	0.2376
S	0.4007	0.3569	0.2376	1

The correlations are considerably reduced, but the correlations of H, T, R with S remain in the same order. Next, consider the elimination of H:

	T	R	S
T	1	0.1772	0.1714
R	0.1722	1	−0.0076
S	0.1714	−0.0076	1

Now none of the correlations is significant at the 5% level, and $r_{RS.FH}$ is actually negative. On the basis of these data, one might conclude that the correlation between stature and radius length is completely explained by their correlations with femur length and humerus length. For estimation of stature, it even seems doubtful whether tibia length adds any information when femur and humerus lengths have been included, at least if a simple linear relation is appropriate.

The multivariate normal distribution

2.7 The multivariate normal distribution is given by

$$f(\boldsymbol{x}) = (2\pi)^{-p/2}|\boldsymbol{\Sigma}|^{-\frac{1}{2}} \exp\{-\frac{1}{2}(\boldsymbol{x}-\boldsymbol{\mu})'\boldsymbol{\Sigma}^{-1}(\boldsymbol{x}-\boldsymbol{\mu})\}. \tag{2.25}$$

It has the same role in multivariate statistics as the univariate normal distribution in univariate statistics. The multivariate central limit theorem may be stated:

Suppose $\boldsymbol{y}$ is distributed with mean $\boldsymbol{\mu}$ and covariance matrix $\boldsymbol{\Sigma}$. If $\bar{\boldsymbol{y}}$ is the mean of a sample of n independent observations, $(\bar{\boldsymbol{y}}-\boldsymbol{\mu})\sqrt{n}$ has zero mean, covariance matrix $\boldsymbol{\Sigma}$, and tends to the multivariate normal distribution as $n \to \infty$. As with the univariate central limit theorem, the conditions may be relaxed somewhat. The $\boldsymbol{y}$ values need not be independent; if they constitute a stationary time series, the theorem still holds, though the approach to normality may be slower. The $\boldsymbol{y}$ values need not be identically distributed, or have the same dispersion matrix; the distribution of the mean still tends to multivariate normality provided only that, as $n \to \infty$ the distribution is not dominated by a few observations with high variances.

The practical conclusion is that inference about means based on the assumption of multivariate normality is unlikely to be misleading, provided distributions are not obviously skew or long-tailed, samples are reasonably large, and caution is exercised in making statements involving very small probabilities.

In equation (2.25) and hereafter, it is assumed that $\boldsymbol{\Sigma}$ is positive definite. If it is singular, $\boldsymbol{x}$ will still have a degenerate multivariate normal distribution, in which $k < p$ variables have a distribution of the form of (2.19), and the remaining $p-k$ are linear functions of them. In practice, redundant variables are simply omitted.

The properties of the multivariate normal distribution are discussed at length in Stuart and Ord (1991), Chapter 15. The following sections summarise the most important.

2.8 The cumulant generating function of the multivariate normal distribution is

$$K(\boldsymbol{t}) = \boldsymbol{\mu}'\boldsymbol{t} + \frac{1}{2}\boldsymbol{t}'\boldsymbol{\Sigma}\boldsymbol{t}. \tag{2.26}$$

The distribution is defined by the p means, p variances, and $\frac{1}{2}p(p-1)$ covariances. All cumulants of order greater than 2 are zero. Variables that are uncorrelated are independent, and variables that are conditionally uncorrelated are conditionally independent.

Sample means are unbiased estimates of the elements of $\boldsymbol{\mu}$, and the variances and covariances have unbiased estimators of the form

$\{\sum(x_i - \bar{x}_i)(x_j - \bar{x}_j)\}/(n-1)$. Further, the sums, sums of squares and sums of products are sufficient statistics for the parameters.

All marginal and conditional distributions are multivariate normal. Specifically, if $\boldsymbol{y}, \boldsymbol{z}$ are any linear functions of $\boldsymbol{x}$, $f(\boldsymbol{y}|\boldsymbol{z})$ is multivariate normal (but possibly degenerate). If $\boldsymbol{y} = \boldsymbol{Bx}$, where $\boldsymbol{B}$ is a $q \times p$ matrix, $\boldsymbol{y}$ is normally distributed with mean $\boldsymbol{B\mu}$ and covariance matrix $\boldsymbol{B\Sigma B}'$. This property characterises the distribution. It is, of course, not true that normal marginal distributions of $x_1, \ldots, x_p$ imply multivariate normality; see exercise (2.2).

All regressions are linear. Suppose $\boldsymbol{x}$ is partitioned into $\boldsymbol{x}_A$ and $\boldsymbol{x}_B$ as in equation (2.10), and the corresponding partition of $\boldsymbol{\Sigma}$ is

$$\boldsymbol{\Sigma} = \begin{pmatrix} \boldsymbol{\Sigma}_{AA} & \boldsymbol{\Sigma}_{AB} \\ \boldsymbol{\Sigma}'_{AB} & \boldsymbol{\Sigma}_{BB} \end{pmatrix} \tag{2.27}$$

where $\boldsymbol{\Sigma}_{AA}, \boldsymbol{\Sigma}_{AB}$ and $\boldsymbol{\Sigma}_{BB}$ are $q \times q, q \times (p-q)$ and $(p-q) \times (p-q)$ matrices respectively. Then

$$E(\boldsymbol{x}_A|\boldsymbol{x}_B) = \boldsymbol{\mu}_A + \boldsymbol{\Sigma}_{AB}\boldsymbol{\Sigma}_{BB}^{-1}(\boldsymbol{x}_B - \boldsymbol{\mu}_B) \tag{2.28}$$

$$\text{cov}(\boldsymbol{x}_A|\boldsymbol{x}_B) = \boldsymbol{\Sigma}_{AA} - \boldsymbol{\Sigma}_{AB}\boldsymbol{\Sigma}_{BB}^{-1}\boldsymbol{\Sigma}'_{AB} \tag{2.29}$$

and the distribution is multivariate normal.

2.9 The problem of integrating the multivariate normal distribution over a 'box' $a_i \leqslant x_i \leqslant b_i$ is a complicated piece of numerical analysis. Schervish (1984) gives an efficient algorithm, but as p increases the execution time quickly becomes prohibitive. Dunnett (1989) gives an algorithm that is much faster for the special case when $\rho_{ij} = \beta_i\beta_j$; Lohr (1993) gives an algorithm for general correlation matrix and for 'star-shaped' regions, so that radii from the origin meet the boundary only once.

Fortunately, this type of integral is not often required. It is much easier, and more useful, to calculate the probability of lying within surfaces of equal density. If

$$D^2 = (\boldsymbol{X} - \boldsymbol{\mu})'\boldsymbol{\Sigma}^{-1}(\boldsymbol{X} - \boldsymbol{\mu}), \tag{2.30}$$

D^2 is distributed as χ^2 with p degrees of freedom. D^2 is known as the squared generalised distance.

It is worth noting how sparse the distributions become for large p. $\Pr(D^2 \leqslant 3.84) = 0.95$ for $p = 1$, but for $p = 10$ the probability is nearly 0.05.

Spherical and elliptical distributions

2.10 Spherical distributions may be generated by the rotation of univariate distributions about a point of symmetry or about an end of the range. Consider a distribution $f(x)$, symmetrical about zero. Rotation of this distribution in p dimensions about the origin gives a volume

$$V = \omega_p \int_0^\infty x^{p-1} f(x)dx, \qquad \omega_p = \frac{2(\pi)^{\frac{p}{2}}}{\Gamma(\frac{p}{2})} \tag{2.31}$$

where ω_p is the surface of the p-dimensional hypersphere. Provided the integral is finite, $Cf(\sqrt{\boldsymbol{x}'\boldsymbol{x}})$ is a properly normalised distribution if $C = V^{-1}$.

Example 2.3
If

$$f(x) = \frac{1}{\sqrt{2\pi}} \exp(-x^2/2),$$

$$\int_0^\infty x^{p-1} f(x) dx = \frac{2^{\frac{p}{2}-1}\Gamma(\frac{p}{2})}{\sqrt{2\pi}}$$

and

$$V^{-1}\frac{1}{\sqrt{2\pi}} \exp(-\frac{\boldsymbol{x}'\boldsymbol{x}}{2}) = \frac{1}{(2\pi)^{\frac{p}{2}}} \exp(-\frac{\boldsymbol{x}'\boldsymbol{x}}{2}),$$

the standardised spherical multivariate normal distribution.

Examples of distributions generated in this way include:
(i) The spherical normal distribution (example 2.3).
(ii) The uniform distribution in a p-dimensional sphere, generated by rotating a uniform distribution.
(iii) The uniform distribution on the surface of a sphere, generated by rotating a 2-point distribution. It is important in the theory of directional distributions.
(iv) A rotated Laplace distribution. This is not, however, the distribution generally referred to as the spherical Laplace distribution—that has marginal Laplace distributions.
(v) Spherical t distributions. The t distribution with v degrees of freedom has a finite moment of order $v - 1$, so that the rotated distribution exists only if $v \geqslant p$. The case $v = p$ is known as the spherical Cauchy distribution.

The general spherical distribution centred at $\boldsymbol{\mu}$ has a density $f(\boldsymbol{x})$ that is a function of $(\boldsymbol{x} - \boldsymbol{\mu})'(\boldsymbol{x} - \boldsymbol{\mu})$. The characteristic function is $e^{i\boldsymbol{\mu}'\boldsymbol{t}}\phi(\boldsymbol{t}'\boldsymbol{t})$. The mean is $\boldsymbol{\mu}$ and the covariance matrix is a multiple of the unit matrix (when the mean and variances exist). The distribution has point symmetry about $\boldsymbol{\mu}$. The variables are uncorrelated; the only spherical distribution for which they are independent is the spherical normal distribution.

2.11 A generalisation of the class of spherical distributions is the class of elliptically contoured distributions, or elliptical distributions, given by replacing $\boldsymbol{x}-\boldsymbol{\mu}$ by $\boldsymbol{H}(\boldsymbol{x}-\boldsymbol{\mu})$, where $\boldsymbol{H}$ is a non-singular $p \times p$ matrix. The density function $f(\boldsymbol{x})$ is a function of $(\boldsymbol{x} - \boldsymbol{\mu})'\boldsymbol{H}'\boldsymbol{H}(\boldsymbol{x} - \boldsymbol{\mu})$. The covariance matrix, if it exists, is proportional to $(\boldsymbol{H}'\boldsymbol{H})^{-1}$, and in this case we may write

$$f(\boldsymbol{x}) = |\boldsymbol{\Sigma}|^{-\frac{1}{2}} g\{(\boldsymbol{x} - \boldsymbol{\mu})'\boldsymbol{\Sigma}^{-1}(\boldsymbol{x} - \boldsymbol{\mu})\} \tag{2.32}$$

where $\boldsymbol{\Sigma}$ is the covariance matrix. The contours of equal density are ellipsoids of the form

$$(\boldsymbol{x} - \boldsymbol{\mu})'\boldsymbol{H}'\boldsymbol{H}(\boldsymbol{x} - \boldsymbol{\mu}) = A \tag{2.33}$$

and the characteristic function has the form

$$\psi(\boldsymbol{t}) = e^{i\boldsymbol{\mu}'\boldsymbol{t}}\phi\{\boldsymbol{t}'(\boldsymbol{H}'\boldsymbol{H})^{-1}\boldsymbol{t}\}. \tag{2.34}$$

One important application of distributions of this type is in examining the robustness of procedures based on the normal distribution. This involves, typically, examining the performance of these procedures with elliptical distributions with longer tails than the normal.

There has also been some progress in developing the theory of the class of elliptical distributions, as a generalisation of multivariate methods based on the multivariate normal distribution. Koutras (1986) discussed generalisations of the non-central chi-squared distributions based on elliptical laws. Mitchell and Krzanowski (1985) derived measures of distance between elliptical distributions. Fang and Zhang (1990) give a general account of the subject.

The following sections summarise some of the most important types of elliptical distributions.

2.12 Kotz (1975) (see also Fang *et al*, 1990) introduced the family of elliptical distributions

$$f(\boldsymbol{x}) = C|\boldsymbol{\Sigma}|^{-\frac{1}{2}}Q^{N-1}\exp(-rQ^s), \quad r, s > 0, \quad 2N + p > 2 \tag{2.35}$$

where

$$Q = (\boldsymbol{x} - \boldsymbol{\mu})'\boldsymbol{\Sigma}^{-1}(\boldsymbol{x} - \boldsymbol{\mu}) \tag{2.36}$$

and

$$\begin{aligned} C &= \Gamma(\frac{p}{2})\pi^{-\frac{p}{2}}\left[\int_0^\infty u^{N+\frac{p}{2}-2}\exp(-ru^s)du\right]^{-1} \\ &= \frac{s\Gamma(\frac{p}{2})}{\pi^{\frac{p}{2}}\Gamma(\frac{2N+p-2}{2s})}r^{\frac{2N+p-2}{2s}}. \end{aligned}$$

This is a very general family of elliptical distributions, with finite moments and covariance matrix equal to $\boldsymbol{\Sigma}$ (the factor r is introduced to ensure this). The distributions with $N > 1$ are of little practical interest; they have zero value at $\boldsymbol{\mu}$, and the maximum density lies on an ellipsoid centred at $\boldsymbol{\mu}$. The case $N = 1, s = 1, r = \frac{1}{2}$ is the multivariate normal distribution, and in general distributions with $s < 1$ are heavier tailed than the multivariate normal. The case $N = 1, s = \frac{1}{2}, r = \frac{1}{2}$ is the elliptical version of the rotated Laplace distribution.

2.13 Various multivariate generalisations of the t distribution have been proposed. The most familiar and useful was introduced by Cornish (1954). Each variable in a multivariate normal distribution is divided by *the same* random variable y, where vy^2 is distributed as χ^2 with v degrees of freedom. The centre is then transferred to $\boldsymbol{\mu}$. This construction is analogous to that of the univariate t distribution, and gives the density

$$f(\boldsymbol{x}) = \frac{\Gamma\left[\frac{1}{2}(v+p)\right]}{(\pi v)^{\frac{p}{2}}\Gamma(\frac{v}{2})|\boldsymbol{\Sigma}|^{\frac{1}{2}}}[1 + (\boldsymbol{x} - \boldsymbol{\mu})'\boldsymbol{\Sigma}^{-1}(\boldsymbol{x} - \boldsymbol{\mu})]^{-\frac{1}{2}(v+p)}. \tag{2.37}$$

The marginal distributions are then t distributions with ν degrees of freedom (in contrast to the rotated t distribution described above). The matrix $\boldsymbol{\Sigma}$ represents the covariance matrix of the underlying normal distribution; the covariance matrix of $\boldsymbol{x}$ is $\frac{\nu}{\nu-2}\boldsymbol{\Sigma}$, provided that $\nu > 2$.

The derivation given above implies that ν is an integer, but the distribution exists for all $\nu > 0$; the form with non-integer ν is sometimes known as the multivariate Type VII distribution. The case $\nu = 1$ is the multivariate Cauchy distribution. These distributions have no importance in sampling theory—Hotelling's T^2 distribution is the univariate generalisation of t used for inference about multivariate normal distributions—but provide another set of long-tailed distributions for comparison with the multivariate normal. An example is given by Sutradher (1990), who studies discrimination between t distributions, using a modified form of the multivariate t, based on the actual covariance matrix.

2.14 Many other elliptical distributions have been discussed; see, for example, Johnson and Kotz (1972); Fang *et al* (1990). Most of these are of little practical importance.

The distribution

$$f(\boldsymbol{x}) = \frac{2}{(2\pi)^{\frac{p}{2}}|\boldsymbol{\Sigma}|^{\frac{1}{2}}\Gamma(\frac{p}{2})}K_0\{[2(\boldsymbol{x}-\boldsymbol{\mu})'\boldsymbol{\Sigma}^{-1}(\boldsymbol{x}-\boldsymbol{\mu})]^{\frac{1}{2}}\} \tag{2.38}$$

where K_0 is a Bessel function, is known as the multivariate Laplace distribution. It has marginal distributions of Laplace form. It is a special case of a family of elliptical Bessell distributions.

Jensen, in Kotz and Johnson (1985), gives an elliptical logistic distribution

$$f(\boldsymbol{x}) = C\,\frac{\exp[-(\boldsymbol{x}-\boldsymbol{\mu})'\boldsymbol{\Sigma}^{-1}(\boldsymbol{x}-\boldsymbol{\mu})]}{\{1+\exp[-(\boldsymbol{x}-\boldsymbol{\mu})'\boldsymbol{\Sigma}^{-1}(\boldsymbol{x}-\boldsymbol{\mu})]\}^2} \tag{2.39}$$

where

$$C = \frac{\pi^{\frac{p}{2}}}{|\boldsymbol{\Sigma}|^{\frac{1}{2}}\Gamma(\frac{p}{2})}\int_0^\infty y^{\frac{p}{2}-1}\frac{e^{-y}}{(1-e^{-y})^2}dy. \tag{2.40}$$

The Dirichlet distribution

2.15 The simplest generalisation of the Beta distribution is the Dirichlet distribution.

$$f(\boldsymbol{x}) = \frac{\Gamma(\Sigma_i\alpha_i)}{\prod_{i=1}^p\Gamma(\alpha_i)}\prod_{i=1}^p x_i^{\alpha_i-1}d\boldsymbol{x}, \qquad \Sigma x_i = 1. \tag{2.41}$$

The constraint implies that the distribution is $(p-1)$ dimensional; x_p is redundant and may be replaced by $1-\sum_1^{p-1}x_i$. Suppose $\Sigma\alpha_i = \alpha$. The values of α_i determine the means, variances and covariances:

$$E(x_i) = \frac{\alpha_i}{\alpha}, \qquad \text{var}(x_i) = \frac{\alpha_i(\alpha-\alpha_i)}{\alpha^2(\alpha+1)}, \qquad \text{cov}(x_ix_j) = \frac{-\alpha_i\alpha_j}{\alpha^2(\alpha+1)}. \tag{2.42}$$

The constraint induces a negative correlation between the x values. This correlation, however, is a fixed value determined by the means. The distribution can be derived as the joint distribution of *independent* χ^2 values as a proportion of their sum (see Exercise 2.4).

The most important application of the Dirichlet distribution is as a prior for Bayesian analysis of multinomial data. Eigenvalue distributions are closely related—see Appendix (**A.11**).

There are other distributions referred to in the literature as generalised Dirichlet distributions, or generalised multivariate beta distributions. For details, see Johnson and Kotz (1972).

The inverted Dirichlet distribution (Tiao and Guttman, 1965) has the form

$$f(\boldsymbol{x}) = \frac{\Gamma(\theta)\prod_{i=1}^{p} x_i^{\theta_i-1}}{\prod_{i=1}^{p}\{\Gamma(\theta_i)\}(1+\sum_{i=1}^{p} x_i)^{\theta/2}} \qquad (0 \leqslant x_i < \infty) \tag{2.43}$$

where $\theta = \sum_{i=1}^{p} \theta_i$.

This is a generalisation of the beta distribution of type II (which includes the variance ratio distribution).

Distributions for compositional data

2.16 The Dirichlet distribution is an example of a distribution that gives rise to 'compositional data', that is, to a set of non-negative variables constrained to sum to unity. The distribution of $x_1, \ldots, x_{p-1}$ lies within the simplex $x_i \geqslant 0, \sum_{i=1}^{p-1} x_i \leqslant 1$. Distributions of this type arise naturally in many situations. The chemical composition of a substance, the proportions of time spent in different activities, the proportion of soil-particles in different size ranges, are examples of data of this sort. Aitchison (1986) lists 40 data sets exhibiting these features. Interpretation of such data is difficult; in particular, there are inevitably negative correlations among components with large means, induced by the constraint.

Modelling compositional data requires special distributions. The Dirichlet distribution itself is clearly too inflexible for general use. It depends only on the $(p-1)$ dimensional mean, and the correlations are determined by the mean. In the terminology of Connor and Mosimann (1969) the x_i are all 'neutral'; that is, the distribution of $x_j/(1-x_i)$ is independent of x_i. This concept brings out the relationship between compositional data and problems of size and shape (see Volume 2). If the sum of a set of measurements represents 'size', and the distribution of proportions defines 'shape', neutrality implies that there is no structure in shape variation, or that proportions interact only because of the constraint.

The Liouville distribution is discussed by Fang *et al* (1990). It is a generalisation of the Dirichlet distribution. If $\boldsymbol{x}$ follows a Dirichlet distribution, $\boldsymbol{y} = r\boldsymbol{x}$, where r is a random variable, follows the Liouville distribution. The distribution has been proposed by Ng (unpublished; see Fang *et al*, 1990) as a model for compositional data, but Aitchison (1986) regards it as inadequate, having less flexibility than distributions involving transformations of the multivariate normal distribution.

Connor and Mosimann (1969) introduced a generalisation of the Dirichlet distribution of the form

$$f(x_1,\ldots,x_p) = x_p^{b_{p-1}-1} \prod_{i=1}^{p-1} \frac{x_i^{a_i-1} \sum_{j=1}^{p} x_j^{b_{i-1}-(a_i+b_i)}}{B(a_i, b_i)} \tag{2.44}$$

where $\sum_{i=1}^{p} x_i = 1$.

This distribution has $2(p-1)$ parameters, and is somewhat less restrictive than the Dirichlet distribution. Nevertheless, it is complex and intractable as far as statistical analysis is concerned. The dependence on the sequence of variables is also a drawback in the general problem—in the example in the original paper the x_i had a natural sequence. Finally, the distribution 'retains a strong independence structure' (Aitchison, 1986) and is not sufficiently flexible to model general compositional data.

Other generalisations of the Dirichlet distribution appear to have similar drawbacks.

2.17 The idea of representing data in the simplex by a suitable transformation of a general multivariate distribution was introduced by Aitchison (Aitchison and Shen, 1980; Aitchison, 1982; Aitchison, 1986), although Obenchain (1970) used this approach in an unpublished technical report. Aitchison and Shen introduced the logistic-normal distribution. If $\boldsymbol{y} = (y_1,\ldots,y_{p-1})$ has a $p-1$ variate normal distribution, the transformation

$$x_i = \frac{\exp(y_i)}{1+\sum \exp(y_i)}, \qquad i = 1,\ldots,p-1$$

$$x_p = \frac{1}{1+\sum \exp(y_i)} \tag{2.45}$$

gives a distribution for $\boldsymbol{x} = (x_1,\ldots,x_p)$, with $x_i > 0$, $\sum x_i = 1$. Further, the inverse transformation $y_i = \log \frac{x_i}{x_p}$ gives the underlying normal distribution, and standard statistical analysis on the transformed variables is possible.

This approach, referred to as a log-ratio analysis, has been widely used and constitutes a major advance in the analysis of compositional data. It should be noted that the asymmetrical form of the transformation is largely immaterial; if another x_i is chosen as divisor, the derived variables are a *linear* transformation of the ys, and inferential properties are invariant under such transformations.

The explicit form of the distribution of $\boldsymbol{x}$ is unimportant; all analysis depends on the approximate normality (perhaps conditional on covariates) of $\boldsymbol{y}$. This should, of course, be checked; for tests of multivariate normality, see Chapter 3. If it does not hold, it may be that a different transformation, or perhaps a further transformation, will be satisfactory.

There is one major difficulty, apparently common to all forms of compositional distribution—the occurrence of zero values. Where zero implies 'a trace too small to measure', it may reasonably be replaced by a suitable small value without seriously distorting the distribution. Often, though, this is not the case. In biochemical data, a component may be absent because an organism is incapable of synthesising it, the zero and non-zero values clearly not belonging to a single continuous distribution. In this situation, the model breaks down, and it becomes necessary to model the zeros explicitly. The problem is discussed at length in Aitchison (1986).

Aitchison (1982, 1986) describes two other transformations of logistic type, which he calls multiplicative logistic and hybrid, or partitioned, logistic. These provide alternative models for compositional data, but are less easy to handle and interpret.

Generalisations of the Gamma distribution

2.18 Various multivariate generalisations of the Gamma distribution (including the chi-squared and exponential distributions) are possible. For inferential purposes, the most important is the Wishart distribution, the joint distribution of the elements of an estimated dispersion matrix based on a multivariate normal distribution. This and other sampling distributions are discussed in the Appendix.

The additive property of the Gamma distribution makes it easy to construct generalisations with Gamma marginal distributions and positive correlations. Suppose $y_1, \ldots, y_k$ are independent Gamma variates with parameters $\theta_1, \ldots, \theta_k$. Now construct $x_1, \ldots, x_p, \quad (p < k)$ as sums of subsets of the ys, linearly independent, and with some y variates in common. The resulting distribution is easily simulated, but is mathematically intractable.

A special case is discussed in Johnson and Kotz (1972). Suppose $y_0, \ldots, y_p$ are independent Gamma variates, and $x_i = y_i + y_0, i = 1, \ldots, p$. The joint density of $y_0, x_1, \ldots, x_p$ is

$$\left[\prod_{j=0}^{p} \Gamma(\theta_j)\right]^{-1} y_0^{\theta_0 - 1} \prod_{j=0}^{p} [(x_j - y_0)^{\theta_j - 1}] \exp\left[(p-1)y_0 - \sum_{j=1}^{p} x_j\right]. \tag{2.46}$$

Even in this simplified case, integrating out y_0 is possible only in very special cases. The marginal distribution of x_i is Gamma, with mean and variance $\theta_i + \theta_0$, and the covariance of x_i, x_j is θ_0.

Multivariate generalisations of the exponential distribution have been proposed for modelling lifetime distributions of components with related failures. Marshall and Olkin (1967) considered a Poisson process in which each event has a certain probability of causing the failure of one or more components. Thus lifetimes are exponentially distributed, and are independent conditionally on there being no simultaneous failures. Weinman (1966), developing an idea due to Freund (1961), suggested a model in which the conditional failure time distribution of each component was exponential with parameter dependent on the number of components that had previously failed. Moran (1967) discussed the distribution of the sum of squares of pairs of multivariate normal variables, each pair independent, but with cross correlations.

There are other possibilities, but the applications are rather specialised and not relevant to general problems of multivariate analysis.

2.19 There has also been some study of bivariate extreme value distributions. This type of distribution is defined as the distribution of $(\max x_1, \max x_2)$ in a sample of n from the bivariate distribution of (x_1, x_2)—note that the extreme value is not, in general, an observation of the bivariate sample. Tiago de Oliveira (1980) gives a general account of the types of distribution that can arise, with a mention of the extension to multivariate extreme values.

These distributions are not to be confused with the univariate distribution of the larger of (x_1, x_2), or of the largest of a set of correlated variables. This problem was first studied by Clark (1961), who derived the first four moments of the larger of bivariate normal variables. The general case has applications in connection with 'record values' in time series.

Multivariate discrete distributions

2.20 Most univariate discrete distributions can be generalised, in some way, to give multivariate discrete distributions with properties and applications related to those of the corresponding univariate distributions. The most important are the simplest. The numbers of independent events in certain categories follow the multinomial distribution. If these categories constitute a contingency table with some fixed marginal totals, the distribution is multivariate hypergeometric.

Categorical data are usually represented by binary variables. Thus if there are p categories, define $x_i = 1$ if an item falls in category i, otherwise $x_i = 0$. Since $\sum_{i=1}^{p} x_i = 1$ for each observation, the variable x_p is redundant. This particular choice of variables is purely arbitrary; any set of $p - 1$ variables that are constant for each category and linearly independent could be used. Ordered categories present special problems; scores chosen to represent roughly the linear, quadratic ... effects of order may help interpretation. The choice does not affect inference about the relationship of the categories with other aspects of the data, but may clarify the interpretation of the effect of the categories. Techniques to be described later, such as correspondence analysis and canonical analysis, derive scores from aspects of the data. Bloomfield (1974) discusses the linear transformation of binary data, particularly in the context of log-linear models.

The multinomial distribution

2.21 Suppose data fall independently into p categories with probability $\pi_i, i = 1, \ldots, p$. Define $x_i = 1$ for an item in category i, $x_i = 0$ otherwise. Then

$$E(x_i) = \pi_i, \qquad \operatorname{var}(x_i) = \pi_i(1 - \pi_i), \qquad \operatorname{cov}(x_i x_j) = -\pi_i \pi_j.$$

The distribution of counts in each category in a sample of size n is known as the multinomial distribution, a natural extension of the binomial distribution, to which it reduces if $p = 2$. The cumulants of the counts are those of $\boldsymbol{x}$ multiplied by n, and the cumulants of the observed proportions are those of $\boldsymbol{x}$ divided by n. The cumulant generating function of $\boldsymbol{x}$ is $\log \sum \pi_i \exp(t_i)$.

The probability of counts

$$n_1, \ldots, n_p, \qquad \sum_{i=1}^{p} n_i = n \qquad \text{is} \qquad n! \prod_{i=1}^{p} \frac{\pi_i^{n_i}}{n_i!}.$$

The multivariate central limit theorem shows that for large n the distribution can be approximated by the multivariate normal distribution, but this is not a very useful result for evaluating the probability of a range of possible sets of counts, because of the difficulties of the multivariate normal integral. It suggests, however, that the quadratic form

$$(\boldsymbol{n} - n\boldsymbol{\pi})' \boldsymbol{V}^{-1} (\boldsymbol{n} - n\boldsymbol{\pi}),$$

where $\boldsymbol{n}' = (n_1, \ldots, n_{p-1})$, $\boldsymbol{\pi}' = (\pi_1, \ldots, \pi_{p-1})$, $\boldsymbol{V}_{ii} = \pi_i(1 - \pi_i)$, $\boldsymbol{V}_{ij} = -\pi_i\pi_j$, is distributed approximately as χ^2 with $p - 1$ degrees of freedom. In fact, this is precisely the usual χ^2 statistic $\sum_{i=1}^{p}(n_i - n\pi_i)^2/n\pi_i$. The approximation is known to be good if no values of $n\pi_i$ are very small, and it may be used to test a postulated set of values of π_i, or to find an approximate confidence region for $\boldsymbol{\pi}$.

As is obvious from the derivation, if categories i and j of a p-category multinomial distribution are merged, the resulting distribution is a $(p - 1)$ category multinomial, with parameter $\pi_i + \pi_j$ for the combined category.

The multivariate hypergeometric distribution

2.22 The multivariate hypergeometric distribution has the same relationship to the multinomial as has the hypergeometric to the binomial. Suppose m items are drawn from p classes with $m_1, m_2, \ldots, m_p$ items in each class. A sample of n (drawn without replacement) contains $n_1, n_2, \ldots, n_p$ in the p classes. Then

$$\Pr(n_1, \ldots, n_p) = \prod_{i=1}^{p} \binom{m_i}{n_i} \Big/ \binom{m}{n}.$$

The marginal distribution of each variable is hypergeometric, with

$$E(n_i) = \frac{nm_i}{m}, \quad \operatorname{var}(n_i) = \frac{nm_i(m - m_i)}{m^2}, \text{ and } \operatorname{cov}(n_i n_j) = \frac{-nm_i m_j}{m^2}.$$

The distribution is, of course, $(p - 1)$ dimensional, since $\sum_{i=1}^{p} n_i = n$.

The main importance of the distribution is in connection with contingency tables with fixed margins. Exact probability calculations are heavy except in special cases, and in practice the analysis of such tables is based on one of two χ^2 approximations. The original Pearson χ^2 test gives

$$X^2 = \sum_{i=1}^{p} \frac{[n_i - E(n_i)]^2}{E(n_i)} \tag{2.47}$$

and the likelihood ratio test gives the 'deviance statistic'

$$\Phi^2 = \sum_{i=1}^{p} n_i \log \frac{n_i}{E(n_i)}. \tag{2.48}$$

These χ^2 statistics, measures of the discrepancy between observed frequencies and the expected values based on some model, are the main tools in the analysis of contingency tables. They are asymptotically equivalent, but there are some important differences for moderate sample sizes—see, for example, McCullagh and Nelder (1990 p127). Log linear models, based on multiplicative effects on probabilities, are the most important class, and are described in a separate book in this series.

The multivariate Poisson distribution

2.23 Many univariate discrete distributions can be generalised to give multivariate discrete distributions usually with the univariate distributions as marginals; see Johnson and Kotz (1969). Most of these are of interest for modelling observed phenomena, rather than for more general multivariate analysis. The most important is the multivariate Poisson distribution. It is easy to construct a multivariate distribution with Poisson margins and positive correlations—compare the corresponding treatment of the Gamma distribution. This type of distribution is useful for modelling point processes varying with time. An immigration-death process, under suitable conditions, gives a Poisson distribution at time t, and observations at short intervals show positive correlations; see Exercise 2.10.

Suppose $y_1, \ldots, y_q$ are *independent* Poisson distributed variables with means $\lambda_1, \ldots, \lambda_q$. Now construct $x_1, \ldots, x_p$ $(p < q)$ as sums of subsets of the ys. Clearly each x_i is a Poisson variable, and the covariances are given by the sum of the common λ values.

For example, the transformation

$$x_1 = y_1 + y_3, \qquad x_2 = y_2 + y_3$$

yields

$$\begin{aligned} E(x_1) &= \mathrm{var}(x_1) &= \lambda_1 + \lambda_3, \\ E(x_2) &= \mathrm{var}(x_2) &= \lambda_2 + \lambda_3, \\ \mathrm{cov}(x_1 x_2) &= \lambda_3 & \end{aligned}$$

and the cumulant generating function

$$K(t_1, t_2) = \lambda_1(e^{t_1} - 1) + \lambda_2(e^{t_2} - 1) + \lambda_3(e^{t_1+t_2} - 1).$$

2.24 Other discrete multivariate distributions have been suggested for specific applications; see Johnson and Kotz (1969) for a full account.

The negative multinomial (multivariate negative binomial) distribution may be written in the form

$$\Pr(\boldsymbol{n}) = \frac{\Gamma(N+n)b^{-(N+n)}}{(n!)\Gamma(N)} \prod_{i=1}^{p} \frac{a_i^{n_i}}{n_i!} \tag{2.49}$$

where $n = \sum_{i=1}^{p} n_i$, $b = 1 + \sum_{i=1}^{p} a_i$ and N is a parameter, the index of the negative multinomial expansion (not necessarily an integer). The distribution is related to the multivariate Poisson in the same way as the negative binomial is related to the univariate Poisson. In fact, if the multivariate Poisson parameters λ_i have gamma distributions with the same index but different scale parameters, it is easy to see that the negative multinomial distribution results. The marginal distributions are negative binomial, and the counts n_i are positively correlated. The probability generating function is $(b - \boldsymbol{a}'\boldsymbol{t})^{-N}$, and the distribution has applications for counts of clustered events, accident data and traffic flow.

The logarithmic series distribution has a multivariate analogue, derived from the negative multinomial in the same way as the univariate logarithmic series distribution is derived from the negative binomial. As $N \to 0$, $\Pr(n = 0) \to 1$. Conditioning on $n \neq 0$ gives the limiting distribution. Notice that individual values of n_i may be zero. The marginal distributions are not of logarithmic series form. Chatfield *et al* (1966) give an application to purchasing behaviour.

Holgate (1966) has discussed three multivariate versions of the Neyman type A distribution. The univariate Neyman type A distribution is derived from a Poisson distribution in which the mean follows a Poisson distribution. In the first two of these generalisations, either of these Poisson distributions is replaced by a multivariate Poisson distribution. The third is formed from sums of subsets of Neyman type A distributed counts, in the same way as the multivariate Poisson is derived from the univariate form.

Mixed binary and continuous data

2.25 In many situations, multivariate data refer to both continuous and binary variables. The former are measured quantities, or ordered categories that can reasonably be regarded as grouped continuous variates. The latter correspond either to natural dichotomies, or to dummy variables defined to separate natural categories.

Multivariate distributions for a set of binary variates $x_1, \ldots, x_q$ taking values 0 or 1, and a set of continuous variates $y_1, \ldots, y_p$ can be structured in various ways. If the x and y values are independent, each can be represented by an appropriate multivariate distribution, discrete and continuous respectively, and the joint density is given by the product. Otherwise, there are two reasonable approaches:

(i) Define a distribution to represent the distribution of the ys, and for each x_i let $\Pr(x_i = 1)$ be some function of the ys. As a typical example, suppose $\boldsymbol{y} \sim N(\boldsymbol{\mu}, \boldsymbol{\Sigma})$,

$$\Pr(x_i = 1) = \frac{\exp(\alpha_i + \boldsymbol{\beta}_i'\boldsymbol{y})}{1 + \exp(\alpha_i + \boldsymbol{\beta}_i'\boldsymbol{y})}. \tag{2.50}$$

This is the logistic-normal distribution. It arises naturally in many situations; for example, in medical statistics, blood pressure and cholesterol may affect the chances of a heart attack; in ecology, continuous environmental features may affect the presence or absence of various species. With distributions of this type, it is easy to set up a marginal distribution for the ys and derive a distribution for the xs, but the distribution of the ys conditional on some or all of the xs is typically intractable.

(ii) Define a distribution for the binary variables—usually multinomial or hypergeometric—and choose a family for the y variables with parameters that depend on the values of the xs. If $\boldsymbol{y} \sim N(\boldsymbol{\mu}_x, \boldsymbol{\Sigma}_x)$, normally distributed with mean and variance (or perhaps just the mean) dependent on $\boldsymbol{x}$, the distribution is known as 'conditional Gaussian'. Again, the distribution has many natural applications—example 2.1 is a simple case. If the binary variables represent sex and race, and the continuous variables physical measurements, it is reasonable to think of the y means as dependent on the x values. This is the model underlying standard parametric forms of discriminant analysis (Mardia *et al*, 1979, Chapter 11). In this case, the $\boldsymbol{x}$ distribution and the conditional $\boldsymbol{y}$ distributions are straightforward, but the marginal $\boldsymbol{y}$ distributions are awkward distribution mixtures. Conditional independence models for the conditional Gaussian distribution have been studied by Edwards (1990), and are implemented in his computer package MIM (Edwards, 1992). See also Whittaker (1990).

These distributions differ in two respects. In the first place, the simplicity of the marginal distribution in (i), or the conditional distribution in (ii), may suggest the more convenient type to choose for a particular application. Secondly, the structure of the distribution suggests a causal chain; in (i), the continuous variable affects the binary variables, while in (ii) the binary variables affect the continuous. In many applications, both assumptions are oversimplifications. Some binary variables may affect the continuous variables, which in turn affect other binary variables, and still more complex systems are possible.

Cox and Wermuth (1992) introduce the general conditional Gaussian chain model, in which sets of binary and normally distributed variables alternate in a causal chain. The general distributions are intractable, and the authors discuss various possible simplifications. The most promising seems to be the linear (in place of logistic) relation of the binary to the normal variables (cf Armitage, 1966). This linear model makes the distributions simpler and more amenable to statistical analysis, but there are obvious dangers for probabilities taking values near 0 or 1.

Multivariate stable distributions

2.26 The (univariate) normal distribution is closed under convolution. The first investigations of the class of distributions with this property were due to Lévy (1925, 1937). A distribution in this class is a *stable* distribution.

Specifically, writing

$$S_n = x_1 + \ldots + x_n$$

where $x_1, \ldots, x_n$ are independent and identically distributed, the distribution is stable if there exist constants $a_n > 0$ and b_n such that

$$\frac{S_n}{a_n} - b_n$$

has the same distribution as x. The distribution is said to be *stable in the strict sense* if $b_n = 0$; Lévy originally defined stability in this sense, referring to the general case as quasi-stable (Lukacs, 1960). The normal distribution is stable with $a_n = n^{1/2}$, and the Cauchy is stable with $a_n = n$. In the general case, $a_n = n^{1/\alpha}$, where $0 < \alpha \leqslant 2$. The degenerate one-point distribution satisfies the conditions, but is excluded from the class of stable distributions.

The log of the characteristic function has the form

$$K(t) = \log \phi(t) \tag{2.51}$$

$$= i\mu t - c|t|^{\alpha}\{1 + i\beta(t/|t|)\omega(t,\alpha)\} \tag{2.52}$$

where

$$\omega(t,\alpha) = \tan\left(\frac{\pi\alpha}{2}\right), \quad \alpha \neq 1,$$

$$= \left(\frac{2}{\pi}\right)\log|t|, \quad \alpha = 1.$$

Here, μ and c are respectively location and scale parameters, α is the parameter in the relationship $a_n = n^{1/\alpha}$, and β is a skewness parameter; $\beta = 0$ gives the symmetric stable distributions.

The stable distributions are all continuous and unimodal, and all belong to the class of infinitely divisible distributions (Stuart and Ord, 1987, Chapter 4). Unfortunately, densities and distribution functions cannot, in general, be expressed in closed form. Of the symmetric stable distributions, only the normal ($\alpha = 2$) and the Cauchy ($\alpha = 1$) can be so expressed. Only one other stable distribution is known in explicit form. The distribution with $\alpha = 1/2$, $\beta = -1$, standardised so that $\mu = 0$, $c = 1$ has the form

$$f(x) = (2\pi)^{-1/2}x^{-\frac{3}{2}}\exp(-\frac{1}{2x}), \quad 0 \leqslant x < \infty \tag{2.53}$$

and is known as Lévy's distribution. The distribution function is

$$F(x) = 2\{1 - \Phi(\frac{1}{\sqrt{x}})\}. \tag{2.54}$$

It has no finite moments.

Note that the definition of a stable distribution implies that if the variance is finite, then, since the conditions for the central limit theorem apply, the distribution is normal. The normal distribution is thus the only stable distribution with finite variance. Symmetric stable distributions are heavy-tailed, while skew stable distributions are heavy-tailed in one direction.

Other cases of univariate stable distributions are less tractable, although in many cases the inversion of the characteristic function leads to an expression in terms of an infinite series. Such expansions were given by Bergström (1952); see Feller (1966).

The main importance of stable distributions is in the theoretical study of random walk type processes. Feller (1966) discusses the first passage time distribution for Brownian movement, and shows that it follows Lévy's distribution. Holtsmark (1919) studied the gravitational field at a randomly chosen point in a random aggregate of stars, and derived a stable distribution with $\alpha = 3/2$; this work predates Lévy's general study of the stable distributions. Mandelbrot (1963) first applied the theory of stable distributions to price movements and income distributions.

The general univariate stable distributions constitute a four-parameter family, and, since few of the distributions have an explicit form, estimation of the parameters is not straightforward. Press (1972b) first discussed the general problem; earlier work had mainly concentrated on the symmetric stable distributions. The empirical characteristic function

$$\hat{\phi}(t) = \sum_{i=1}^{n} e^{itx_i} = \sum_{i=1}^{n} \{\cos(tx_i) + i\sin(tx_i)\} \tag{2.55}$$

is an estimate of the characteristic function $\phi(t)$, and evaluation of the real and imaginary parts of $\hat{\phi}(t)$ at two values t_1 and t_2 gives four equations for the estimates $\hat{\mu}$, $\hat{c}$, $\hat{\alpha}$ and $\hat{\beta}$. Press gives details of this method, which he describes as 'a version of the method of moments', and goes on to discuss interval estimation for the parameters. This approach is clearly possible only with large samples, and its efficiency depends on the choice of t_1 and t_2. It has, however, the great advantage that it extends to the multivariate case with empirical characteristic function

$$\hat{\phi}(\boldsymbol{t}) = \sum_{i=1}^{n} e^{i\boldsymbol{t}'\boldsymbol{x}_i} = \sum_{i=1}^{n} \{\cos(\boldsymbol{t}'\boldsymbol{x}_i) + i\sin(\boldsymbol{t}'\boldsymbol{x}_i)\}. \tag{2.56}$$

Stable distributions are computationally rather intractable, but an efficient algorithm for generating random samples from stable distributions was developed by Chambers *et al* (1976), and is implemented in S-plus.

The multivariate stable distributions are a natural generalisation of the univariate family. Suppose $\boldsymbol{S}_n$ is a p-element vector consisting of the sums of n independent observations $\boldsymbol{x}_1, \ldots, \boldsymbol{x}_n$ from a p-variate distribution. Then if there are constant vectors $\boldsymbol{a}_n$, $\boldsymbol{b}_n$, such that

$$\frac{\boldsymbol{S}_n}{\boldsymbol{a}_n} - \boldsymbol{b}_n$$

where the division is carried out component by component, has the same distribution as $\boldsymbol{x}$, the distribution of $\boldsymbol{x}$ is multivariate stable. Again, the degenerate one-point distribution is excluded.

For the symmetric multivariate stable distributions, the log characteristic function has the form (Press, 1972b)

$$K(\boldsymbol{t}) = \log \phi(\boldsymbol{t}) \tag{2.57}$$

$$= i\boldsymbol{a}'\boldsymbol{t} - \frac{1}{2}(\boldsymbol{t}'\boldsymbol{\Omega}\boldsymbol{t})^{\alpha/2}. \tag{2.58}$$

Here α, with $0 < \alpha \leqslant 2$, has the same meaning as before, and $\boldsymbol{a}$ is a location parameter. The matrix $\boldsymbol{\Omega}$ is positive semi-definite, and determines the ellipsoidal contours of equal density. The cases $\alpha = 2$ and $\alpha = 1$ correspond to the multivariate normal and Cauchy distributions respectively.

More general forms of the characteristic function when elliptical symmetry does not hold are given by Press (1972b) and Galambos (1985). Further generalisation is possible; see, for example, Hudson and Mason (1981). Applications of these more general forms seem, however, rather limited.

The multivariate stable distributions have stable marginals (provided they are not degenerate) and, apart from the multivariate normal, are heavy-tailed with infinite variances. They arise naturally for simultaneous observations of variables that might be expected to have univariate stable distributions.

Matrix-valued distributions

2.27 Multivariate distributions in which the variates are elements of a matrix arise naturally in two different ways. First, sampling distributions of matrices of sums and products, or estimated variances and covariances, or matrices derived from these are important particularly in inference based on the multivariate normal distribution. The most important of these is the Wishart distribution (see Appendix). This distribution is the multivariate analogue of the χ^2 distribution; the non-central Wishart distribution is similarly related to the non-central χ^2 distribution.

Khatri and Pillai (1965) discuss matrix Beta distributions of type I and II. The former is the distribution of

$$(\boldsymbol{A}+\boldsymbol{B})^{-1/2}\boldsymbol{A}(\boldsymbol{A}+\boldsymbol{B})^{-1/2}$$

and the latter of

$$\boldsymbol{B}^{-1/2}\boldsymbol{A}\boldsymbol{B}^{-1/2}$$

where $\boldsymbol{A}$ and $\boldsymbol{B}$ are independent Wishart matrices. They are the multivariate equivalents of the distributions of R^2 and F respectively.

Secondly, when multivariate distributions are replicated, in time or otherwise, on individuals the q replicates of the p-variate observations can naturally be thought of as a $q \times p$ matrix, with a correlation structure among the p variables and among the q replicates. This sort of formulation may be useful for multivariate repeated measures experiments, multivariate growth curves or multivariate time series.

The most important distribution in this context is the matrix normal distribution. The following brief description follows de Waal (1985).

Suppose $\boldsymbol{X}$ is a $p \times q$ matrix random variable, with mean $\boldsymbol{\mu}$, (also a $p \times q$ matrix) and covariance matrix $\boldsymbol{\Sigma} \otimes \boldsymbol{\Psi}$.

Here, $\boldsymbol{\Sigma}$ and $\boldsymbol{\Psi}$ are positive semi-definite matrices, $p \times p$ and $q \times q$ respectively, and $\otimes$ stands for the Kronecker product; that is, the $pq \times pq$ matrix $\boldsymbol{\Sigma} \otimes \boldsymbol{\Psi}$ can be partitioned into a $p \times p$ array of $q \times q$ matrices of the form

$$\begin{pmatrix} \sigma_{11}\boldsymbol{\Psi} & \sigma_{12}\boldsymbol{\Psi} & \dots & \sigma_{1p}\boldsymbol{\Psi} \\ \sigma_{21}\boldsymbol{\Psi} & \sigma_{22}\boldsymbol{\Psi} & \dots & \sigma_{2p}\boldsymbol{\Psi} \\ \vdots & \vdots & & \vdots \\ \sigma_{p1}\boldsymbol{\Psi} & \sigma_{p2}\boldsymbol{\Psi} & \dots & \sigma_{pp}\boldsymbol{\Psi} \end{pmatrix}.$$

Then the density function of $\boldsymbol{X}$ is given by

$$f(\boldsymbol{X}) = (2\pi)^{-pq/2}|\boldsymbol{\Sigma}|^{-q/2}|\boldsymbol{\Psi}|^{-p/2}\exp(-\tfrac{1}{2}\mathrm{tr}\{\boldsymbol{\Sigma}^{-1}(\boldsymbol{X}-\boldsymbol{\mu})\boldsymbol{\Psi}^{-1}(\boldsymbol{X}-\boldsymbol{\mu})'\}) \quad (2.59)$$

$$-\infty < x_{ij} < \infty, \quad \forall\ i, j.$$

This result follows from considering the distribution of vec$\boldsymbol{X}$, where the vec operator converts the $p \times q$ matrix $\boldsymbol{X}$ into a $pq \times 1$ column vector in sequence by rows. This vector has a multivariate normal distribution with mean vec$\boldsymbol{\mu}$ and covariance matrix $\boldsymbol{\Sigma} \otimes \boldsymbol{\Psi}$.

The matrix-valued normal distribution is no more general than the ordinary multivariate normal distribution. Its advantage is that it specifically models the variation in rows and columns. If the columns of $\boldsymbol{X}$ represent different times, it may well be reasonable to model the rows of $\boldsymbol{\mu}$ by simple trends, such as polynomials, and the covariance matrix $\boldsymbol{\Psi}$ by a structure appropriate for time series, such as a simple autoregressive structure. This possibility makes the matrix-valued distribution particularly suitable for modelling multivariate repeated measures.

Exercises

2.1 If u_1, u_2 are independent $U(0,1)$ variables and

$$\begin{aligned} x_1 &= \sqrt{-2\log(u_1)}\cos(2\pi u_2) \\ x_2 &= \sqrt{-2\log(u_1)}\sin(2\pi u_2) \end{aligned}$$

show that x_1, x_2 are independent standard normal variables.

[This is the Box–Muller (1958) transformation for obtaining random normal deviates from random uniform variates. It is still widely used, but other methods have better numerical properties].

2.2 Construct a bivariate distribution for which x, y, and $x + y$ are normally distributed, but (x, y) is not bivariate normal.

[Stoyanov (1987) gives a number of examples illustrating the danger of inferring multivariate normality from marginal and/or conditional distributions].

2.3 If all correlations between pairs of p variables are equal to ρ, show that every partial correlation of order s is $\rho/(1 + s\rho)$. Hence show that $\rho \geqslant -1/(p-1)$.

2.4 Show that if $x_1, \ldots, x_p$ are independently distributed as χ^2 with degrees of freedom $\nu_1, \ldots, \nu_p$ and $y_i = x_i / \sum_{i=1}^{p} x_i$, then $\boldsymbol{y}$ has a Dirichlet distribution with parameters $\alpha_i = \nu_i/2$.

2.5 A distribution consists of a mixture of two bivariate normal distributions with means $(0,0)$ and (μ_x, μ_y), proportions $1 - \alpha$, α and common covariance matrix $\begin{pmatrix} 1 & \rho \\ \rho & 1 \end{pmatrix}$.

Find the regression of y on x, and show that it is linear only if $\mu_y = \rho\mu_x$. Show that the correlation is

$$\frac{\rho + \alpha(1-\alpha)\mu_x\mu_y}{[(1+\alpha(1-\alpha)\mu_x^2)(1+\alpha(1-\alpha)\mu_y^2]^{\frac{1}{2}}}$$

and show that if μ_x is fixed, the correlation is maximum when $\mu_y = \mu_x/\rho$.

2.6 Verify the statement in **2.21** that $(\boldsymbol{n} - n\boldsymbol{\pi})'V^{-1}(\boldsymbol{n} - n\boldsymbol{\pi})$ gives the ordinary Pearson χ^2 statistic.

[Note that $V = n(\boldsymbol{D} - \boldsymbol{\pi}\boldsymbol{\pi}')$, where $\boldsymbol{D} = \text{diag}(\boldsymbol{\pi})$, and use Bartlett's (1951) matrix identity

$$(\boldsymbol{A} + \boldsymbol{u}\boldsymbol{v}')^{-1} = \boldsymbol{A}^{-1} - \frac{\boldsymbol{A}^{-1}\boldsymbol{u}\boldsymbol{v}'\boldsymbol{A}^{-1}}{1 + \boldsymbol{v}'\boldsymbol{A}^{-1}\boldsymbol{u}}\ ].$$

2.7 Given a method of generating standard $N(0, 1)$ random variables x, it is required to generate p-variate $N(\boldsymbol{0}, \Sigma)$ random variables $\boldsymbol{y}$. Describe how to do this

(a) By generating in turn y_1, $y_2|y_1$, $y_3|(y_1, y_2), \ldots$

(b) By a transformation $\boldsymbol{y} = \boldsymbol{H}\boldsymbol{x}$, where $\boldsymbol{x} \sim N(\boldsymbol{0}, \boldsymbol{I})$ and $\boldsymbol{H}\boldsymbol{H}' = \Sigma$.

2.8 If x_1, x_2 have a bivariate normal distribution with zero mean and correlation ρ, show that

$$\Pr(x_1 > 0, x_2 > 0) = \frac{1}{4} + \frac{1}{2\pi}\arcsin(\rho)$$

(Sheppard, 1898).

Prove the corresponding result for a trivariate normal distribution

$$\Pr(x_1 > 0, x_2 > 0, x_3 > 0) = \frac{1}{8} + \frac{1}{4\pi}(\arcsin \rho_{12} + \arcsin \rho_{13} + \arcsin \rho_{23}).$$

[No simple result holds for $p > 3$].

2.9 Mardia's coefficient of multivariate kurtosis (see **3.16**) is defined as $E\{(\boldsymbol{x} - \boldsymbol{\mu})'\Sigma^{-1}(\boldsymbol{x} - \boldsymbol{\mu})\}^2$.

Show that, for the multivariate t distribution with v degrees of freedom, the value is $p(p+2)(v-2)/(v-4)$.

[Note that $\boldsymbol{\Sigma}$ is the population dispersion matrix, not the dispersion matrix of the underlying normal distribution, as in **2.6**].

2.10 In an immigration-death process, the probability of immigration and death in time δt are respectively $v\delta t$, and $\mu\delta t$ for each individual. Show that the distribution of the number of individuals tends to a Poisson distribution with mean v/μ. Show also that when this stationary distribution has been reached, the joint distribution of the numbers at times τ apart has probability generating function

$$\Pi(z_1, z_2) = \exp\{-\frac{v}{\mu}[(z_1 - 1) + (z_2 - 1) + e^{-\mu\tau}(z_1 - 1)(z_2 - 1)]\}\ ,$$

a bivariate Poisson distribution with equal means and a correlation $e^{-\mu t}$.

2.11 Variables y,u have a bivariate normal distribution with correlation ρ.

A binary variable a takes the value 0 ($u < \alpha$), 1 ($u \geqslant \alpha$). The value of u is unobserved; without loss of generality, assume $U \sim N(0, 1)$. Show that

$$\Pr(a = 1 | y = y^*) = \Phi\left\{\left[\frac{\rho(y^* - \mu_y)}{\sigma_y} - \alpha\right] / (1 - \rho^2)^{\frac{1}{2}}\right\}$$

(Cox and Wermuth, 1992).

[This is the probit-normal distribution, virtually indistinguishable from the logistic-normal].

3

Initial Data Analysis

Graphical displays of multivariate data

3.1 The first step in any statistical analysis is to look at the data and to identify their main features. It has been said that 'a picture is worth a thousand numbers', and indeed simple plots of the data can easily reveal such facets as clustering of individuals, relationships between variables, presence of outliers, and so on. Even if a picture does not answer all the analyst's questions it will generally highlight aspects of interest, provide pointers for the analysis, and perhaps generate hypotheses for future investigation. Consequently, various authors have considered how best to summarise pictorially the information contained in an $n \times p$ data matrix. The problem is thus one of representing p-dimensional information by a picture that is restricted to be in just two dimensions if it is to be presented on the printed page.

3.2 First let us assume that all variables are quantitative. Then the multivariate data matrix can be notionally envisaged as a set of n points (one for each row of the matrix) in p dimensions (one for each column). If $p = 2$ then a scatter plot of one variable against the other is an exact depiction of this 'data space', but when $p > 2$ we need to find an approximate representation. One obvious possibility is to provide the $\frac{1}{2}p(p-1)$ possible scatter plots of each variable against every other. Although this might seem to invite potential confusion, it is possible to build up an overall picture by suitably 'linking' the separate scatter plots. Such linked scatter plots now form a cornerstone of both static (Chambers *et al*, 1983) and dynamic (Becker *et al*, 1987) graphic software packages for computer data analysis.

A second possibility with $p > 2$ is to plot a scatter diagram for two arbitrarily chosen variables and then to incorporate the values of the other variables on the same plot. For example, the values of a third variable can be represented as a line originating from each point, with length proportional to the value and directed eastwards if this value is positive and westwards if negative. Fourth,

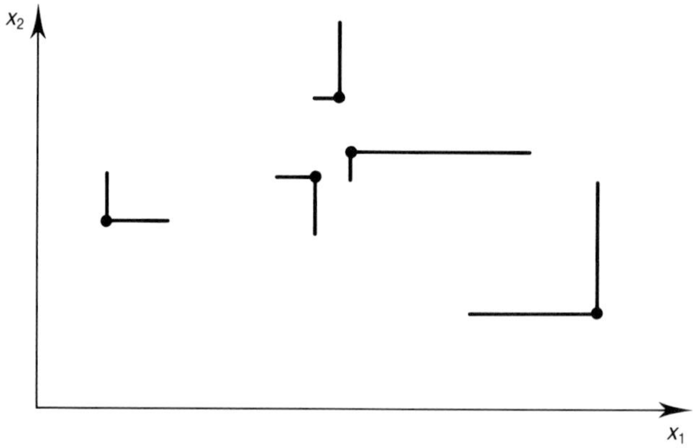

Figure 3.1 A four-dimensional set of data

fifth, sixth and further variables can use the north-south, NE-SW, NW-SE and other such directions (Gower, 1967). An example is shown in Fig. 3.1.

This representation attempts to incorporate all the information in a single plot. An alternative way of doing so is to find a projection of the points from the original p-dimensional space into two dimensions, and then to plot the points in this subspace. Such a procedure will of necessity lose some information, and perhaps introduce some distortion, in the course of projection. The resulting plot will therefore only be an approximation to the true picture, but if the projection is carefully chosen then the amount of information loss will be minimised. Various possible projections will be described in Chapter 4. Modern dynamic statistical graphics packages have built on these concepts to provide very powerful methods of computer inspection of multivariate data. For example, Young and Rheigans (1991) discuss the notion of a 'guided tour' of multivariate data space, and describe a number of tools including subspace projection and axis spinning for effecting guided tours.

3.3 The above methods start with the idea of a 'true' representation in high-dimensional space, for which a two-dimensional approximation is then sought. Instead, one might seek directly to represent the individuals by entities in two dimensions. Arguably the most flexible method in this general class is the one proposed by Andrews (1972), wherein the p-variable observation $\boldsymbol{x}' = (x_1, \ldots, x_p)$ is represented by the Fourier curve

$$f_x(t) = x_1/\sqrt{2} + x_2 \sin t + x_3 \cos t + x_4 \sin 2t + x_5 \cos 2t + \ldots \qquad (3.1)$$

plotted over the region $[-\pi, \pi]$.
A set of multivariate observations will thus appear as a set of curves drawn across the plot. Andrews (1972) has established the following properties of these curves.

(1) The function representation preserves means, i.e. if $\bar{\boldsymbol{x}}$ is the mean of a set of n multivariate observations $\boldsymbol{x}_i$, then at each point t in $-\pi < t < \pi$ the

function corresponding to $\bar{x}$ is the mean of the n functions corresponding to the individual observations.

(2) The function representation preserves Euclidean distances, i.e. $d \propto D$, where $d^2 = \sum_{i=1}^{p}(x_i - y_i)^2$ is the squared Euclidean distance between two observations $\boldsymbol{x}' = (x_1, \ldots, x_p)$ and $\boldsymbol{y}' = (y_1, \ldots, y_p)$ while $D^2 = \int_{-\pi}^{\pi}[f_x(t) - f_y(t)]^2\,dt$ is the squared Euclidean distance between the corresponding functions.

(3) If the variables in the data matrix are uncorrelated with constant variance σ^2, then the variance of the function at any point t is $\frac{1}{2}p\sigma^2$ when p is odd and lies between $\frac{1}{2}(p-1)\sigma^2$ and $\frac{1}{2}(p+1)\sigma^2$ when p is even. In either case the relative dependence of the function variance on t is either very slight or non-existent, so the variability of the plotted function is almost constant across the graph. (Goodchild and Vijayan (1974) discuss briefly the extension of these results to the case of correlated variables.)

(4) The function preserves linear relationships. If $\boldsymbol{y}$ lies on the line joining $\boldsymbol{x}$ and z, then $f_y(t)$ lies between $f_x(t)$ and $f_z(t)$ for all t.

(5) For any particular value t_0 of t, the function value $f(t_0)$ is proportional to the length of the projection of the vector $\boldsymbol{x}$ on the vector

$$\boldsymbol{a}_0 = (1/\sqrt{2}, \sin t_0, \cos t_0, \sin 2t_0, \cos 2t_0, \ldots),$$

since $f_x(t_0) = \boldsymbol{x}'\boldsymbol{a}_0$.

Property 2 implies that two observations having similar sets of variable values will yield two curves that are close together over all values of t. Conversely, if the two observations have very different sets of variable values then values of t will occur at which the corresponding curves are far apart. Property 5 provides the appropriate projection of the data that highlights the difference between these observations. Properties 1 and 4 establish the correspondence between facets of the curves and those of the data, while property 3 is useful in calculation of confidence regions and tests of hypotheses for 'true' curves and their differences (see Andrews (1972) and Goodchild and Vijayan (1974) for details). Thus by representing a multivariate data set by means of such Fourier curves we can readily inspect it for the presence of clusters of observations, outliers, or other patterns. For an illustration, see Example 3.1 below.

3.4 Representation of multivariate data by means of Fourier curves is not possible when some or all of the variables are qualitative, but many other graphical methods suitable for categorical or mixed data now exist. An early such display was the *glyph*, devised by Anderson (1957), in which each individual in the sample is represented by a circle of fixed radius and each variable by a ray emanating from this circle. The position of the ray indicates which variable is being represented, and the length of the ray indicates either the value of a quantitative variable or the category of a qualitative variable for the individual represented. Ordered categories (e.g. small, medium, large) can be represented by progressively longer rays, the lowest category often being indicated by absence of a ray. If the categories are unordered the lengths of rays can be assigned to them arbitrarily. For quantitative data the length of ray is usually proportional to the value of the variable, the entire set of

Table 3.1 Five variables observed on three individuals

	Variables				
Unit	1	2	3	4	5
A	0	g	n	5.2	-2.0
B	0	r	l	3.6	4.2
C	1	b	h	-1.6	0.8

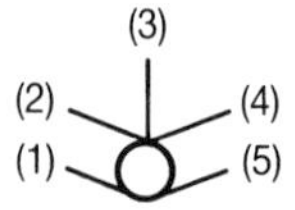

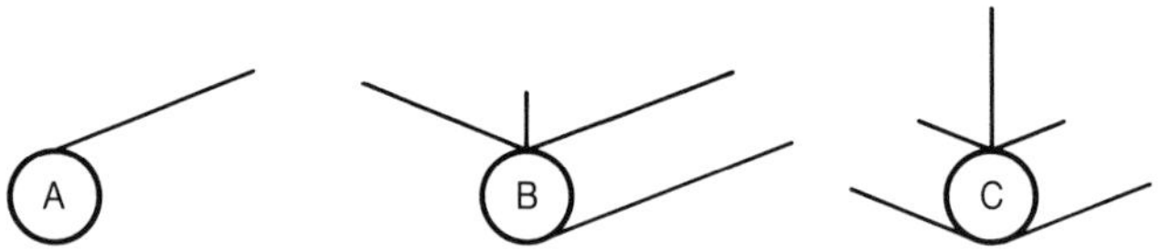

Figure 3.2 Glyphs for data in Table 3.1

quantitative data having first been scaled so that the smallest value is at zero. As an example, consider the small data set given in Table 3.1 where values are given for five variables on each of three individuals. Variable 1 is binary, with values 0 or 1; variable 2 is three-state with categories green (g), blue (b) and red (r); variable 3 is also three-state but with categories none (n), low (l) and high (h) while variables 4 and 5 are both quantitative. This data set is represented by glyphs in Fig. 3.2. Note that for this representation all values of variables 4 and 5 in Table 3.1 first had 2.0 added to them (to make the smallest value in the table zero). The correspondence of rays and variate values is: ray absent for 0 and ray present for 1 (variable 1); ray absent for g, short ray for b and long ray for r (variable 2); ray absent for n, short ray for l and long ray for h (variable 3); rays proportional to $x + 2.0$ for variables 4 and 5.

Two variations of this representation are popular. If there are at least two quantitative variables in the data set, then the glyphs can be plotted as points in a two-dimensional scatter diagram for two of these variables. The result then resembles Fig. 3.1, and only $p - 2$ rays are required for a p-variable data set. The second variation is to space the rays equally around the circle and to join up the ends of the rays to form polygons. The resulting pictures are known as 'Stars'; an example is shown on page 49. Many other variations on the theme have appeared sporadically in the literature, including the plotting of triangles (Pickett and White, 1966), p-sided polygons (Siegel *et al*, 1971), weather-vanes (Cleveland and Kleiner, 1974), boxes (Hartigan,

Table 3.2 Permanent first lower premolar : canonical variate means for eight groups (Reproduced with permission from Ashton *et al*, 1957; Andrews, 1972)

	Canonical variate							
Group	1	2	3	4	5	6	7	8
A West African	-8.09	0.49	0.18	0.75	-0.06	-0.04	0.04	0.03
B British	-9.37	-0.68	-0.44	-0.37	0.37	0.02	-0.01	0.05
C Aboriginal	-8.87	1.44	0.36	-0.34	-0.29	-0.02	-0.01	-0.05
D Gorilla(m)	6.28	2.89	0.43	-0.03	0.10	-0.14	0.07	0.08
E Gorilla(f)	4.82	1.52	0.71	-0.06	0.25	0.15	-0.07	-0.10
F Orangutan(m)	5.11	1.61	-0.72	0.04	-0.17	0.13	0.03	0.05
G Orangutan(f)	3.60	0.28	-1.05	0.01	-0.03	-0.11	-0.11	-0.08
H Chimpanzee(m)	3.46	-3.37	0.33	-0.32	-0.19	-0.04	0.09	0.09
I Chimpanzee(f)	3.05	-4.21	0.17	0.28	0.04	0.02	-0.06	-0.06

1975b), constellations (Wakimoto and Taguri, 1978), and trees and castles (Kleiner and Hartigan, 1981).

3.5 One other related technique that merits some mention is the suggestion by Chernoff (1973) that multivariate observations be represented by human faces. This is done by associating each variable with a different characteristic of the face (e.g. length of nose, shape of face, size and slant of eyes, curvature of mouth, and so on). To simplify matters it may be necessary to categorise the quantitative variables before producing a face to represent a given multivariate observation. On the other hand, there is scope for matching highly correlated variables to highly correlated facial features and thereby bringing out the most from the data. This technique needs the most sophisticated software of all the methods discussed so far but also has, at least potentially, the most promise given the extensive experience that we all have in reacting to and recognising human faces; see Flury and Riedwyl (1988) for some good examples. Unfortunately, despite a few contributions such as improvement of software (Wainer, 1981) and the use of asymmetric faces (Flury and Riedwyl, 1981), the technique does not yet appear to have been widely taken up.

Example 3.1

To illustrate some of these ideas, consider the data given in Table 3.2. These data are taken from Ashton *et al* (1957), who used canonical variate analysis (see **4.10** and **4.11**) to study differences between various human and ape populations from measurements on their teeth. The values in Table 3.2 are the means on all eight canonical variates for these populations as obtained from analysis of eight measurements made on the permanent first premolar. Andrews (1972) used these values to illustrate his Fourier curve technique, obtaining the plot shown in Fig. 3.3.

This plot shows a clear separation of the three human populations from the six ape populations, across the whole range of t. Additionally, several projections of interest can be obtained at specified t values. At t_2 and t_4 the human populations have a common value; at t_1 the chimpanzees have a single value, the gorillas and orangutans have a different common value, and the humans have a third, almost constant, value; while at t_3

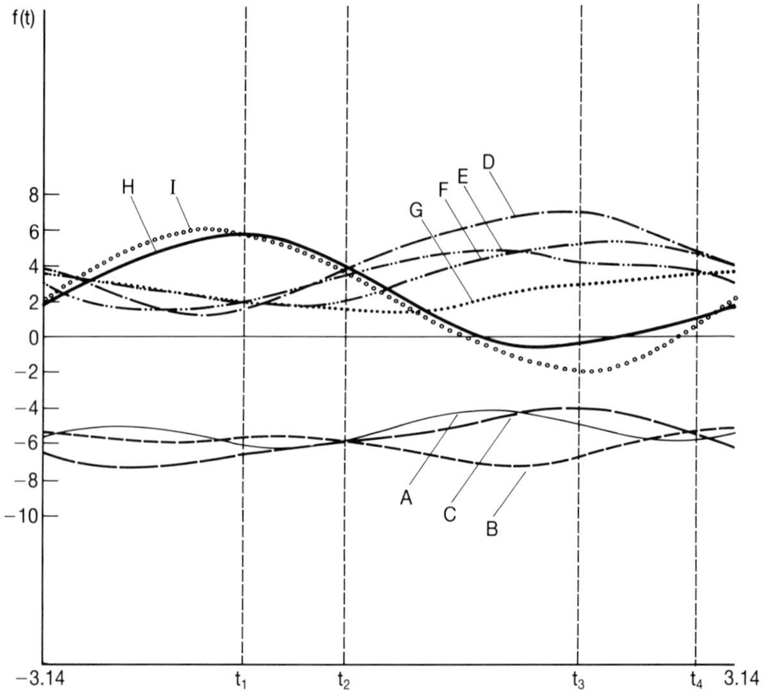

Figure 3.3 Andrews' curves for data of Table 3.2. Reproduced with permission from Andrews (1972).

the group members have their widest possible separation. From property 5 of **3.3** we would therefore deduce that the projection on the vector

$$\boldsymbol{a}_1 = (1/\sqrt{2}, \sin t_1, \cos t_1, \sin 2t_1, \cos 2t_1, \ldots)$$

gives the best discrimination between the three groups 'humans', 'chimpanzees' and 'gorillas plus orangutans'. Replacing t_1 by either t_2 or t_4 gives appropriate projections for distinguishing 'humans' from 'apes', while using t_3 gives the best projection for separating all nine populations.

Fienberg (1979) used the same data to illustrate both stars and faces; his diagrams are reproduced in Figs. 3.4 and 3.5 respectively. Consider first the stars. Each canonical variate is associated with one of the eight rays, beginning with variate one located at three o'clock and running anticlockwise. The length of each ray gives $x + 9.37$ (since 9.37 is the largest negative entry in the table) for the corresponding variate in a specified row of the table. Examination of the plot suggests that the humans (A, B, C) form one group, the gorillas and orangutans (D, E, F, G) a second group and the chimpanzees (H, I) a third. It is also evident that it is variates one and two that heavily influence this categorisation into groups.

Next consider the faces. Fienberg comments that it took considerable trial and error to get the program working and to produce a reasonable

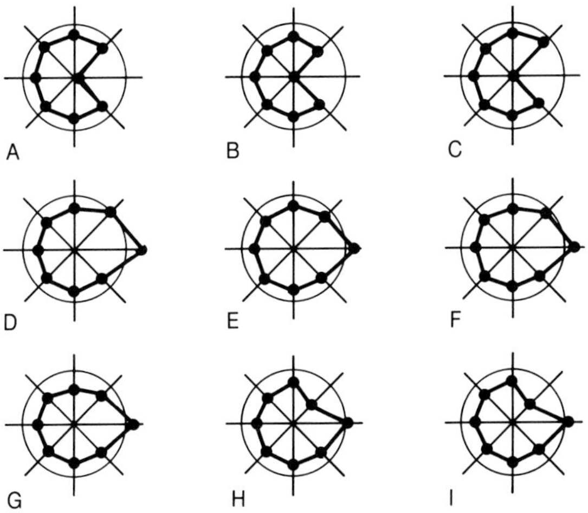

Figure 3.4 Stars for data of Table 3.2. Reproduced with permission from Fienberg (1979), *The American Statistician* by the American Statistical Association. All rights reserved.

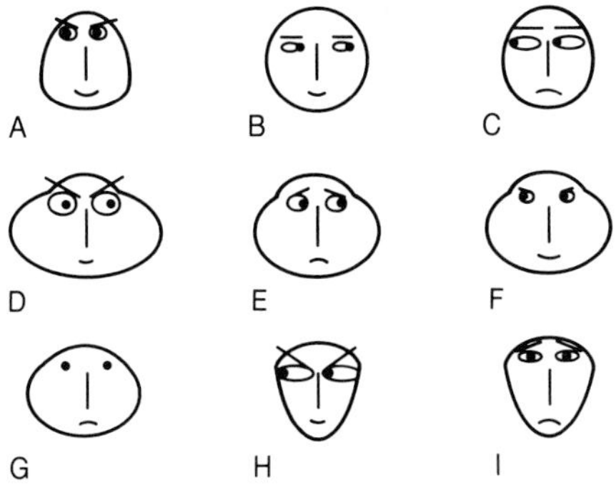

Figure 3.5 Chernoff's faces for data of Table 3.2. Reproduced with permission from Fienberg (1979), *The American Statistician* by the American Statistical Association. All rights reserved.

display! This diagram is the final outcome, the eight canonical variates (in order) being represented by the following facial features : (a) face shape, (b) jaw shape, (c) eye size, (d) eye position, (e) pupil position, (f) forehead shape, (g) eyebrow slant, and (h) mouth shape. The resulting picture does a moderately good job of producing the same groupings as with the other techniques.

3.6 While the above techniques are all undoubtedly useful in representing multivariate data, it is also obvious that interpretation of the resulting pictures entails a considerable element of subjectivity. Different people may come to very different conclusions on viewing the same set of stars or faces, say. Perhaps a more serious objection to the techniques, however, is that the impression conveyed by a picture depends considerably on the order in which the variates are presented. Permuting the variables before applying equation (3.1) can produce a very different looking set of Andrews' curves, as can rescaling the variables. Embrechts and Herzberg (1991) explore these and other variations of Andrews' plots. Similarly, very different patterns might emerge if variables are assigned differently to the rays of a set of stars or to the facial features of a set of Chernoff's faces. Some further investigations and examples are provided by Chernoff and Rizvi (1975), Fienberg (1979) and Jacob (1983).

Note that in the case of Andrews' curves the low frequencies (i.e. x_1, x_2, x_3) are distinguished more readily than the high frequencies (i.e. x_{p-2}, x_{p-1}, x_p), so if possible the 'most important' variables should be entered into equation (3.1) first. Thus Andrews' curves are particularly successful if the data have first been subjected to a technique such as principal component analysis or canonical variate analysis (Chapter 4), where a ranking of variables in 'order of importance' has taken place; this is why the data of Example 3.1 were represented so well. Note, however, that large data sets may need to be analysed in subsets: including too many Fourier curves in a single diagram will lead to confusion.

The detection of outliers

3.7 One of the main purposes of initial data analysis is to screen the data for possible anomalous values. If such values are present, then they should be investigated before any detailed analysis of the data is undertaken. For example, checks should be made to see if any recording errors have been made and, if they have, then the values should be corrected. If, on the other hand, the rogue values are genuine then some thought must be given as to whether or not they should be retained when analysing the data. Such considerations belong within the context of the study in question; here we will only concern ourselves with the problem of identifying anomalous values, or 'outliers'.

While the graphical techniques described above might allow such identification, it should be remembered that these techniques have been designed to highlight many different facets of a multivariate data set so the chance of missing a few anomalous values is not negligible. Consequently, much effort has been devoted over the years to providing simple statistics for the identification of outliers. Intuitively, the problem is the seemingly simple one of isolating any individuals whose values are atypical of those in the rest of the data set. The trouble is that, in multivariate data, atypicality can arise in a number of different ways; different aspects of atypicality will in general require different techniques for their detection. We will first consider various informal procedures for detection of anomalous observations, and then survey briefly the more formal hypothesis tests that have been proposed. Comprehensive texts devoted to outlier detection are those by Barnett and Lewis (1978) and Hawkins (1980).

3.8 An intuitive notion of an outlier is as an 'extreme' observation that is 'far away' from the rest of the data values. In univariate analysis there is a natural ordering of the data, which enables extremes of a data set to be identified and the distance of these extremes from the centre to be computed readily. Multivariate situations offer no such clear-cut solution. Barnett (1976) discusses the ordering of multivariate data, and identifies four different types : marginal *(M-ordering)*, reduced *(R-ordering)*, partial *(P-ordering)* and conditional *(C-ordering)*. Of these, R-ordering is the one most suitable for definition of 'extremes' as here each multivariate observation is reduced to a single value by means of some combination of the component sample values. These single values are then amenable to univariate ordering, so that if the method of combination of the component values is through a measure of 'distance' then we have a natural mechanism for identification of outliers. Siotani (1959) bases his definition of extremeness of a multivariate observation $\boldsymbol{x}$ on its 'distance value' $(\boldsymbol{x}-\boldsymbol{\alpha})'\boldsymbol{\Gamma}^{-1}(\boldsymbol{x}-\boldsymbol{\alpha})$ where $\boldsymbol{\alpha}$ is a location parameter and $\boldsymbol{\Gamma}$ is a dispersion parameter. These parameters can be given arbitrary values such as $\boldsymbol{\alpha}=\boldsymbol{0}$ and $\boldsymbol{\Gamma}=\boldsymbol{I}$, or they can be assigned population location ($\boldsymbol{\mu}$) and dispersion ($\boldsymbol{\Sigma}$) settings. Alternatively, if $\boldsymbol{x}_1, \boldsymbol{x}_2, \ldots, \boldsymbol{x}_n$ is a random sample of observations from a population with unknown location and dispersion parameters $\boldsymbol{\mu}$ and $\boldsymbol{\Sigma}$ then suitable quantities to use would be the standard estimates (see **3.20**)

$$\bar{\boldsymbol{x}} = \frac{1}{n}\sum_{i=1}^{n}\boldsymbol{x}_i \qquad (3.2)$$

and

$$\boldsymbol{S} = \frac{1}{n-1}\boldsymbol{A} \qquad (3.3)$$

where $\boldsymbol{A}=\sum_{i=1}^{n}(\boldsymbol{x}_i-\bar{\boldsymbol{x}})(\boldsymbol{x}_i-\bar{\boldsymbol{x}})'$.

3.9 Gnanadesikan and Kettenring (1972) list the following statistics within this general class. We assume here that $(\boldsymbol{x}_1, \boldsymbol{x}_2, \ldots, \boldsymbol{x}_n)$ is a multivariate sample and that summary statistics have been calculated as in equations 3.2 and 3.3.

$$q_j^2 = (\boldsymbol{x}_j-\bar{\boldsymbol{x}})'(\boldsymbol{x}_j-\bar{\boldsymbol{x}}) \quad (j=1,\ldots,n) \qquad (3.4)$$

$$t_j^2 = (\boldsymbol{x}_j-\bar{\boldsymbol{x}})'\boldsymbol{S}(\boldsymbol{x}_j-\bar{\boldsymbol{x}}) \quad (j=1,\ldots,n) \qquad (3.5)$$

$$u_j^2 = \frac{(\boldsymbol{x}_j-\bar{\boldsymbol{x}})'\boldsymbol{S}(\boldsymbol{x}_j-\bar{\boldsymbol{x}})}{(\boldsymbol{x}_j-\bar{\boldsymbol{x}})'(\boldsymbol{x}_j-\bar{\boldsymbol{x}})} \quad (j=1,\ldots,n) \qquad (3.6)$$

$$v_j^2 = \frac{(\boldsymbol{x}_j-\bar{\boldsymbol{x}})'\,\boldsymbol{S}^{-1}(\boldsymbol{x}_j-\bar{\boldsymbol{x}})}{(\boldsymbol{x}_j-\bar{\boldsymbol{x}})'(\boldsymbol{x}_j-\bar{\boldsymbol{x}})} \quad (j=1,\ldots,n) \qquad (3.7)$$

$$d_{j0}^2 = (\boldsymbol{x}_j-\bar{\boldsymbol{x}})'\boldsymbol{S}^{-1}(\boldsymbol{x}_j-\bar{\boldsymbol{x}}) \quad (j=1,\ldots,n) \qquad (3.8)$$

$$d_{jk}^2 = (\boldsymbol{x}_j-\boldsymbol{x}_k)'\boldsymbol{S}^{-1}(\boldsymbol{x}_j-\boldsymbol{x}_k) \quad (j<k=1,\ldots,n) \qquad (3.9)$$

Each of these statistics identifies the contribution of the individual observations (or combinations of observations) to specific effects as follows: q_j^2 isolates observations which excessively inflate the overall scale; t_j^2 determines which observations have the greatest influence on the orientation and scale of the first few principal components (Chapter 4) of $\boldsymbol{S}$; u_j^2 is similar in spirit but puts more emphasis on orientation and less on scale; v_j^2 measures the relative contributions of the observations on the orientations of the last few principal components; d_{j0}^2 uncovers those observations which lie far away from the general scatter of points, and d_{jk}^2 has the same objective but provides far more detail of inter-object separation. Corresponding statistics for standardised data are obtained by replacing $\boldsymbol{S}$ by the correlation matrix of the sample, $\boldsymbol{R}$, in all the above formulae. Note, however, that this is not necessary for either d_{j0}^2 or d_{jk}^2 as they are invariant under non-singular transformations of the data matrix.

3.10 Gnanadesikan and Kettenring (1972) suggest probability plotting (Seber, 1984 p542) of these statistics as an informal way of identifying outliers, which should show up as rogue points on such graphs. They recommend gamma-type probability plots with estimated shape parameters as reasonable starting points for $q_j^2, t_j^2, d_{j0}^2, d_{jk}^2$, and either beta- or F-type probability plots for u_j^2, v_j^2. If the $\boldsymbol{x}_i$ are additionally assumed to have come from a normal population, then Cox (1968) and Healy (1968) have suggested either a χ_p^2 probability plot for the d_{j0}^2 or a normal probability plot for the cube roots of the d_{j0}^2. Alternatively, (Exercise 3.3) the exact distributions of

$$\frac{n}{(n-1)^2} d_{j0}^2$$

and

$$\frac{1}{2(n-1)} d_{jk}^2$$

are both beta with parameters $\frac{1}{2}p$ and $\frac{1}{2}(n-p-1)$, where p is the number of elements of $\boldsymbol{x}_j$. Thus the distances can be transformed into F variables for probability plotting. Note two drawbacks inherent in the application of such probability plotting, however. The first is that there is correlation present between any two values for the data set, e.g. between u_j^2 and u_k^2 for all $j \neq k$, but all probability plots assume that independent entities are being plotted. The second is that if outliers *are* present in the data then $\bar{\boldsymbol{x}}$ and $\boldsymbol{S}$ are not the best estimates of location and dispersion for the data (since they will be adversely affected by the outliers). Correlations among the statistics are generally felt to be minor problems, particularly if the sample is a large one. The problem of inappropriate parameter estimates can be overcome by using robust estimates of location and scale (see **3.22** below). Finally, note that the statistics which measure influence on the first few principal components (such as t_j^2, u_j^2 or either d^2) tend to detect those outliers which inflate variances, covariances or correlations in the data, while the statistics such as v_j^2 which measure influence on the last few principal components will detect those outliers that add insignificant dimensions to, or obscure singularities in, the data. An example of the first sort of outlier is the point at the top right-hand corner of Fig. 3.6 while an example of the second type of outlier is the point near the bottom of the same figure. For a number of examples of these probability plots, see Gnanadesikan and Kettenring (1972) and Gnanadesikan (1977).

3.11 A more formal approach to the detection of outliers provides a model for the data, encompassing the possibility of outliers, and sets up tests of hypotheses that certain observations are outliers against the alternative that

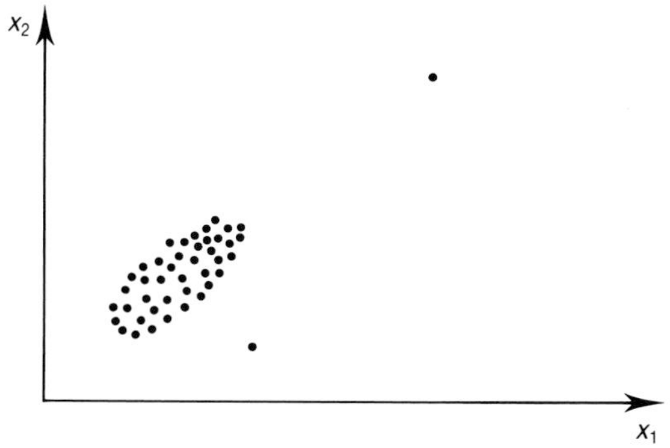

Figure 3.6 Two types of bivariate outlier

they are part of the main body of data. Hawkins (1980) identifies two basic mechanisms which give rise to samples that appear to have outliers. In the first mechanism the data come from some heavy-tailed distribution such as Student's t; there is no question here that any observation is in any way erroneous. In the second mechanism the data come from two distributions. The first distribution provides the majority of observations, while the second one provides a small minority. If this second distribution has heavier tails than the first, then there will be a tendency for the minority of observations to contain outliers; observations from the first distribution are then sometimes called 'inliers'.

Formal tests for outliers build on this second mechanism, generally by assuming normal distributions. Suppose that $\boldsymbol{x}_1, \boldsymbol{x}_2, \ldots, \boldsymbol{x}_n$ are the data vectors under consideration. The null hypothesis considers these vectors to be a random sample from some arbitrary normal distribution,

$$H_0 : \boldsymbol{x}_i \sim N_p(\boldsymbol{\mu}, \boldsymbol{\Sigma}) \quad (i = 1, \ldots, n) \tag{3.10}$$

while a k-outlier alternative hypothesis would postulate that $n - k$ of the $\boldsymbol{x}_i$ come from this distribution but the remaining k come from a different distribution (or distributions). Formally this can be specified by assuming that there is some unknown permutation $\boldsymbol{x}_{[1]}, \boldsymbol{x}_{[2]}, \ldots, \boldsymbol{x}_{[n]}$ of the $\boldsymbol{x}_i$ such that

$$\boldsymbol{x}_{[j]} \sim N_p(\boldsymbol{\mu}, \boldsymbol{\Sigma}) \quad (j = k+1, \ldots, n) \tag{3.11}$$

while $\boldsymbol{x}_{[1]}, \ldots, \boldsymbol{x}_{[k]}$ follow some other distribution or distributions. The most likely possibilities are

$$H_1 : \boldsymbol{x}_{[j]} \sim N_p(\boldsymbol{\mu}_j, \boldsymbol{\Sigma}) \quad (j = 1, \ldots, k), \tag{3.12}$$

$$H_2 : \boldsymbol{x}_{[j]} \sim N_p(\boldsymbol{\mu}, a_j\boldsymbol{\Sigma}) \quad (j = 1, \ldots, k), \tag{3.13}$$

or

$$H_3 : \boldsymbol{x}_{[j]} \sim N_p(\boldsymbol{\mu}, \boldsymbol{\Sigma}_j) \quad (j = 1, \ldots, k), \tag{3.14}$$

and simplifications of these three hypotheses are obtained by setting

$$\begin{aligned} \boldsymbol{\mu}_1 &= \boldsymbol{\mu}_2 = \ldots = \boldsymbol{\mu}_k, \\ a_1 &= a_2 = \ldots = a_k, \\ \boldsymbol{\Sigma}_1 &= \boldsymbol{\Sigma}_2 = \ldots = \boldsymbol{\Sigma}_k, \end{aligned}$$

respectively. In practice, attention has focused on H_1 and H_2, as H_3 gives rise to a number of severe difficulties (Hawkins, 1980).

3.12 In the case $k = 1$, the forms of H_0, H_1 and H_2 suggest that we are essentially in the realm of two-sample hypothesis tests (Chapter 6). If we have identified a potential outlier $\boldsymbol{x}_i$, then suitable test statistics for H_0 versus H_1 are either the two-sample T^2 statistic

$$T_i^2 = (\boldsymbol{x}_i - \bar{\boldsymbol{x}}_i)' \boldsymbol{A}_i^{-1} (\boldsymbol{x}_i - \bar{\boldsymbol{x}}_i)(n-1)(n-2)/n \tag{3.15}$$

or Wilks's lambda statistic

$$\Lambda_i = \mid \boldsymbol{A}_i \mid / \mid \boldsymbol{A} \mid \tag{3.16}$$

where $\bar{\boldsymbol{x}}_i = \frac{1}{n-1} \sum_{j \neq i} \boldsymbol{x}_j$, $\boldsymbol{A}_i = \sum_{j \neq i} (\boldsymbol{x}_j - \bar{\boldsymbol{x}}_i)(\boldsymbol{x}_j - \bar{\boldsymbol{x}}_i)'$ and $\boldsymbol{A}$ is given by equation (3.3). To obtain the distribution of T_i^2 under H_0 we use standard theory (**6.27** and Appendix **A.1**) for groups of size 1 and $n-1$ respectively. If we haven't a particular $\boldsymbol{x}_i$ in mind, then $T_{max}^2 = \max_i T_i^2$ will identify the best candidate and simultaneously provide the test statistic; this statistic also turns out to be good for H_2 as the alternative hypothesis. One could alternatively use Λ_{min}, while Ferguson (1961) proposed the statistic D_{max}^2 where $D_i^2 = (\boldsymbol{x}_i - \bar{\boldsymbol{x}})' \boldsymbol{A}^{-1} (\boldsymbol{x}_i - \bar{\boldsymbol{x}})$ with $\bar{\boldsymbol{x}}$ and $\boldsymbol{A}$ given by equations (3.2) and (3.3). Note therefore that $D_i^2 = d_{i0}^2/(n-1)$, where d_{i0}^2 is defined in equation (3.8). The null hypothesis is rejected for small values of Λ_{min} and for large values of T_{max}^2, D_{max}^2 or $d_{max}^2 = \max_i d_{i0}^2$. In fact, some straightforward matrix manipulations (Press, 1972a p23) and standard distribution theory (Appendix) establish equivalence of all these statistics. Asymptotic null distributions can be obtained from the work of Siotani (1959), which leads to formal tests of a single outlier. For example, tables of critical values of d_{max}^2 are given by Seber (1984, table D12).

3.13 The case $k > 1$ does not provide such a tidy state of affairs. Assume first that we have k candidate observations $\boldsymbol{x}_1, \ldots, \boldsymbol{x}_k$ in mind as outliers, and that the general forms of equations 3.12 and 3.13 are adopted. By analogy with the $(k+1)$-group MANOVA situation (Chapter 7 and Appendix), there are now various non-equivalent test statistics available. If we write $\bar{\boldsymbol{x}}_{(k)} = \frac{1}{n-k} \sum_{i=k+1}^{n} \boldsymbol{x}_i$ and $\boldsymbol{A}_{(k)} = \sum_{i=k+1}^{n} (\boldsymbol{x}_i - \bar{\boldsymbol{x}}_{(k)})(\boldsymbol{x}_i - \bar{\boldsymbol{x}}_{(k)})'$, and denote the ith largest eigenvalue of $\boldsymbol{A}\boldsymbol{A}_{(k)}^{-1}$ by $1 + \lambda_i$ for $i = 1, \ldots, p$ some possible test statistics are:

(1) $\Lambda = \prod_{i=1}^{p} (1 + \lambda_i)^{-1}$ (Wilks's lambda);
(2) $\lambda_1/(1 + \lambda_1)$ (Roy's largest root);
(3) $T_0^2 = \sum_{i=1}^{p} \lambda_i$ (Hotelling's generalised T^2).

The null hypothesis is rejected for small values of Λ and large values of λ_1 or T_0^2; null distributions and hence critical values are obtained from standard theory (Appendix **A.8**) with k groups of size one and one group of size k. If it is not known *a priori* which of the n observations are outliers, then the chosen test statistic is computed for each of the $r = n!/k!(n-k)!$ possible sets of k from n observations. The most extreme of these r values identifies the likely set of outliers and also provides the test statistic. Appropriate distributional results are summarised by Hawkins (1980).

Recent increases in computer power have revived interest in procedures for the detection of multiple outliers, and various methods have been suggested. Rousseeuw and van Zomeren (1990) propose the use of distances based on robust estimates of location and covariance (see **3.22** below), but Cook and Hawkins (1990) show that this procedure may select a plethora of outliers, the identities of which depend critically on the parameters chosen for the robust estimation algorithm. They recommend instead using a sequential approach, in which outliers are detected and deleted individually starting from the full set of observations. This can be termed a *backward* selection procedure; Hadi (1992) and Atkinson and Mulira (1993) propose a *forward* procedure, which starts by using a small random subset of the data for the estimation phase and the size of the subset is then increased in such a way as to exclude outliers. It is evident that this is still very much an open area, and more developments can be expected in the future.

Example 3.2

Ryan *et al* (1985) list a number of data sets, which they also make available to users of the MINITAB statistical software package. Consider the two variables weight and height in the data set concerned with the study of long-term environmental changes on the blood pressure of Peruvian Indians. The weights in kilograms and the heights in millimetres of the thirty-nine Indians in the study are shown in columns two and three of Table 3.3. Values of d_{i0}^2, D_i^2, T_i^2 and Λ_i were calculated for each individual and these values are listed in columns four to seven of the table. Ranking the values of d_{i0}^2 and plotting the ranked values against the abscissae corresponding to Chi-squared (2 d.f.) cumulative distribution function values $(i - 0.5)/39$ for $i = 1, \ldots, 39$ is easily accomplished in MINITAB using commands SORT, INVCDF and PLOT. The resulting Chi-squared probability plot is shown in Fig. 3.7.

It is evident from this plot that there is one anomalous observation, far to the right and above all the other points on the diagram. The largest values of D_i^2, d_{i0}^2, T_i^2, and the smallest value of Λ_i, all occur for the last individual in Table 3.3. The critical value of d_{max}^2 for a test at the one percent significance level is 13.4 when $n = 40$ and $p = 2$, using table D12 in Seber (1984). The observed value of 17.422 is well in excess of this critical value, identifying individual 39 as an outlier. Removing this individual from the data set and repeating all the calculations would yield a new largest value of 5.41 for d_{i0}^2, much less than any of the critical values. We thus conclude that individual 39, and only this individual, is an outlier.

Tests of normality

3.14 Before embarking on any analysis that makes distributional assumptions about the data, it is prudent to check that those assumptions are reasonable for the data under consideration. The majority of techniques to be described rely on the assumption of multivariate normality of data, so testing this assumption is often an important aspect of initial data analysis. Very many techniques exist

Table 3.3 Weights and heights of Peruvian Indians, together with various statistics for outlier detection

Unit	Weight	Height	D_i^2	d_{i0}^2	T_i^2	Λ_i
1	71.0	1629	0.039	1.477	1.538	0.960
2	56.5	1569	0.025	0.949	0.973	0.974
3	56.0	1561	0.027	1.033	1.062	0.972
4	61.0	1619	0.029	1.103	1.136	0.970
5	65.0	1566	0.006	0.232	0.233	0.994
6	62.0	1639	0.049	1.874	1.973	0.949
7	53.0	1494	0.085	3.221	3.526	0.913
8	53.0	1568	0.060	2.288	2.437	0.938
9	65.0	1540	0.026	0.985	1.011	0.973
10	57.0	1530	0.029	1.115	1.149	0.970
11	66.5	1622	0.018	0.681	0.694	0.982
12	59.1	1486	0.083	3.172	3.466	0.914
13	64.0	1578	0.001	0.020	0.020	0.999
14	69.5	1645	0.045	1.708	1.789	0.954
15	64.0	1648	0.053	1.998	2.110	0.946
16	56.5	1521	0.038	1.454	1.513	0.961
17	57.0	1547	0.021	0.811	0.828	0.978
18	55.0	1505	0.061	2.304	2.455	0.938
19	57.0	1473	0.106	4.042	4.535	0.891
20	58.0	1538	0.021	0.781	0.798	0.979
21	59.5	1513	0.041	1.568	1.636	0.958
22	61.0	1653	0.081	3.078	3.355	0.919
23	57.0	1566	0.021	0.779	0.795	0.979
24	57.5	1580	0.021	0.816	0.834	0.978
25	74.0	1647	0.073	2.790	3.015	0.925
26	72.0	1620	0.042	1.611	1.683	0.956
27	62.5	1637	0.043	1.650	1.726	0.955
28	68.0	1528	0.066	2.499	2.678	0.932
29	63.4	1647	0.054	2.045	2.164	0.945
30	68.0	1605	0.013	0.509	0.516	0.986
31	69.0	1625	0.026	0.995	1.022	0.973
32	73.0	1615	0.051	1.926	2.030	0.948
33	64.0	1640	0.041	1.548	1.614	0.958
34	65.0	1610	0.009	0.348	0.351	0.991
35	71.0	1572	0.045	1.716	1.798	0.954
36	60.2	1534	0.019	0.728	0.742	0.980
37	55.0	1536	0.038	1.432	1.488	0.961
38	70.0	1630	0.034	1.288	1.333	0.965
39	87.0	1542	0.458	17.422	32.885	0.529

for assessing univariate normality of a sample of values on a single variable. A popular informal approach is the Q-Q plot (Wilk and Gnanadesikan, 1968), while commonly used statistics for a formal hypothesis test are the sample coefficients of skewness and kurtosis (Bowman and Shenton, 1973a, 1973b, 1975; Shenton and Bowman, 1977), Wilk and Shapiro's W (Shapiro and Wilk, 1965), the Anderson–Darling statistic A_n^2 (Dyer, 1974), and D'Agostino's D (D'Agostino, 1971, 1972). See D'Agostino (1986) for a survey. One possible approach in a multivariate situation would be to test the marginal normality of each variable separately, using one of these statistics. However, this approach

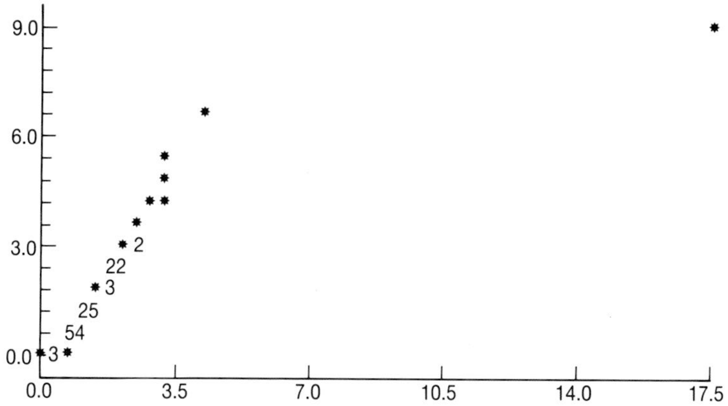

Figure 3.7 Chi-squared probability plot of d_{i0}^2 values from Table 3.3

would ignore the covariances between the variables in its execution. Also, marginal normality of all variables does not ensure joint normality of the ensemble (see **2.8** and Exercise 2.2). Thus we will here restrict attention to tests of joint multivariate normality only.

3.15 As with the detection of outliers, the assumption of multivariate normality can be investigated either through informal plots of the data or by applying formal hypothesis testing procedures. Among the informal plotting ideas, the most popular appear to be the probability plots of the d_{i0}^2 described in **3.10** and by Healy (1968). If the underlying data have a multivariate normal distribution then these plots will be linear; any systematic departure from linearity signifies departure from multivariate normality of the data. Note that $d_{i0}^2 = (\boldsymbol{x}_i - \bar{\boldsymbol{x}})'\boldsymbol{S}^{-1}(\boldsymbol{x}_i - \bar{\boldsymbol{x}}) = \boldsymbol{z}_i'\boldsymbol{z}_i$ where $\boldsymbol{z}_i = \boldsymbol{S}^{-1/2}(\boldsymbol{x}_i - \bar{\boldsymbol{x}})$ is a 'scaled residual'. Transforming the elements of $\boldsymbol{z}_i$ to polar coordinates (Mardia *et al*, 1979 p36) yields a 'radius' d_{i0} and $p-1$ independent angles θ_{ij} for each individual i; the transformation is given explicitly by $z_{ik} = d_{i0} \cos\theta_{ik} \prod_{l=0}^{k-1} \sin\theta_{il}$ for $i = 1, \ldots, n$ and $k = 1, \ldots, p$, where $\sin\theta_{i0} = \cos\theta_{ip} = 1$. Under the null hypothesis of multivariate normality, the scaled residuals are approximately spherically symmetrically distributed (**2.10**), any one arbitrarily chosen angle has an approximate uniform distribution over $(0, 2\pi)$, and the remaining $p-2$ independent angles have distributions whose densities are proportional to $\sin^{p-1-j}\theta_j$ for $0 \leqslant \theta_j \leqslant \pi$ and $j = 1, \ldots, (p-2)$ (Gnanadesikan, 1977). To supplement the probability plot of the d_{i0}^2, Gnanadesikan thus suggests plotting the n ordered values of the jth angles against the n corresponding quantiles of the appropriate distribution for $j = 1, \ldots, (p-2)$. Underlying normality of data again induces linearity of these plots. Moreover, under the null hypothesis the squared radius and the $(p-1)$ angles are mutually independent. Thus bivariate scatter plots over the unit square of probability integral transforms of any two chosen angles, or of one angle and the radii, should be uniform for multivariate normal data.

3.16 Turning now to more formal procedures for testing the null hypothesis that the data come from a multivariate normal distribution, we find a number of generalisations of the univariate statistics mentioned in **3.14**.

Mardia (1970,1974,1975) defines the following measure of multivariate skewness:

$$\beta_{1,p} = E[\{(\boldsymbol{x} - \boldsymbol{\mu})'\boldsymbol{\Sigma}^{-1}(\boldsymbol{y} - \boldsymbol{\mu})\}^3], \tag{3.17}$$

where $\boldsymbol{y}$ is independent of $\boldsymbol{x}$ but has the same distribution. He also provides a corresponding generalisation of multivariate kurtosis,

$$\beta_{2,p} = E[\{(\boldsymbol{x} - \boldsymbol{\mu})'\boldsymbol{\Sigma}^{-1}(\boldsymbol{x} - \boldsymbol{\mu})\}^2]. \tag{3.18}$$

Natural sample estimates of these quantities are

$$b_{1,p} = \frac{1}{n^2}\sum_{i=1}^{n}\sum_{j=1}^{n}[(\boldsymbol{x}_i - \bar{\boldsymbol{x}})'\boldsymbol{S}^{-1}(\boldsymbol{x}_j - \bar{\boldsymbol{x}})]^3 \tag{3.19}$$

and

$$b_{2,p} = \frac{1}{n}\sum_{i=1}^{n}[(\boldsymbol{x}_i - \bar{\boldsymbol{x}})'\boldsymbol{S}^{-1}(\boldsymbol{x}_i - \bar{\boldsymbol{x}})]^2. \tag{3.20}$$

When $\boldsymbol{x} \sim N_p(\boldsymbol{\mu}, \boldsymbol{\Sigma})$ then $\beta_{1,p} = 0$, $\beta_{2,p} = p(p+2)$, $\frac{1}{6}nb_{1,p}$ has an asymptotic chi-squared distribution with $\frac{1}{6}p(p+1)(p+2)$ degrees of freedom, and $b_{2,p}$ has an asymptotic normal distribution with mean $p(p+2)$ and variance $\frac{8}{n}p(p+2)$. These results enable large-sample tests of multivariate normality to be conducted, but sample sizes in excess of 50 are needed for the approximations to be accurate. Mardia (1974) provides tables of approximate percentiles for $p = 2$ and $n \geqslant 10$ as well as some alternative large-sample approximations.

Malkovich and Afifi (1973) suggest alternative approaches to multivariate skewness and kurtosis, by finding values of $\boldsymbol{a}$ to maximise the univariate skewness and kurtosis of $\boldsymbol{a}'\boldsymbol{x}$. This enables an informal approach to tests of normality to be conducted, but the distributional problems seem to be too formidable for tests of hypothesis to be constructed. The authors also propose a similar generalisation of the Wilk–Shapiro W statistic. Cox and Small (1978) and Hensler *et al* (1977) base tests of normality on properties of the conditional distribution of a subset of multivariate variables given values of the rest (see **2.4**). Andrews *et al* (1973) suggest using the transformation technique to be described in **3.19** below for testing multivariate normality, Rohlf (1975) has drawn on graph-theoretic ideas in tests for normality based on minimum spanning trees of the data, while Mudholkar *et al* (1992) give a test of multivariate normality based on Healy's plotting technique as described above.

Example 3.3

Returning to the Peruvian Indian data of Example 3.2, we calculate Mardia's sample kurtosis measure $b_{2,2}$ by finding the average of the squares of the d_{i0}^2 values in column five; this yields the value 10.876. Referring to the table in Mardia (1974), we see that the lower and upper critical values of kurtosis for a test of normality at the 5 percent level with $n = 40$ are 6.14 and 10.11. The calculated value exceeds the upper critical value and hence we reject the hypothesis of bivariate normality of the data. Looking at Fig. 3.7, of course, this conclusion is unsurprising in view of the obvious outlier in the sample. However, the other points in the diagram appear to be reasonably linear so we might ask whether the 38 observations left after omitting the outlier could have come from a bivariate normal population. Removing the outlier and recomputing the sample statistics we obtain the following values of d_{i0}^2:

2.00, 1.30, 1.35, 1.37, 0.60, 2.23, 3.18, 3.47, 1.82, 1.07, 0.68, 3.58, 0.12 , 1.77, 2.14, 1.40, 0.85, 2.23, 4.24, 0.74, 1.71, 3.90, 1.01, 1.15, 3.66, 2.57 , 1.90, 4.71, 2.27, 0.84, 1.22, 3.33, 1.63, 0.33, 3.70, 0.78, 1.58, 1.60.

The new value of $b_{2,2}$ is 5.14, and we now see that it falls below the lower critical value quoted earlier. Hence we still reject the hypothesis of normality of the data, even without the outlier. The Chi-squared probability plot of these 38 d_{i0}^2 values is shown in Fig. 3.8; the distinct evidence of curvature in the centre of the plot is consistent with the formal rejection of the hypothesis of normality.

Plotting histograms of weight and height suggests that the latter have come from a bimodal distribution which has a 'gap' at 1600mm. Taking this as an arbitrary cut-off value, the data were divided into two groups. This produced one group of 21 individuals with heights less than or equal to 1600mm, and a second group containing the remaining 17 individuals. All the above calculations were repeated for each group separately, yielding kurtosis measures of 6.13 and 5.23 respectively. The former value is well within the range of normal values for a test at even the ten percent significance level, the critical values from Mardia's table for $n = 20$ being 5.71 and 9.47. Thus the individuals having heights below 1600mm are consistent with a sample from a bivariate normal distribution. Interpolating in Mardia's table for $n = 17$ shows the significance level of the value 5.23 to be about 3 percent. Thus there is some evidence of non-normality for the second group of individuals, but this evidence is not very strong. A reasonable conclusion would therefore be that the 39 original observations came from a mixture of two bivariate normal populations, and contained one outlying individual.

Transformations of data

3.17 If initial inspection of the data suggests that they do not satisfy the necessary assumptions made by a particular method of analysis, one possible way forward is to seek a transformation of the data such that the transformed values do satisfy the assumptions. The method can then be applied to the transformed data and, if appropriate, the results can be back-transformed so that conclusions are presented in relation to the original units of measurement. In general, there are various ways in which data can fail to satisfy assumptions made by a statistical model. The most common ones are non-additivity,

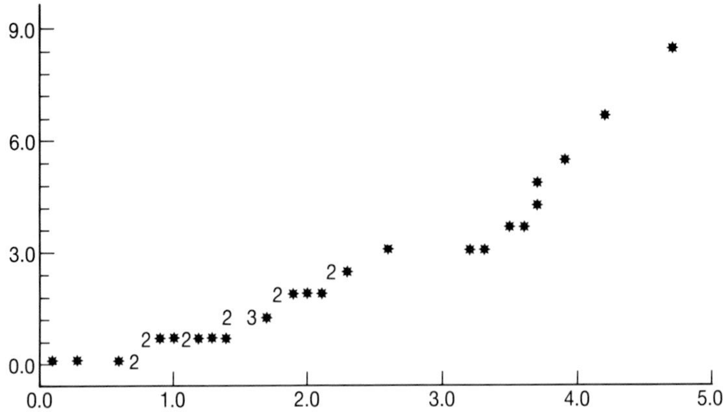

Figure 3.8 Chi-squared probability plot of Peruvian Indian d_{i0}^2 values after omitting the outlier

heteroscedasticity, and breakdown of distributional assumptions. Theoretical approaches to the problem of heteroscedasticity lead to the well-known variance stabilising transformations for the binomial, the Poisson, the correlation coefficient, and others. Here we will concentrate on the breakdown of distributional assumptions, and consider ways of transforming data so that they are more nearly normal. This in general requires a data-based transformation to be found. An early contribution in this line was by Tukey (1957), and the idea was developed in the univariate case by Box and Cox (1964). It was then generalised to multivariate data by Andrews *et al* (1971).

3.18 Consider first the univariate case. A general family of transformations of the variable x, including the log, square root and inverse transformations, is given by

$$x^{(\lambda)} = \begin{cases} x^{\lambda}, & \lambda \neq 0, \\ \log x, & \lambda = 0 \text{ and } x > 0. \end{cases} \tag{3.21}$$

This family was studied for $|\lambda| \leqslant 1$ by Tukey (1957). To avoid a discontinuity at $\lambda = 0$, Box and Cox (1964) modified it to

$$x^{(\lambda)} = \begin{cases} \frac{x^{\lambda}-1}{\lambda}, & \lambda \neq 0, \\ \log x, & \lambda = 0 \text{ and } x > 0. \end{cases} \tag{3.22}$$

They then suggested finding the value of λ which makes the transformed observations as nearly normal as possible. One way of achieving this is by maximum likelihood. If the transformed values $x_i^{(\lambda)}$ are independent $N(\mu, \sigma^2)$, then the likelihood function for the untransformed data is

$$(2\pi\sigma^2)^{-n/2} \left[\exp\left\{ -\sum_{i=1}^{n} \frac{(x_i^{(\lambda)} - \mu)^2}{2\sigma^2} \right\} \right] \left[\prod_{i=1}^{n} x_i^{\lambda-1} \right], \tag{3.23}$$

the last term in square brackets being the Jacobian of the transformation. If λ is fixed, this expression is maximised at

$$\bar{x}(\lambda) = \frac{1}{n}\sum_{i=1}^{n} x_i^{(\lambda)} \tag{3.24}$$

and

$$s^2(\lambda) = \frac{1}{n}\sum_{i=1}^{n}(x_i^{(\lambda)} - \bar{x}^{(\lambda)})^2. \tag{3.25}$$

The maximised value of the log likelihood is thus proportional to

$$\mathscr{L}_{max}(\lambda) = -\frac{n}{2}\log s^2(\lambda) + (\lambda - 1)\sum_{i=1}^{n}\log x_i \tag{3.26}$$

The maximum likelihood estimate $\hat{\lambda}$ is the value that maximises $\mathscr{L}_{max}(\lambda)$. The maximisation can be done numerically using one of the standard function optimisation routines that is provided with many software packages. Alternatively, a useful approach is to evaluate and plot $\mathscr{L}_{max}(\lambda)$ for λ ranging in small increments over a suitable interval such as $-2.5 \leqslant \lambda \leqslant 2.5$. This enables the behaviour of $\mathscr{L}_{max}(\lambda)$ to be investigated, as well as identifying $\hat{\lambda}$. A simple MINITAB macro for doing this, kindly provided by Dr A. G. Munford, is shown in Fig. 3.9. Further investigations of the Box–Cox family of transformations have been reported by Draper and Cox (1969), Draper and Hunter (1969), Andrews (1971), Hinkley (1975), Lindsey (1975), Hernandez and Johnson (1980), Bickel and Doksum (1981), Box and Cox (1982), and Linnet (1988). Modifications to equation (3.22) to allow for negative x values have been proposed by Manly (1976) and John and Draper (1980).

3.19 Turning now to the multivariate case, we can identify three ways in which the above approach can be adapted: for seeking *marginal*, *joint*, or *directional* normality.

For marginal normality, we simply need to apply equation (3.22) and the associated maximisation procedure to each variable separately. While this has the same drawbacks as were outlined for testing normality (see **3.14**), Gnanadesikan (1977) points out that many of the standard multivariate techniques work satisfactorily in the presence merely of symmetry of data. Transforming to marginal normality may achieve such symmetry even if it does not produce full normality, so may still be worthwhile.

If full normality is required, however, then we need to treat the variables jointly. The way to do this is to use the same transformation equation (3.22), but now to use joint normality of the transformed variables as the criterion to optimise. Consider the $n \times p$ matrix $\boldsymbol{X} = (x_{ij}), i = 1, \ldots, n; j = 1, \ldots, p$, the rows $\boldsymbol{x}'$ of which are the multivariate observations, and assume that after some transformations of the variables of the form of equation (3.22) the rows of the transformed data $\boldsymbol{X}^{(\lambda)}$ are consistent with observations from a multivariate normal distribution with mean $\boldsymbol{\mu}$ and dispersion matrix $\boldsymbol{\Sigma}$. Note that the superscript $(\boldsymbol{\lambda})$ here is a vector $\boldsymbol{\lambda} = (\lambda_1, \ldots, \lambda_p)$, as we can in general allow each variable to have its own transformation parameter λ_i. The Jacobian of

```
#         Name :    BOX.MTB (calls BOX1.MTB)

#  Description :    Minitab macro for Box-Cox transformation
#                   Data are assumed to be in column   c1

#    Variables :

#                   k1    loop counter
#                   k2    sum log(y)
#                   k3    current lambda
#                   k4    standard deviation of observations
#                   k5    log likelihood
#                   k6    number of lambda's
#                   k7    number of data values

#                   c1    data
#                   c2    values of lambda
#                   c3    values of transformed y's
#                   c4    values of log likelihood

   oh = 0                              # prevents paging
   let k1 = 1                          # initialise loop counter
   let k2 = sum(log(c1))               # get sum of log y's
   set c2                              # load lambda values
   -25 : 25 / 5                        # desired range of lambda -
   let c2 = c2/100                     # transformed to fine grid
   let k6 = count(c2)                  # get the number of lambdas
   let k7 = count(c1)                  # get the number of observations
   exec 'box1' k6                      # do the estimation k6 times
   name  c2 'lambda' c4 'Log(L)'       #
   plot  c4  c2                        # plot the data
   oh 24                               # turns paging back on
```

```
#          Name :  BOX1.MTB (called from BOX.MTB)

   let k3 = c2(k1)                     # get current lambda
   let k7 = (k3=0)                     # k7 is 1 if lambda = 0
   let c3 = k7*log(c2) + (1-k7)*(c2**k3 - 1)/(k3+k7)
                                       # trick prevents division by 0
   let k4 = stdev(c1)                  # get standard deviation
   let k5 = -k7*log(k4) + k3*k2        # log likelihood
   let c4(k1) = k5                     # store in array
   print  k3  k5                       # Something to look at!
   let k1 = k1 + 1                     # increment k1 for the next pass
```

Figure 3.9 MINITAB macro for evaluating and plotting $\mathscr{L}_{max}(\lambda)$ over a range of values of λ

the transformation is $\prod_{j=1}^{p} \prod_{i=1}^{n} x_{ij}^{\lambda_j - 1}$. Hence if we write $\boldsymbol{\Upsilon} = \mathbf{1}\boldsymbol{\mu}'$ then the log-likelihood of $\boldsymbol{\mu}$, $\boldsymbol{\Sigma}$ and $\boldsymbol{\lambda}$ is proportional to

$$-\frac{n}{2}\log|\boldsymbol{\Sigma}| - \frac{1}{2}\mathrm{tr}\ \boldsymbol{\Sigma}^{-1}(\boldsymbol{X}^{(\lambda)} - \boldsymbol{\Upsilon})'(\boldsymbol{X}^{(\lambda)} - \boldsymbol{\Upsilon}) + \sum_{j=1}^{p}[(\lambda_j - 1)\sum_{i=1}^{n}\log x_{ij}]. \quad (3.27)$$

For specified values of λ_j, $j = 1, \ldots, p$, the maximum likelihood estimates of $\boldsymbol{\mu}$ and $\boldsymbol{\Sigma}$ are given by

$$\hat{\boldsymbol{\mu}} = \frac{1}{n}\mathbf{1}'\boldsymbol{X}^{(\lambda)}, \quad (3.28)$$

and

$$\hat{\boldsymbol{\Sigma}} = \frac{1}{n}(\boldsymbol{X}^{(\lambda)} - \hat{\boldsymbol{\Upsilon}})'(\boldsymbol{X}^{(\lambda)} - \hat{\boldsymbol{\Upsilon}}), \quad (3.29)$$

where $\hat{\boldsymbol{\Upsilon}} = \mathbf{1}\hat{\boldsymbol{\mu}}'$. (See also **3.20** below). Substituting these values into equation (3.27), the maximised log-likelihood is proportional to

$$\mathscr{L}_{max}(\lambda_1, \ldots, \lambda_p) = -\frac{n}{2}\log|\hat{\boldsymbol{\Sigma}}| + \sum_{j=1}^{p}[(\lambda_j - 1)\sum_{i=1}^{n}\log x_{ij}]. \quad (3.30)$$

The required values $\hat{\lambda}_1, \ldots, \hat{\lambda}_p$ which yield the optimal transformation can then be obtained by numerically maximising equation (3.30).

As an intermediate stage between marginal and joint normality, Andrews *et al* (1971) and Gnanadesikan (1977) suggest seeking transformations for achieving *directional* normality. The idea here is that sometimes the data might exhibit non-normality in some but not all directions in the space of the original responses. If one can specify such a direction by the vector $\boldsymbol{b}$, say, then the transformation (3.22) can be applied to the projections of the data points on $\boldsymbol{b}$, i. e. to $y_i = \boldsymbol{b}'\boldsymbol{x}_i$. Now any non-normal characteristics of the observations $\boldsymbol{x}_i$ will be reflected in correspondingly non-normal characteristics of the residuals $\boldsymbol{z}_i$ defined in **3.15**. To specify a direction of non-normal clustering of points, Andrews *et al* (1971) suggest considering

$$\boldsymbol{d}_\alpha = \sum_{i=1}^{n} w_i \boldsymbol{z}_i / \parallel \sum_{i=1}^{n} w_i \boldsymbol{z}_i \parallel, \quad (3.31)$$

where $w_i = \parallel \boldsymbol{z}_i \parallel^\alpha$ and $\parallel \boldsymbol{x} \parallel = \boldsymbol{x}'\boldsymbol{x}$. The vector $\boldsymbol{d}_\alpha$ provides a parameterisation of directions in the space of the residuals (and hence in the space of the data) in terms of the single parameter α, and choice of an appropriate value of α can yield a direction of non-normality of the data. On specifying α, we obtain the direction as $\boldsymbol{b} = \boldsymbol{S}^{-1/2}\boldsymbol{d}_\alpha$ and hence can apply (3.22) as outlined above. In general, if $\alpha > 0$ then $\boldsymbol{d}_\alpha$ is a direction in space pointing towards any abnormal clustering of points far from the mean of the data, while if $\alpha < 0$ then $\boldsymbol{d}_\alpha$ points to any abnormal clustering of points near the centre of gravity of the data. Andrews *et al* suggest either $\alpha = 1$ or $\alpha = -1$ as suitable values to choose. If $\alpha = 1$ then $\boldsymbol{d}_\alpha$ becomes sensitive primarily to those observations far from the mean, so that if the $\boldsymbol{z}_i$ are skew in one direction then $\boldsymbol{d}_\alpha$ will tend to point in that direction. Alternatively, if $\alpha = -1$, $\boldsymbol{d}_\alpha$ is a function only of the orientation of the $\boldsymbol{z}_i$ and gives the direction of any clustering.

Table 3.4 Data from experiment on detergent manufacturing process, taken from Roy *et al.* (1971) with permission.

Run	Rate	Stickiness	Run	Rate	Stickiness
1	38.0	5.40	17	37.0	4.60
2	38.0	5.90	18	38.0	5.20
3	35.0	2.95	19	32.0	2.49
4	36.0	5.38	20	39.0	6.10
5	38.0	5.22	21	39.0	3.84
6	37.0	5.33	22	37.0	4.90
7	37.0	4.90	23	35.0	4.30
8	36.0	4.50	24	34.0	3.50
9	34.5	3.15	25	37.0	3.24
10	38.0	3.06	26	37.0	3.79
11	36.0	5.70	27	39.0	5.80
12	37.0	4.20	28	39.0	5.30
13	38.5	4.70	29	39.0	5.60
14	38.0	4.20	30	40.0	6.20
15	38.0	5.17	31	40.0	5.47
16	39.0	5.66	32	40.0	4.77

A much more general question concerns the seeking of appropriate projections which highlight specific features of the data, and non-normality might be a feature that we wish to highlight. This general area is known as *projection pursuit* and is discussed further in Chapter 4.

Example 3.4; *Andrews et al, 1971*
The data in Table 3.4 give two of the variables, rate and stickiness, obtained in a 2^{7-2} experiment concerned with 7 factors which affect the operation of a detergent manufacturing process (see Roy *et al*, 1971, for details). Chi-squared probability plots of squared treatment effects on each of the two original response scales indicated the presence of considerable distributional peculiarities (Andrews *et al*, 1971, figures 5a and 5b). Applying each of the above methods in turn yielded $\hat{\lambda}_1 = 8.88, \hat{\lambda}_2 = 2.06$ from the marginal transformations, $\hat{\lambda}_1 = 7.22, \hat{\lambda}_2 = 1.88$ from the joint transformation, and $\hat{\lambda} = 0.451$ from the directional transformation in the direction $\boldsymbol{d}' = (-0.7, -0.7)$. Re-estimating treatment effects for each set of transformed data and obtaining chi-squared and gamma probability plots (figures 5c, 5d, 6a and 6b, *op cit*) showed improvement with each transformation, but best results with the joint normality.

Descriptive statistics for multivariate data

3.20 If $\boldsymbol{x}_1, \ldots, \boldsymbol{x}_n$ is a random sample from a multivariate normal distribution with mean $\boldsymbol{\mu}$ and (positive definite) dispersion matrix Σ, then these two parameters completely specify the distribution (see **2.7**) and so an adequate summary of the data will be provided by estimates of $\boldsymbol{\mu}$ and Σ. Now the likelihood

$L(\boldsymbol{\mu}, \boldsymbol{\Sigma})$ is given by

$$\log L(\boldsymbol{\mu}, \boldsymbol{\Sigma}) = -\frac{np}{2}\log(2\pi) - \frac{n}{2}\log|\boldsymbol{\Sigma}| - \frac{1}{2}\sum_{i=1}^{n}[(\boldsymbol{x}_i - \boldsymbol{\mu})'\boldsymbol{\Sigma}^{-1}(\boldsymbol{x}_i - \boldsymbol{\mu})]. \quad (3.32)$$

This can be re-expressed as

$$\log L(\boldsymbol{\mu}, \boldsymbol{\Sigma}) = -\frac{np}{2}\log(2\pi) - \frac{n}{2}\log|\boldsymbol{\Sigma}| - \frac{1}{2}\mathrm{tr}[\boldsymbol{\Sigma}^{-1}\sum_{i=1}^{n}(\boldsymbol{x}_i - \boldsymbol{\mu})(\boldsymbol{x}_i - \boldsymbol{\mu})'], \quad (3.33)$$

and by adding and subtracting $\bar{\boldsymbol{x}}$ within each bracket inside the summation this expression can be reduced to

$$\log L(\boldsymbol{\mu}, \boldsymbol{\Sigma}) = -\frac{np}{2}\log(2\pi) - \frac{n}{2}\log|\boldsymbol{\Sigma}| - \frac{1}{2}\mathrm{tr}[\boldsymbol{\Sigma}^{-1}\boldsymbol{A} + n\boldsymbol{\Sigma}^{-1}(\bar{\boldsymbol{x}} - \boldsymbol{\mu})(\bar{\boldsymbol{x}} - \boldsymbol{\mu})'], \quad (3.34)$$

where $\boldsymbol{A}$ is defined after equation (3.3). Since $\boldsymbol{\Sigma}$ is positive definite, the second term in square brackets must be greater than or equal to zero and hence if $\hat{\boldsymbol{\mu}} = \bar{\boldsymbol{x}}$ then $L(\hat{\boldsymbol{\mu}}, \boldsymbol{\Sigma}) \geqslant L(\boldsymbol{\mu}, \boldsymbol{\Sigma})$ for all positive definite $\boldsymbol{\Sigma}$.

Substituting $\hat{\boldsymbol{\mu}}$ into (3.33), we find

$$\log L(\hat{\boldsymbol{\mu}}, \boldsymbol{\Sigma}) = -\frac{np}{2}\log(2\pi) - \frac{n}{2}\left(\log|\boldsymbol{\Sigma}| + \mathrm{tr}\left[\frac{\boldsymbol{\Sigma}^{-1}\boldsymbol{A}}{n}\right]\right). \quad (3.35)$$

Now writing $f(\boldsymbol{\Sigma}) = \log|\boldsymbol{\Sigma}| + \mathrm{tr}[\boldsymbol{\Sigma}^{-1}\boldsymbol{A}]$, then $f(\boldsymbol{\Sigma}) - f(\boldsymbol{A}) = -\log|\boldsymbol{\Sigma}^{-1}\boldsymbol{A}| + \mathrm{tr}[\boldsymbol{\Sigma}^{-1}\boldsymbol{A}] - p$. Let $\lambda_1, \ldots, \lambda_p$ be the eigenvalues of $\boldsymbol{\Sigma}^{-1}\boldsymbol{A}$, and hence also of $\boldsymbol{\Sigma}^{-1/2}\boldsymbol{A}\boldsymbol{\Sigma}^{-1/2}$. Using the fact that $\boldsymbol{A}$ is positive definite with probability one (cf Exercise 3.2), it follows that the λ_i are all positive and hence $f(\boldsymbol{\Sigma}) - f(\boldsymbol{A}) = \sum_{i=1}^{p}(-\log\lambda_i + \lambda_i - 1) \geqslant 0$. Applying this result to equation (3.35), it follows that the maximum of $\log L(\hat{\boldsymbol{\mu}}, \boldsymbol{\Sigma})$ is achieved at $\hat{\boldsymbol{\Sigma}} = \frac{1}{n}\boldsymbol{A}$. Thus $\log L(\hat{\boldsymbol{\mu}}, \hat{\boldsymbol{\Sigma}}) \geqslant \log L(\hat{\boldsymbol{\mu}}, \boldsymbol{\Sigma}) \geqslant \log L(\boldsymbol{\mu}, \boldsymbol{\Sigma})$ for all $\boldsymbol{\mu}, \boldsymbol{\Sigma}$, and the maximum likelihood estimates of $\boldsymbol{\mu}$ and $\boldsymbol{\Sigma}$ are $\hat{\boldsymbol{\mu}} = \bar{\boldsymbol{x}}$ and $\hat{\boldsymbol{\Sigma}} = \frac{1}{n}\boldsymbol{A} = \frac{1}{n}\sum_{i=1}^{n}(\boldsymbol{x}_i - \bar{\boldsymbol{x}})(\boldsymbol{x}_i - \bar{\boldsymbol{x}})'$. By standard properties of maximum likelihood estimates (Stuart and Ord, 1991), these are therefore sufficient statistics for $\boldsymbol{\mu}$ and $\boldsymbol{\Sigma}$ so are the best summary values of the multivariate sample. However, by analogy with the univariate situation, while $\bar{\boldsymbol{x}}$ is an unbiased estimator of $\boldsymbol{\mu}$, $\hat{\boldsymbol{\Sigma}}$ is a biased estimate of $\boldsymbol{\Sigma}$. The unbiased version is $\boldsymbol{S} = \frac{1}{n-1}\boldsymbol{A}$, so the most commonly used summary statistics for the data are $\bar{\boldsymbol{x}}$ and $\boldsymbol{S}$.

3.21 The above theory has established the optimality of $\bar{\boldsymbol{x}}$ and $\boldsymbol{S}$ as summary statistics for a sample from a normal distribution. By extension, these statistics are generally used to summarise *any* multivariate distribution. In practice, however, it is common to encounter samples which have come from distributions with much heavier tails than the normal, or samples which contain a few outliers, or samples which have become contaminated by having a significant proportion α of members from a different distribution than the one of interest. In all these cases, a number of anomalous observations will be present in the sample, usually ‘far away’ from the typical sample member. Consequently statistics such as $\bar{\boldsymbol{x}}$ and $\boldsymbol{S}$ will be distorted by these observations and will not be accurate estimates of $\boldsymbol{\mu}$ or $\boldsymbol{\Sigma}$. It is therefore of some practical importance to devise estimation methods which are insensitive to a small proportion of anomalous values in a sample, and the last twenty years has seen vigorous activity in the area of *robust* estimation. For a brief introduction to the general topic see Hogg (1979), and for a comprehensive survey of univariate theory see Huber (1981). Here we restrict ourselves merely to the most common robust measures of location and dispersion for a multivariate sample.

3.22 As with all the other topics in this chapter, robust estimation in the multivariate case can be tackled either in a *marginal* or in a *joint* fashion. In the former case we would use as a robust measure of location the vector of robust measures for each variable separately (such as, say, the vector of medians), and as a robust measure of dispersion the matrix of robust measures for all pairwise combinations of variables (see Devlin *et al*, 1975). However, anomalous observations will often only show up in a multivariate context when the values for each variable are considered in relation to all the other variables. Moreover, location, scale and dispersion are closely interrelated when searching for multivariate outliers; adjusting an estimate of location to allow for an outlier will inevitably lead to the necessity of adjustment to estimates of dispersion and orientation. These two aspects suggest that not only is a *joint* approach necessary, but that additionally any sensible procedure will be an iterative one. At any stage of the process we have 'current estimates' $\boldsymbol{\mu}^*$ and $\boldsymbol{\Sigma}^*$ of the parameters of interest, and these estimates are used to identify anomalous observations which leads to the next iteration and improved estimates of the parameters.

To implement such a scheme we need to decide on:

(1) initial values of $\boldsymbol{\mu}^*$ and $\boldsymbol{\Sigma}^*$ to start the process off;
(2) how to identify anomalous observations at any stage of the iteration;
(3) how to treat these anomalous values in the estimation of the population parameters.

The first two decisions can be made using results given above. An obvious pair of starting values are the standard estimates $\boldsymbol{\mu}^* = \bar{\boldsymbol{x}}$ and $\boldsymbol{\Sigma}^* = \boldsymbol{S}$, while identification of anomalous observations can be made using any of the statistics discussed in **3.9**. In practice, the most popular choice is the appropriate version of equation (3.8), which in the present case becomes

$$d_i^2 = (\boldsymbol{x}_i - \boldsymbol{\mu}^*)'(\boldsymbol{\Sigma}^*)^{-1}(\boldsymbol{x}_i - \boldsymbol{\mu}^*). \tag{3.36}$$

The third decision has provoked a number of alternative suggestions in the literature. One possibility, known as 'multivariate trimming', is to rank the observations using the d_i^2 values and then to use only a portion of the observations in computation of $\boldsymbol{\mu}^*$ and $\boldsymbol{\Sigma}^*$. Typically either those observations which exceed some critical value of d_i^2 or a fixed proportion, say 0.1, of those observations with the largest d_i^2 values would be ignored, and $\boldsymbol{\mu}^*$, $\boldsymbol{\Sigma}^*$ would be calculated as the mean and dispersion matrix of the remainder. The whole procedure could either continue for a fixed number of iterations, or until some pre-specified convergence criterion was satisfied; see, for example, Devlin *et al* (1981).

A second possibility, instead of deleting observations with large values of d_i^2, is to assign each observation a weight depending on its value of d_i^2 and to downweight those observations with large d_i^2 in the computation of $\boldsymbol{\mu}^*$ and $\boldsymbol{\Sigma}^*$. It is generally appropriate to allow different weights in computation of the mean from those in the computation of the dispersion matrix, so the estimating equations can be written

$$\boldsymbol{\mu}^* = \sum_{i=1}^{n} w_{1i}\boldsymbol{x}_i / \sum_{i=1}^{n} w_{1i}, \tag{3.37}$$

and

$$\boldsymbol{\Sigma}^* = \sum_{i=1}^{n} w_{2i}(\boldsymbol{x}_i - \boldsymbol{\mu}^*)(\boldsymbol{x}_i - \boldsymbol{\mu}^*)' / \sum_{i=1}^{n} w_{2i}. \tag{3.38}$$

The denominator of (3.38) is sometimes varied, with some authors preferring to use n or $(\sum_{i=1}^{n} w_{2i}) - 1$. Also, the w_{2i} should be standardised so that $E(\boldsymbol{\Sigma}^*) = \boldsymbol{\Sigma}$ for the multivariate normal distribution (at least asymptotically), but the appropriate scaling constant is generally unknown. Consequently, equations (3.37) and (3.38) are used as they stand. Such estimates can be derived formally from solution of systems of equations of the form

$$n^{-1} \sum_{i=1}^{n} u_1[\{(\boldsymbol{x}_i - \boldsymbol{\mu})'\boldsymbol{\Sigma}^{-1}(\boldsymbol{x}_i - \boldsymbol{\mu})\}^{1/2}](\boldsymbol{x}_i - \boldsymbol{\mu}) = \boldsymbol{0}$$

and

$$n^{-1} \sum_{i=1}^{n} u_2[(\boldsymbol{x}_i - \boldsymbol{\mu})'\boldsymbol{\Sigma}^{-1}(\boldsymbol{x}_i - \boldsymbol{\mu})](\boldsymbol{x}_i - \boldsymbol{\mu})(\boldsymbol{x}_i - \boldsymbol{\mu})' = \boldsymbol{\Sigma},$$

where u_1, u_2 are functions satisfying the conditions set out by Maronna (1976). They are called *M-estimates* of the mean and dispersion matrix.

Various suggestions have been put forward for the weight functions to apply in equations (3.37) and (3.38). A simple weighting is given by

$$w_{1i} = w_{2i} = \frac{1+p}{1+d_i^2},$$

where the weight of each observation depends directly on its d_i^2 value. Alternatively, one can give observations in the main part of the data full weight, and only downweight those observations that are extreme. This can be achieved for example by the weighting

$$w_{1i} = \begin{cases} 1 & \text{if } d_i \leqslant a \\ \frac{a}{d_i} & \text{if } d_i > a \end{cases}$$

and

$$w_{2i} = w_{1i}^2.$$

The above weighting functions are discussed by Maronna (1976) and Devlin *et al* (1981); the latter recommend taking a to be the square root of the 90 percent quantile of the χ_p^2 distribution. Another possibility was provided by

Campbell (1980), who suggested the more complicated weighting

$$w_{1i} = \begin{cases} 1 & \text{if } d_i \leqslant a \\ \frac{1}{d_i}(\sqrt{p} + c_1/\sqrt{2})\exp\{-\frac{1}{2c_2^2}(d_i - [\sqrt{p} + c_1/\sqrt{2}])^2\}, & \text{if } d_i > a \end{cases}$$

along with

$$w_{2i} = w_{1i}^2,$$

where $a = \sqrt{p} + c_1/\sqrt{2}$ and c_1, c_2 are to be chosen by the experimenter. Campbell suggests from practical experience that one of the following three selections should prove acceptable in most applications.

(1) $c_1 = \infty, c_2$ immaterial;

(2) $c_1 = 2, c_2 = \infty$;

(3) $c_1 = 2, c_2 = 1.25$.

The first choice yields $w_{1i} = w_{2i} = 1$ for all i, the second choice gives a step function with two possible values, while the third choice leads to a full descending set of weights over the whole sample. (Note also that Campbell uses the variant $\sum_{i=1}^{n} w_{2i} - 1$ in the denominator of (3.38)).

Example 3.5
Campbell (1980) discusses a data set taken from a study of geographical variation in the whelk *Thais lamellosa.* Measurements were made on twenty variables, and the whelks came from twelve distinct groups on the west coast of North America. Preliminary analysis had identified seven of the variables as providing most of the between-group discrimination, so Campbell restricted attention to just these variables and to one of the groups that contained ninety-nine individuals. Fig. 3.10a shows Campbell's probability plot of $d_{j0}^{2/3}$ values for this group against Normal order statistics (see **3.10**), where the d_{j0}^2 values were calculated using the usual mean and covariance matrix (i.e. equations (3.2) and (3.3)). One atypical observation (number 79) seems to be indicated. Robust M-estimation using $c_1 = 2$ and $c_2 = 1.25$ gave zero weight to this observation and also to a second observation (number 97). Fig. 3.10b shows the probability plot when the d_{j0}^2 were recomputed using robust estimates of the mean and covariance matrix, with $c_1 = 2$ and $c_2 = 1.25$. The two observations 79 and 97 are clearly atypical. Inspection of the data showed the atypicality to reside in the second variable; the first individual was discrepant by 100 units and the second by 50 units (the recording dial on the calipers used to measure the whelks being marked in 50-unit divisions). When these two individuals had the discrepant values corrected, the Normal probability plot of the robust distances (Fig. 3.10c) became linear, and none of the weights was now less than 0.35.

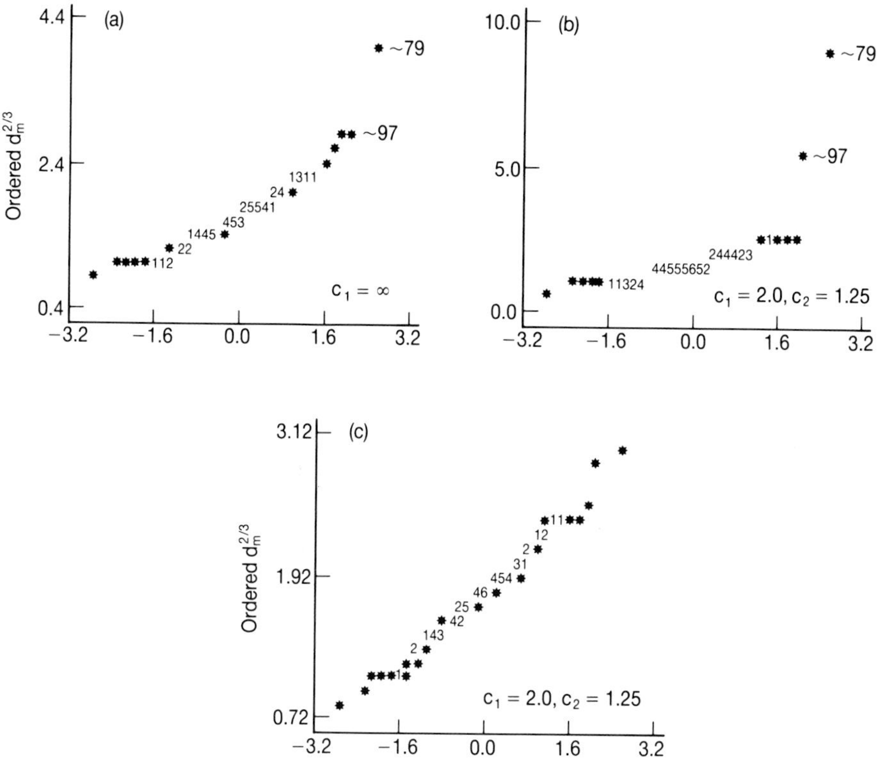

Figure 3.10 Normal probability plots of ordered $d_{j0}^{2/3}$ values, for various estimates of mean and covariance matrix in a group of whelks, reproduced with permission from Campbell (1980)

Similarity, dissimilarity and distance

3.23 The above summary statistics are designed to capture in a simple way the overall features, such as location, dispersion and orientation, of a multivariate distribution. Their focus of interest is therefore on the *variables* in the sample. It is often important additionally to summarise and investigate interrelationships between the *units*, i.e. *individuals* in the sample, and to do this it is necessary to compute the *similarity* either between specified pairs of individuals or, more generally, between all pairs of individuals in the sample. In fact it is more useful to think in terms of dissimilarity rather than similarity between individuals, because many multivariate techniques result in a pictorial representation of the sample individuals as points in space; there is then a natural correspondence linking the dissimilarity between two individuals and the distance between the points representing them. We shall explore such techniques fully in chapter 5 and Volume 2; the purpose of these last sections of the present chapter is merely to survey the possible measures of dissimilarity that can be used.

3.24 The definition of a measure of dissimilarity depends critically on the type of data from which the computation is to be made. Suppose first that all variables are quantitative/continuous, and that x_{ik} is the value of the kth variable for the ith individual. The following are the most common measures of dissimilarity d_{ij} between individuals i and j.

(1) Euclidean distance : $d_{ij} = \{\sum_{k=1}^{p}(x_{ik} - x_{jk})^2\}^{1/2}$.

(2) Minkowski metric : $d_{ij} = \{\sum_{k=1}^{p} \mid x_{ik} - x_{jk} \mid^{\lambda}\}^{1/\lambda}$ for some integer λ.

(3) Canberra metric : $d_{ij} = \sum_{k=1}^{p} \frac{|x_{ik}-x_{jk}|}{(x_{ik}+x_{jk})}$ (for non-negative variables only).

(4) Czekanowski coefficient : $d_{ij} = 1 - \dfrac{2\sum_{k=1}^{p} \min(x_{ik}, x_{jk})}{\sum_{k=1}^{p}(x_{ik}+x_{jk})}$

(also for non-negative variables only).

If the variables under study are on very different scales or of very different quantities, then it would make sense to standardise the data before applying any of these formulae. This ensures that the importance of each variable is equalised in the calculation and no single variable predominates. Note that such standardisation is equivalent to application of *weighted* versions of each of the above formulae, the weight on variable k being the appropriate power (depending on which formula is used) of the inverse standard deviation of that variable. Range is an acceptable substitute for standard deviation in standardisation. None of the above measures makes any allowance for the correlations between variables; the Mahalanobis-like (see Appendix **A.1**) distance of equation (3.9) can be used if such allowance is felt to be important, but use of this distance in the techniques of chapters 5 and 10 (Volume 2) can have problems. Finally, if there are many missing values in the data it is not advisable to adopt the standard procedures of imputing estimates for the missing values, as this procedure will lead to overstated similarity between those individuals which have high proportions of missing values. Rather, the dissimilarity d_{ij} should be calculated from the h variables that exhibit values for both individuals, and the resulting value scaled up by the factor p/h.

3.25 Now suppose that the variables are all categorical. Then the simplest measure of dissimilarity between two individuals is the proportion of variables for which the individuals exhibit different categories. This is known as the matching coefficient. A special case occurs when all the variables are binary, i.e. categorical with just two categories each. If we denote the two categories 0 and 1, then for any two individuals we can count up the number a of variables that are 0 for both individuals, the number b that are 0 for the first and 1 for the second individual, the number c that are 1 for the first and 0 for the second, and the number d that are 1 for both. Then the above dissimilarity in this case is given by $d_{ij} = (b+c)/p$, where $p = a+b+c+d$; this is known as the simple matching coefficient. Variations of this coefficient have been proposed to deal with particular problems. For example, if 1 indicates 'presence' of some attribute and 0 its 'absence', then it is often felt that two 'absences' should not contribute anything towards the similarity between the respective individuals. In this case it may be more appropriate to use either $d_{ij} = \frac{b+c}{b+c+d}$ (the Jaccard coefficient) or $d_{ij} = \frac{b+c}{b+c+2d}$ (the Czekanowski coefficient).

Finally, the situation most often encountered in practice is where some of the variables are quantitative and some are categorical. Here one possibility is to calculate separate values, d_{1ij} from the quantitative variables and d_{2ij} from the categorical variables, and then to produce an overall measure as a (weighted) average of d_{1ij} and d_{2ij}. Alternatively, one can use the all-purpose measure of dissimilarity defined by Gower (1971a), which is the measure implemented in the statistical computer package GENSTAT.

Exercises

3.1 Suppose that the variables $x_1, \ldots, x_p$ are independently distributed such that $x_i \sim N(\mu_i, \sigma^2)$ for $i = 1, \ldots, p$, and let $f_x(t)$ be given by equation (3.1). Show that, if σ^2 is known, then for all $t \in [-\pi, \pi]$

$$\Pr\{| f_x(t) - f_{\boldsymbol{\mu}}(t) |^2 \leqslant \tfrac{1}{2}\sigma^2(p+1)\chi^2_{p,\alpha}\} = 1 - \alpha,$$

where $\boldsymbol{\mu} = (\mu_1, \ldots, \mu_p)$ and $\chi^2_{p,\alpha}$ is the $100(1-\alpha)$ percentage point of the χ^2 distribution on p degrees of freedom.

(Andrews, 1972)

Suppose now that the x_i are not independent, but that their covariance matrix is $\boldsymbol{W}$. Obtain the variance of $f_{\boldsymbol{x}}(t)$ and suggest how you would test the hypothesis that the expectation of $f_{\boldsymbol{x}}(t)$ at a particular t is $f_{\boldsymbol{\mu}_0}(t)$, where $\boldsymbol{\mu}_0$ is a hypothesised known constant.

(Goodchild and Vijayan, 1974)

3.2 Let $\boldsymbol{X}' = (\boldsymbol{x}_1, \ldots, \boldsymbol{x}_n)$, where the $\boldsymbol{x}_i$ are n independent p-dimensional vectors of random variables, and let $\boldsymbol{B}$ be a positive semidefinite $n \times n$ matrix of rank r ($\geqslant p$). Suppose that for each $\boldsymbol{x}_i$ and all $\boldsymbol{b} \neq \boldsymbol{0}$ and c, $\Pr[\boldsymbol{b}'\boldsymbol{x}_i = c] = 0$. Show that $\boldsymbol{X}'\boldsymbol{B}\boldsymbol{X}$ is positive definite with probability one.

(Das Gupta, 1971, Theorem 5)

(Eaton and Perlman, 1973, Theorem 2.3)

By considering $\boldsymbol{b}'\boldsymbol{x}_i$, where the $\boldsymbol{x}_i$ are independent normal vectors with common positive definite dispersion matrix $\boldsymbol{\Sigma}$, apply the above result to show that $\boldsymbol{A} = \sum_{i=1}^{n} (\boldsymbol{x}_i - \bar{\boldsymbol{x}})(\boldsymbol{x}_i - \bar{\boldsymbol{x}})'$ is positive definite with probability one when $p \leqslant n - 1$.

(Dykstra, 1970)

3.3 Let c_i, $\boldsymbol{l}_i$ for $i = 1, \ldots, p$ be the eigenvalues and eigenvectors of

$$\boldsymbol{S} = \frac{1}{n-1} \sum_{i=1}^{n} (\boldsymbol{x}_i - \bar{\boldsymbol{x}})(\boldsymbol{x}_i - \bar{\boldsymbol{x}})'.$$

Show that

$$t_j^2 = \sum_i c_i [\boldsymbol{l}_i'(\boldsymbol{x}_j - \bar{\boldsymbol{x}})]^2,$$

$$u_j^2 = \sum_i c_i \left[\frac{\boldsymbol{l}_i'(\boldsymbol{x}_j - \bar{\boldsymbol{x}})}{\| \boldsymbol{x}_j - \bar{\boldsymbol{x}} \|} \right]^2,$$

$$v_j^2 = \sum_i c_i^{-1} \left[\frac{\boldsymbol{l}_i'(\boldsymbol{x}_j - \bar{\boldsymbol{x}})}{\| \boldsymbol{x}_j - \bar{\boldsymbol{x}} \|} \right]^2,$$

$$d_{j0}^2 = \sum_i c_i^{-1} [\boldsymbol{l}_i'(\boldsymbol{x}_j - \bar{\boldsymbol{x}})]^2,$$

$$\sum_j t_j^2 = (n-1) \sum_i c_i^2,$$

where $t_j^2, u_j^2, v_j^2, d_{j0}^2$ and d_{jk}^2 are defined by equations (3.5) to (3.9).

(Gnanadesikan and Kettenring, 1972)

Show also that $\frac{n}{(n-1)} d_{j0}^2$ and $\frac{1}{2(n-1)} d_{jk}^2$ are beta variables with parameters $\frac{1}{2}p$ and $\frac{1}{2}(n-p-1)$.

(Wilks, 1962, p562)

3.4 For T_i^2, D_i^2 and Λ_i defined in **3.12**, show that

$$\Lambda_i^{-1} = 1 + T_i^2/(n-2)$$

and

$$D_i^2 = T_i^2/(n - 2 + T_i^2).$$

(Hawkins, 1980, p107)

3.5 Prove that the coefficients $b_{1,p}$ and $b_{2,p}$ of equations (3.19) and (3.20) are invariant under the transformation $\boldsymbol{y} = \boldsymbol{C}\boldsymbol{x} + \boldsymbol{d}$, where $\boldsymbol{C}$ is nonsingular. Hence verify that these coefficients do not depend on the mean $\boldsymbol{\mu}$ and dispersion matrix $\boldsymbol{\Sigma}$ of $\boldsymbol{x}$.

3.6 Let $\boldsymbol{x}_1, \ldots, \boldsymbol{x}_n$ be a random sample from a normal distribution with mean $\boldsymbol{\mu}$ and dispersion matrix $\boldsymbol{\Sigma}$. Consider the M-estimates of $\boldsymbol{\mu}$ and $\boldsymbol{\Sigma}$ given by equations (3.37) and (3.38) with Campbell's weights

$$w_{1i} = \begin{cases} 1 & \text{if } d_i \leqslant d_0 \\ \frac{d_0}{d_i} \exp\{-\frac{1}{2c_2^2}(d_i - d_0)^2\}, & \text{if } d_i > d_0 \end{cases}$$

and

$$w_{2i} = w_{1i}^2,$$

where $d_0 = \sqrt{p}+c_1/\sqrt{2}$ and d_i^2 is given by equation (3.36). Show that, asymptotically, $E(d_i^2) = p$ when $c_1 = \infty$ and $E(d_i^2) = p\chi(d_0^2; p+2) + d_0^2\{1 - \chi(d_0^2; p)\}$ when $c_1 = 2, c_2 = \infty$, where $\chi(.; p)$ is the cumulative Chi-squared distribution function on p degrees of freedom.

Campbell (1980)

4

Projections and Linear Transformations

Principal components

4.1 Karl Pearson (1901) first discussed principal components as 'lines and planes of closest fit' to data, considering two- and three-dimensional cases. The mathematical problem was already well known, from studies of the axes of inertia of physical objects and the principal axes of ellipsoids. The extension to higher dimensional cases, however, involving the calculation of eigenvalues and eigenvectors of larger matrices, seems to have discouraged much development of the idea. Hotelling (1933) introduced the method in the context of factor analysis, and first described an iterative method for finding the principal components in the general case.

The underlying idea is to represent the main structural features of a multivariate data set in terms of a smaller number of variables, so that they may be better understood and displayed graphically, while those features of the data that are lost will, it is hoped, consist of irrelevant 'noise'. The method is to project the data into a lower dimensional space chosen to include as much as possible of the variability in the data.

Suppose $\boldsymbol{X}$ is an $n \times p$ data matrix, centred about the mean so that column totals are zero, consisting of n independent observations of the variables $\boldsymbol{x}' = (x_1, \ldots, x_p)$. The variance–covariance matrix of $\boldsymbol{x}$ is estimated as $\boldsymbol{V} = \boldsymbol{X}'\boldsymbol{X}/(n-1)$, and any linear combination $\boldsymbol{a}'\boldsymbol{x}$, where $\boldsymbol{a}$ and $\boldsymbol{x}$ are $p \times 1$ vectors, has estimated variance $\boldsymbol{a}'\boldsymbol{V}\boldsymbol{a}$. Now the first principal component is defined as the variable $\boldsymbol{a}'\boldsymbol{x}$ that has maximum variance, subject to $\boldsymbol{a}'\boldsymbol{a} = 1$. This involves solving the equation

$$\frac{d}{d\boldsymbol{a}}\{\boldsymbol{a}'\boldsymbol{V}\boldsymbol{a} - \lambda\boldsymbol{a}'\boldsymbol{a}\} = \boldsymbol{0} \qquad (4.1)$$

where λ is a Lagrange multiplier. The values of λ must satisfy

$$\boldsymbol{V}\boldsymbol{a} = \lambda\boldsymbol{a} \qquad (4.2)$$

and are thus the p eigenvalues of $\boldsymbol{V}$. To each of the eigenvalues $\lambda_1, \lambda_2, \ldots, \lambda_p$, arranged in decreasing order of magnitude, there corresponds an eigenvector $\boldsymbol{a}_i$, and $\text{var}\,\boldsymbol{a}_i'\boldsymbol{x} = \lambda_i$. The vectors $\boldsymbol{a}_i'\boldsymbol{x}$ are known as the principal components, with the first principal component corresponding to λ_1, and so on. The standardisation ensures that $\boldsymbol{a}_i'\boldsymbol{a}_i = 1$, and the construction implies $\boldsymbol{a}_i'\boldsymbol{a}_j = 0, i \neq j$. The vector $\boldsymbol{a}_i$ contains the *coefficients* of the ith principal component, and $\boldsymbol{X}\boldsymbol{a}_i$ gives the *scores* of the n individuals on the ith principal component.

Another derivation of the principal components is by way of the singular value decomposition. Suppose $\boldsymbol{X}$ is a mean-centred data matrix, so that $\mathbf{1}'\boldsymbol{X} = \mathbf{0}'$, where $\mathbf{1}$ and $\mathbf{0}$ are vectors with elements 1 and 0 and orders n and p respectively. Now the singular value decomposition of $\boldsymbol{X}$ has the form

$$\boldsymbol{X} = \boldsymbol{U}\boldsymbol{D}\boldsymbol{V}' \tag{4.3}$$

where $\boldsymbol{U}$ and $\boldsymbol{V}$ are orthogonal matrices, $n \times n$ and $p \times p$ respectively, and $\boldsymbol{D}$ is an $n \times p$ matrix containing the singular values of $\boldsymbol{X}$—the square roots of the eigenvalues of $\boldsymbol{X}'\boldsymbol{X}$—in the leading diagonal, and zero elsewhere. Then $\boldsymbol{U}\boldsymbol{D}$ contains the principal component scores, and the rows of $\boldsymbol{V}'$ are the vectors $\boldsymbol{a}_i'$ giving the coefficients of the ith principal component. Note that in this standard notation $\boldsymbol{V}$ has no correspondence to the variance–covariance matrix, also sometimes written $\boldsymbol{V}$.

Plotting the first few principal components in pairs may now show at least some of the structure in the data. Further, the coefficients $\boldsymbol{a}_i$ of the ith principal component may admit of some physical interpretation or 'reification' (see **1.5**). The variance of the ith principal component is λ_i, and, in a rather loose sense, it is often said that this component 'accounts for' a proportion $\lambda_i / \sum_{j=1}^{p} \lambda_j$ of the total variance.

Another application is in regression. If there are many regressor variables, and they are strongly correlated, there are well known problems of variable selection and interpretation. A possible solution is to replace the regressor variables by principal components, and fit them in order. The problem of collinearity disappears, since the components are uncorrelated by construction, and often the first few components give an excellent fit.

Unfortunately, the advantage gained is largely illusory. The resulting regression involves all the original variables, and can be difficult to understand. The method gives a real insight into the factors that affect the dependent variable only if the components used can themselves be interpreted.

The chief interest in principal components is as a data-analytic device for displaying the main features of a set of observations. Nevertheless, they can be regarded as estimates of a set of population axes, and inferential arguments about population values or components in different samples are possible. This aspect is discussed in a later section.

In many applications the original variables are not measured in comparable units, and scaling is necessary. Scaling is discussed in the next section.

Example 4.1

A study of Central American pines was carried out by members of the forestry department at Oxford University. The data consisted of observations on 100 trees in a forest area of Honduras, and were analysed by Fernandez de la Reguera (1983). Figure 4.1 shows a plot of the first

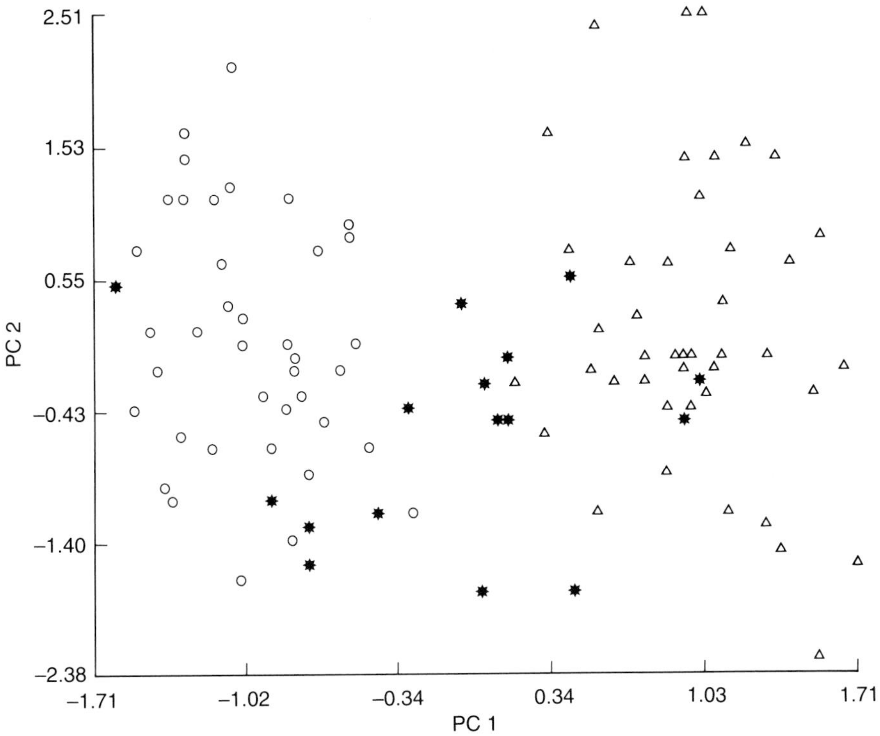

Figure 4.1 Principal component analysis of data on pines. Taxonomist's classification: △ *Pinus caribaea*; ○ *Pinus oocarpa*; ★ uncertain. PC 1 is related to needle length and chemical composition of the resin. PC 2 represents cone size. Reproduced from Fernandez de la Reguera (1983).

two principal components, calculated from measurements on the needles, cones and chemical composition of the resin.

The pines were classified by B.T. Styles as *P. caribaea* or *P. oocarpa*, with a number of doubtful cases unclassified. One of the aims of the study was to check the possibility of hybridisation between the species.

The principal components were calculated from the correlation matrix, without, of course, any reference to the taxonomic classification. The first principal component was a combination of stomata rows and the quantity of two components of the resin, myrcene and limonene. *P. caribaea* has typically long, wide needles in bunches of about three, while *P. oocarpa* has smaller needles in bunches of five or more. The first principal component quite effectively separates the two species.

The second component represents cone size, and is almost unrelated to the specific classification. The species differ in cone shape—rather than size—and this is also strongly represented in the first component. Notice that the two components have, by construction, exactly zero correlation.

The plot of the first two components shows two distinct groups, and the classification confirms that these groups correspond to what are recognised as two species. Most of the trees not classified are close to the boundary between the two groups. This is not unexpected; the information about needles, with characteristics of the cones, was used in deciding the classification.

This example illustrates the ability of principal components to reveal structure in data, and the possibility of interpreting the components. The first two components represented 42% and 12% of the total variance, the trace of the standardised covariance matrix, respectively. The plot does not shed much light on the question of hybridisation; it possibly suggests that there are some trees not typical of either species, but these are not exclusively the ones that were not definitely classified.

Scaling

4.2 In many multivariate data sets, the variates are of quite different types, often measured in different units and not comparable in scale. Principal components are scale dependent. If one variate has a much higher variance than the others, it will dominate the first principal component, and this is clearly undesirable in most situations. Nearly always, it is necessary to scale the original variates before calculating principal components.

The only exception to this is when all variates are of the same type, and of comparable scatter. The most familiar example is in studies on plants or animals when all the variates are log lengths. Other possible examples are when the variates are scores, all on the same range and supposedly comparable in scale. Generally, however, some preliminary standardisation is needed.

Usually, all variates are scaled by dividing by their standard deviations. The variance–covariance matrix is then replaced by the correlation matrix. In this case the first principal component will be dominated by the variates that are strongly—positively or negatively—correlated. The trace of the correlation matrix, and the sum of the eigenvalues, is then p.

Other methods of scaling are possible. Occasionally variates are standardised by range, but this seems to have no advantages. Scaling using robust estimates of variance avoids the possibility of distortion by outliers. After scaling, the variance–covariance matrix $\boldsymbol{V}$ may be calculated by robust methods (for details, see **3.22**). The resulting matrix may, with certain estimates, not be positive semi-definite, and the principal component analysis may give some negative eigenvalues. This is not important; the first few components may still give a good impression of the main features of the data set.

In multivariate inference, the inclusion of very highly correlated variates has little effect on the conclusions. The information in a pair of highly correlated variates is almost unchanged if one of them is omitted from the analysis. In principal components, however, such variates tend to dominate the early components, and the inclusion of redundant variates may substantially alter the component structure.

Size and shape

4.3 There are many situations in which most, or all, of the correlations among a set of multivariate observations are positive. One example is the log lengths of different parts of organisms; usually, large objects tend to be large in all their measurements. Another example arises in educational psychology. Spearman (1904a, b) noticed that examination results among schoolchildren are nearly always positively correlated, and discussed the relation of this observation to the concept of 'general intelligence'. This insight was the first step in the development of factor analysis.

In a principal component analysis, if the variables are scaled to have equal variance, and all the correlations are equal and positive, the first principal component is just the sum of the scaled variables. In this case, the first component is a measure of 'size', in the obvious sense when the observations are physical measurements, and in a slightly more general sense when they are not. If the correlations are strictly equal, the remaining components are undefined; if they are roughly equal, the remaining components are contrasts among the variables, uncorrelated with the first component representing size, and so naturally interpreted as measures of 'shape'.

This interpretation of the first component as size, when most correlations are positive, goes back at least to Penrose (1947). It was further developed, in biological applications, by Jolicoeur and Mosimann (1960). Rao (1964) discussed the interpretation of principal components in terms of size and shape, arguing that the interpretation outlined above is oversimplified, and that what is naturally interpreted as shape is not necessarily uncorrelated with size.

Nevertheless, the tradition has grown, particularly in taxonomy and biological morphology, that the first component may be relatively unimportant in classification, as it is often dominated by size. There is therefore a tendency to rely more on the second and third components for the study of relationships among organisms.

Allometry is the study of changes in shape as an organism grows. Thompson (1917) stimulated interest in the problem. Suppose $x_1, \ldots, x_p$ are the logarithms of linear measurements on organisms at different stages of growth. Isometry implies that the first principal component has coefficients $(1/\sqrt{p}, 1/\sqrt{p}, \ldots, 1/\sqrt{p})$. A likelihood ratio test of the general hypothesis that the coefficients of the ith principal component take the specified values $\boldsymbol{\alpha}_{io}$ has the form (Morrison, 1976 p250)

$$\chi^2_{p-1} = n\left(\lambda_i \boldsymbol{\alpha}'_{io} \boldsymbol{V}^{-1} \boldsymbol{\alpha}_{io} + \frac{1}{\lambda_i} \boldsymbol{\alpha}'_{io} \boldsymbol{V} \boldsymbol{\alpha}_{io} - 2\right).$$

Here, λ_i is the ith sample eigenvalue and $\boldsymbol{V}$ is the sample variance–covariance matrix. This test of course assumes p-variate normality. As a test of isometry, based on the first principal component, it was suggested by Jolicoeur (1963).

Mosimann (1970) discussed more general definitions of size and shape variables. The geometric mean is the only measure of size that is truly scale independent, in the sense that changing the scale of one of the variables merely multiplies it by a constant, or adds a constant to its logarithm. It is therefore the only measure appropriate for describing size when the variables are measures differing in order of magnitude. Often, though, another measure, such as the arithmetic mean, may seem a suitable measure of size. Mosimann showed that, given any measure of size (of dimension one in the variables) it is possible to define a shape vector by dividing each variable by that measure.

The idea of shape analysis has been further developed recently. Bookstein (1986) discussed the analysis of 'landmark' data. Observations consist of the positions of p reference points or landmarks defining the position of an object in k dimensions; thus each object is characterised by a $p \times k$ matrix. The shapes of the n objects are unaffected by translation, scaling, rotation, and in some applications reflection. Kendall and Kendall (1980) studied two-dimensional alignments, particularly with reference to lines of standing stones, and the development of significance tests for hypotheses about collinearity. Kendall (1989) reviewed the subject, and Goodall (1991) discussed the application of Procrustes methods (Chapter 5) in handling landmark data. See Part 2 for some further discussion.

Population principal components

4.4 For any multivariate distribution with finite variances and covariances, population principal components exist. They are defined in terms of the variance–covariance matrix $\boldsymbol{\Sigma}$ in exactly the same way as sample components are calculated from the sample variance–covariance matrix. The calculation is equivalent to the familiar geometric problem of finding the principal axes of a quadric surface, and for elliptically symmetrical distributions (see **2.11**), the principal components are these principal axes.

The principal components calculated from a set of data can be regarded as estimates of the population values, but some care is necessary. The ith vector $\boldsymbol{a}_i$ and the corresponding eigenvalue λ_i are consistent estimates of the ith direction and weight in the population only if (a) the variance and covariance estimates are consistent, and (b) the ith population eigenvalue is unique. Of course, if there are equal eigenvalues in the population the corresponding directions are undefined, and the sample eigenvectors will be arbitrarily determined by random variation.

Further, when population eigenvalues are not very different, the corresponding sample eigenvectors can become confused. Inference based on principal components is thus complicated. Sometimes rotation of components may assist interpretation. The question of rotation will be covered in more detail in volume 2, in the discussion of factor analysis. Here it may be noted that, while in factor analysis the factors are completely undefined and may be chosen arbitrarily in the estimated factor space, here the components are estimates—except in the extreme case when population axes are exactly equal—of the corresponding directions, and are confused by sampling variation, rather than by essential unidentifiability.

Some asymptotic results on the distribution of eigenvalues and the coefficients of principal components are known for the case when the underlying distribution is multivariate normal and the eigenvalues of the population covariance matrix are distinct. For details, see Morrison (1976) Chapter 7, or Anderson (1984), Chapter 11. These are of limited value; even when the distribution is strictly multivariate normal, the approach to the limiting distribution may be very slow, particularly when the population eigenvalues are not very different, so that the sample eigenvectors may become confused.

Common principal components

4.5 A question related to the idea of population principal components is whether samples from two populations can be regarded as having the same principal components. Of course this is so if the covariance matrices—or the correlation matrices if the principal components are based on standardised variates—are the same. The hypothesis to be investigated is less restrictive than that, however; population covariance matrices may have the same eigenvectors, but different eigenvalues, so that the related ellipsoids have parallel axes, but not necessarily the same shape nor the magnitude of the axes in the same order.

This idea of comparing the principal components in different groups is interesting, but has certain limitations. In the first place, a model that postulates parallel axes but unequal covariance matrices is difficult to justify except on the assumption that there are unobservable effects operating in all the groups, but with different strengths. Essentially this implies a factor model, and if such a model holds the question may perhaps be better investigated by confirmatory factor analysis. Secondly, a significance test based on the assumption of multivariate normality within the groups is likely to be very sensitive to that assumption. As with all tests of equality of variances or covariance matrices, the results depend heavily on the behaviour of the higher order moments, and long-tailed distributions are likely to give high rejection rates.

Krzanowski (1979) first investigated the problem. He examined the angles between subsets of principal components based on different groups; first, the angles between the first principal components, next between the planes of the first pair, and so on. The analysis was extended to the case of more than two groups by finding the vector closest to the spaces spanned by the sets of principal components, in the sense of minimising

$$V = \sum_{i=1}^{g} \cos^2 \delta_i$$

where δ_i is the angle between the vector and the closest vector in the space of the principal component space of group i. This procedure is repeated with vectors orthogonal to the first, to find the subspace of dimension k most closely approximating the g subspaces of the sets of principal components. The angles between each of these components and the corresponding component in each subgroup are then examined.

Krzanowski does not attempt a formal significance test, though he mentions a Monte Carlo study, not described in detail. As an illustration, he examined a principal component analysis of examination results in eight subjects in three colleges. The individual components—particularly the second and third components—had apparently very different coefficients in the colleges, but Krzanowski showed that in fact two components could be regarded as common to the three colleges, whereas the third showed considerable differences and the fourth contrasted one college clearly with the other two.

Flury (1984, 1986) investigated the null hypothesis that there exists an orthogonal matrix $\boldsymbol{\beta}$ such that

$$\boldsymbol{\beta}'\boldsymbol{\Sigma}_i\boldsymbol{\beta} = \boldsymbol{\Lambda}_i$$

for all i, where $\boldsymbol{\Sigma}_i$ is the covariance matrix for group i, and $\boldsymbol{\Lambda}_i$ is diagonal. This hypothesis is that the principal components are the same for all groups, but not necessarily with the same eigenvalues. He developed a likelihood ratio test, based on the multivariate normal distribution, for this hypothesis. In a later paper (Flury, 1987) he extended this test to the case where $\boldsymbol{\beta}$ is $k \times p$, to test whether the first k principal components can be regarded as the same. This is the problem investigated by Krzanowski. Flury suggests that it can be studied using the likelihood ratio test, though he adds that, since in practice k is unknown, the investigation should be regarded as exploratory data analysis rather than formal inference.

Choosing subsets of variables

4.6 Two problems that are often discussed in connection with principal components are concerned with selection or rejection of variables. In the first, the aim is to separate 'informative' components from those regarded as 'noise'; where is the division, and how many components should be retained? In the second, principal component analysis may suggest that some of the original variables are redundant (highly correlated with other variables) or uninformative, because they feature only weakly in the first few components. In this case, it may be that they can be discarded, and further analysis, by principal components or otherwise, can be based on a subset of the original variables with gain of clarity. A great deal of discussion has been devoted to both these questions. Essentially, both depend on subjective judgement; no statistical test can decide whether a variable is interesting or not, but further examination of the data may guide such decisions.

Various criteria have been suggested for the first problem; for detailed discussion see Jolliffe (1986) or Jackson (1991). Some options are as follows:

(1) The proportion of variance explained may be a guide. If the first two or three components account for 90% or more of the total variance, it may be felt that further components are irrelevant. The decision is subjective, and can quite easily be misleading; in particular, a single 'size' component can account for most of the variance, while most of the interesting information is contained in other components.
(2) Components with variances below a certain level may be rejected. In particular, if components are calculated on the basis of the correlation matrix, components with variances less than 1 are often discarded. There seems no logical reason for this suggestion; if one variable is virtually independent of the rest, it will appear as a component with variance slightly less than 1, but there is no reason to suppose it is uninformative.
(3) Sometimes, particularly in non-biological applications, the accuracy of

observations is known approximately *a priori*. If this is so, it seems reasonable to stop extracting components when the residual variance is comparable with that arising from errors of observation. This criterion, however, is often not available.

(4) Bartlett (1950) derived a sphericity test, of the hypothesis that after removing k principal components, the data can be regarded as derived from $p-k$ uncorrelated variables of equal variance. The test is a modified likelihood ratio test, based on the normal distribution and asymptotically valid; it takes the form:

$$\left(n - \frac{2p+11}{6}\right)(p-k)\log\frac{a_0}{g_0} \sim \chi^2_{(p-k+2)(p-k-1)/2} \tag{4.4}$$

(Mardia *et al*, 1979 p236), where a_0 and g_0 are respectively the arithmetic and geometric means of the $p-k$ eigenvalues $\lambda_{k+1}, \ldots, \lambda_p$.
This test was proposed in the context of factor analysis, and can be regarded as a test of the existence of any further common factor. If the data are normally distributed and the sample is large, a non-significant result is certainly an indication that there is no point in extracting further principal components. This does not, however, mean that the remaining components contain no information. Again, independent variables are not necessarily irrelevant.

(5) A 'scree plot' is simply a plot of the eigenvalues λ_i against i. The eigenvalues are in decreasing order, and often the plot will simply fall towards zero with gradually decreasing slope. If, however, the variables are linear functions of a much smaller number of underlying factors with random error, the graph will drop sharply for the first few values, and then much more slowly. The 'elbow' suggests that components corresponding to the eigenvalues from that point on correspond to the random error part of the model. The graph has the form of a mountainside with scree at the bottom—the name is due to Cattell (1966).
This procedure assumes a factor analytic model, and again it is unwise to conclude that principal components in the scree section are not informative. The identification of the break-point is a matter of judgement, and is often by no means clear. Variations are possible. Cattell (1966) actually plotted *differences* between successive eigenvalues. Plotting log-eigenvalues is sometimes advocated, in the hope that the error part of the plot will be approximately linear. Attempts have been made to associate rules for the number of retained components with the plots—see Jackson (1991)—but the reasoning behind them is doubtful.

(6) All the methods disscussed so far depend only on the eigenvalues. There is, however, much more information in the data that may help to decide on the appropriate number of principal components, and *cross-validation* methods attempt to use this information. Wold (1976, 1978) originated the idea, which was developed by Eastment and Krzanowski (1982) and Krzanowski (1983, 1987b). Each element x_{ij} of the data matrix $\boldsymbol{X}$ is left out in turn, and estimated from the reduced rank singular value decomposition. The accuracy of the approximation is then based on the sum of squares of differences between the actual and estimated values.

Define

$$\mathrm{PRESS}(m) = \frac{1}{np}\sum_{i=1}^{n}\sum_{j=1}^{p}(\hat{x}_{ij}^{(m)} - x_{ij})^2 \tag{4.5}$$

where $\hat{x}_{ij}^{(m)}$ is the estimate of x_{ij} based on the first m principal components, omitting that observation. PRESS is an acronym for PREdiction Sum of Squares. The number of components to retain is then determined by the value of

$$W_m = \frac{\mathrm{PRESS}(m-1) - \mathrm{PRESS}(m)}{\mathrm{PRESS}(m)} \, \frac{p(n-1)}{n+p-2m}. \tag{4.6}$$

W_m represents the increase in predictive information supplied by the mth component, divided by the average predictive information in each of the remaining components, Then if W_m is small, the inclusion of the mth principal component has little effect on the approximation. If $W_m < 1$ the mth principal component appears to carry less information than the average of the remaining components, but to allow for bias and sampling error Krzanowski (1983) suggests a cut off at $W_m = 0.9$.

The main problem here is the calculation of $\hat{x}_{ij}^{(m)}$. The method given by Eastment and Krzanowski (1982) (see also Krzanowski 1987b, 1988b) depends on two singular value decompositions, omitting respectively the ith row and the jth column of $\boldsymbol{X}$. This method uses all the information available and is strictly independent of the observation x_{ij} itself, but is extremely computer intensive. An efficient algorithm is essential; see Moonen *et al* (1992), and references therein.

Another possible question is whether it is possible and useful to base principal components on a subset of the original variables. This problem was investigated by Jolliffe (1972, 1973). The aim is to find a group of variables, often of the same dimension as that chosen for the principal components, to retain as much of the information in the principal components as possible. Various criteria have been suggested. Several of the papers discuss a data set first given by Jeffers (1967), consisting of 19 measurements on 40 specimens of *Alate adelges*, winged aphides, and Jolliffe (1986) (p. 111) compares the variables selected in his earlier papers with those selected by McCabe (1982, 1984) using various criteria based on the eigenvalues of the deleted variables and on their canonical correlations with the retained variables. Krzanowski (1987a) described a different approach based on a Procrustes analysis comparing the k-dimensional principal component scores based on the original p variables and on a subset of q variables; again, the method is applied to the aphis data.

Not surprisingly, the results from the various methods are markedly different. The first principal component is, typically, a 'size' variable with positive coefficients for nearly all the original variables. The choice of one or more of these for inclusion is largely arbitrary, and several subsets of the original variables are nearly equivalent in the information they contain. In these circumstances, the attempt to identify a best subset is of largely academic interest; any subset that adequately represents the data and is easier to interpret than the principal components based on the full set is worth considering.

Three-mode component analysis

4.7 A principal component analysis may be written in the form

$$x_{ij} = \sum_{\alpha=1}^{q} a_{i\alpha} b_{j\alpha} + e_{ij} \tag{4.7}$$

where $i = 1, \ldots, n$, $j = 1, \ldots, p$ and $q < p$ represents the number of retained principal components, leaving error terms e_{ij}. The terms a and b may be the 'scores' of the subjects on the components and the 'loadings' of the variables on the components, and represent scoring of the rows and columns of the data matrix $\boldsymbol{X}$. For further discussion, see **4.9**.

Often, the data matrix is replaced by a three-way array, with elements x_{ijk}. This structure may represent p-variate observations on different groups as in a two-way multivariate analysis of variance, or p-variate observations made at different times, as in multivariate repeated measures or growth curve problems (see Part 2). It is natural to ask whether lower dimensional representations of such data sets, related to principal components, can be found.

This problem has been studied by Tucker (1966). It is related to the multidimensional scaling problems for three-dimensional arrays discussed in **5.13**. Tucker suggested a number of models of considerable complexity and flexibility; these are rather a generalisation of factor analysis than of principal components, and will be discussed in Part 2.

The simplest generalisation of equation (4.7), which can be regarded as a special case of the models proposed by Tucker, is known as Harshman's model (Harshman *et al*, 1977). The equation is replaced by

$$x_{ijk} = \sum_{\alpha=1}^{q} a_{i\alpha} b_{j\alpha} c_{k\alpha} + e_{ijk}. \tag{4.8}$$

This model has three sets of scores, relating to the individuals, variates and groups or occasions. Each set is clearly defined only up to a multiplying factor. The model is fitted by alternating least squares (see **5.13**), and for given q, the solution is unique, though the ordering of the q triplets is arbitrary. The computer programme PARAFAC was written by Harshman for fitting such models.

Comparison with other techniques

4.8 *Projection pursuit* is the name given to a collection of techniques aimed at finding 'interesting' projections, usually in two dimensions, of multidimensional data sets. This typically involves maximising or minimising some objective function chosen to reveal the data structure. Principal components can be regarded as a particular case of projection pursuit, in which the objective function is the variance. It is by far the oldest technique of this sort, and computationally much the simplest; it is only since the development of computers and computer expertise that other methods, claimed to be more effective at revealing interesting features, have been evolved. Applications of projection pursuit are discussed later in the chapter, from **4.12** onwards.

Factor analysis (see Part 2) is a statistical idea almost as old as principal components, dating back to the work of Spearman (1904b). The model postulates that the correlation structure is derived from $k(< p)$ unobservable factors. The observations are linear functions of the factors, with independent errors. The covariances are due entirely to the factors common to the different variates.

It is easy to see that if the errors were absent, or even if they all had the same variance, the principal components, calculated from the correlation matrix, would be equivalent to the factors. In the factor analysis model, this is a completely implausible assumption. Nevertheless, one of the popular methods of fitting the factor model consists in iteratively fitting principal components, and adjusting the diagonal terms of the correlation matrix to make it approximate one of lower rank. The details are given in Part 2. Although the concepts and aims of factor analysis are completely different, the calculation of principal components is implicit in this particular method. In fact, in certain computer packages (notably SPSS) principal components are calculated using the factor analysis program, without adjustment of the diagonal or iteration.

Canonical variables (**4.10**) are also linear functions of the original variates, and sometimes consist of a reduced set of linear combinations intended to show particular features of the data, but the canonical variables associated with a data matrix $\boldsymbol{X}$ are defined in terms of its relationship with another data matrix $\boldsymbol{Y}$, which may either be another set of random variables or a design matrix defining a grouping. Principal components and canonical analysis are sometimes referred to respectively as the internal and external analysis of the data matrix $\boldsymbol{X}$.

Principal coordinate analysis (Gower, 1966a), also known as *metric scaling* is a method of finding the best low-dimensional fit to a set of data expressed as a similarity or dissimilarity matrix. If a data matrix $\boldsymbol{X}$, $n \times p$, is transformed to a $n \times n$ dissimilarity matrix by calculating Euclidean distances between each pair of rows, the principal coordinates calculated from it are the principal component scores of the original data matrix $\boldsymbol{X}$. See **5.8**.

Correspondence analysis is another technique for reduced dimensional representation of a $n \times p$ data matrix. Devised originally for categorical data, it is based on the singular value decomposition, and the same technique applied to a centred matrix of data derived from continuous variables gives principal component analysis as a special case. See **5.19**; for a full analysis of the relationships of correspondence analysis with other multivariate techniques, see Greenacre (1984).

Biplots

4.9 The calculation of principal components can be approached from a rather different viewpoint. Consider a data matrix $\boldsymbol{X}$, $n \times p$. The singular value decomposition of the centred data matrix X gives

$$X = U\Lambda V' \tag{4.9}$$

where the columns of U, $n \times p$, are orthogonal, Λ is a $p \times p$ diagonal matrix containing the singular values of X—the positive square roots of the eigenvalues of $X'X$—and V is an orthogonal $p \times p$ matrix. This equation is a slightly different form of the singular value decomposition from that given in equation (4.3). The singular values in Λ are arranged in decreasing order. Consider approximating the matrix X by a matrix of lower rank. Now any unitarily invariant norm of X is a symmetric function of the singular values (see Rao, 1980) and so the best rank k approximation to X, in the sense of having maximum unitarily invariant norm, is given by replacing Λ by Λ^* with diagonal elements $\lambda_1, \ldots, \lambda_k, 0, \ldots, 0$. Suppose X is a data matrix with zero column totals. The rows of $U\Lambda$ are the principal component scores, and the columns of V are the coefficients $\boldsymbol{a}$ of the original variables in the successive components.

A plot of the first few principal components can then show something of the data structure, as has been discussed. There is also the possibility of plotting the first few vectors of coefficients, indicating which variates are given high and low weightings in the different components. With suitable choice of scales, these coefficients can be plotted on the same axes as the component scores. Then the positions of individual observations close to particular variates suggests that those individuals have high scores on the variates.

That is an example of a *biplot*, a graph in which row and column scores of a matrix are shown in the same diagram. The plot may be in one or more dimensions; the prefix *bi*- refers to the the two dimensions of the original matrix, and the dimensions of the plot reflect the rank of the approximation $U\Lambda^* V'$. Biplots are usually two-dimensional merely because of the convenience of plotting.

The idea of a reduced rank representation using the singular value decomposition goes back to Eckart and Young (1936). The biplot was introduced by Gabriel (1971), and developed in subsequent papers, particularly Bradu and Gabriel (1976) and Gabriel (1981).

The reduced rank representation $U\Lambda^* V'$ can be regarded as an optimal way of deriving a lower dimensional approximation X^* of the data matrix X. The next step is to reduce X^* to a product, say GH', in which the rows of G and the columns of H' are scores for rows and columns. Generally, we can write $G = U(\Lambda^*)^\alpha, H' = (\Lambda^*)^{1-\alpha} V'$. When $\alpha = 1$, H' and G are the coefficients and values of the principal components, and this is perhaps the most natural choice for displaying a data matrix in which the rows are cases and the columns variables. When $\alpha = 0$, the vector lengths corresponding to the variates have lengths approximately equal to their standard deviations. This is sometimes referred to as a $J'K$ biplot.

Example 4.2

In a study of car-buyers in France (Bertier and Bouroche, 1975) buyers of nine types of car were asked to indicate which of ten characteristics they considered important in choosing a car. The responses were binary, and the resulting contingency table can be summarised in a biplot, Figure 4.2.

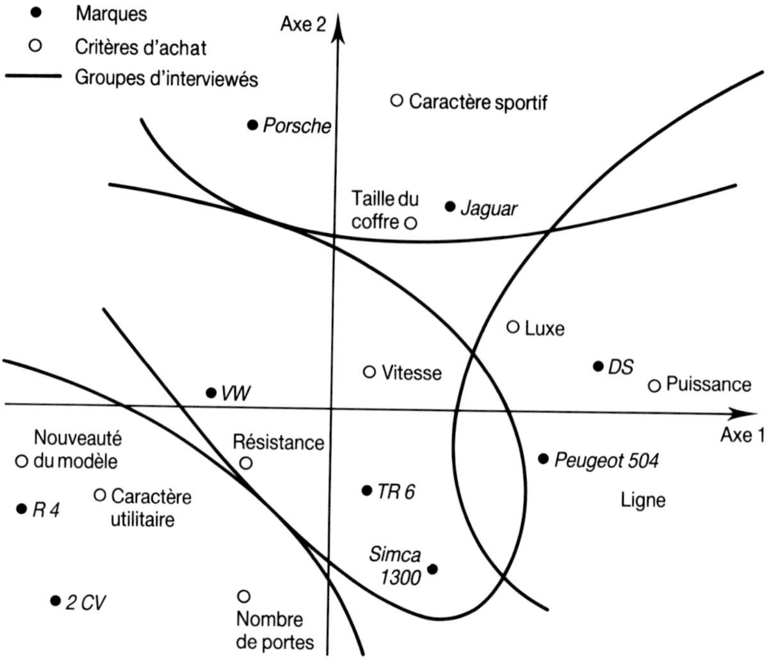

Figure 4.2 Biplot of criteria for car purchase. Reproduced from Bertier and Bouroche (1975).

The curves show a subjective grouping of buyers, with the cars chosen and the characteristics judged important. The first axis clearly separates large, medium and small cars, with luxury and power contrasted with utilitarian character. The second separates off the sports cars, Jaguar and Porsche, from the rest. On the whole, the models are associated with the criteria as might be expected, but there are some features—such as the position of the Triumph TR 6, a small sports car—that suggest that a third axis may be needed.

Canonical variables

4.10 Suppose $\boldsymbol{x}$ and $\boldsymbol{y}$ are vectors of p and q variates respectively, and suppose the variance–covariance matrix $\boldsymbol{V}$ of $\boldsymbol{z}' = (\boldsymbol{x}', \boldsymbol{y}')$ is partitioned:

$$\boldsymbol{V} = \begin{pmatrix} \boldsymbol{V}_{11} & \boldsymbol{V}_{12} \\ \boldsymbol{V}_{21} & \boldsymbol{V}_{22} \end{pmatrix} \tag{4.10}$$

so that $\boldsymbol{V}_{11}, p \times p$, and $\boldsymbol{V}_{22}, q \times q$, are the variance–covariance matrices of $\boldsymbol{x}$ and $\boldsymbol{y}$ respectively, while $\boldsymbol{V}_{12}, p \times q$, and its transpose $\boldsymbol{V}_{21}$ contain the covariances between the variates in $\boldsymbol{x}$ and those in $\boldsymbol{y}$.

Now consider the correlation between two linear combinations of $\boldsymbol{x}$ and $\boldsymbol{y}$ respectively, say $\boldsymbol{a}'\boldsymbol{x}$ and $\boldsymbol{b}'\boldsymbol{y}$. This correlation may be written

$$\rho = \boldsymbol{a}'\boldsymbol{V}_{12}\boldsymbol{b}/\sqrt{\boldsymbol{a}'\boldsymbol{V}_{11}\boldsymbol{a}\boldsymbol{b}'\boldsymbol{V}_{22}\boldsymbol{b}}. \tag{4.11}$$

Next, choose $\boldsymbol{a}$ and $\boldsymbol{b}$ to maximise this correlation. (Of course, the values of the coefficients are determined only up to a multiplying factor). This is equivalent to maximising

$$\boldsymbol{a}'\boldsymbol{V}_{12}\boldsymbol{b} - \tfrac{1}{2}\lambda\boldsymbol{a}'\boldsymbol{V}_{11}\boldsymbol{a} - \tfrac{1}{2}\mu\boldsymbol{b}'\boldsymbol{V}_{22}\boldsymbol{b}$$

where λ and μ are Lagrange multipliers.

Differentiating with respect to $\boldsymbol{a}$ and $\boldsymbol{b}$ gives

$$\boldsymbol{V}_{12}\boldsymbol{b} - \lambda\boldsymbol{V}_{11}\boldsymbol{a} = 0, \qquad (4.12)$$

$$\boldsymbol{a}'\boldsymbol{V}_{12} - \mu\boldsymbol{b}'\boldsymbol{V}_{22} = 0. \qquad (4.13)$$

Substituting for $\boldsymbol{b}$ gives

$$\boldsymbol{V}_{12}\boldsymbol{V}_{22}^{-1}\boldsymbol{V}_{21}\boldsymbol{a} - \lambda\mu\boldsymbol{V}_{11}\boldsymbol{a} = 0. \qquad (4.14)$$

This equation has non-trivial roots only if

$$|\boldsymbol{V}_{12}\boldsymbol{V}_{22}^{-1}\boldsymbol{V}_{21} - l\boldsymbol{V}_{11}| = 0, \qquad (4.15)$$

writing l for $\lambda\mu$. The values of l are the roots of the determinantal equation, or the eigenvalues of $\boldsymbol{V}_{12}\boldsymbol{V}_{22}^{-1}\boldsymbol{V}_{21}\boldsymbol{V}_{11}^{-1}$. This is not a symmetric matrix, but it is known to have non-negative eigenvalues. If we assume, without loss of generality, that $p \leqslant q$ and that $\boldsymbol{V}_{11}$ is non-singular, there are exactly p non-zero roots, say $l_1, \ldots, l_p$ in decreasing order of magnitude. To each value l_i there correspond vectors $\boldsymbol{a}_i$ and $\boldsymbol{b}_i$, and the correlation between $\boldsymbol{a}_i'\boldsymbol{x}$ and $\boldsymbol{b}_i'\boldsymbol{y}$ is $l_i^{1/2}$. These correlations, the positive square roots of the eigenvalues, are known as the *canonical correlations* between $\boldsymbol{x}$ and $\boldsymbol{y}$, and the corresponding variables are the *canonical variables.*

The construction gives p pairs of variables, and if $q > p$ it is possible to define a further set of $q-p$ orthogonal combinations of the y variables, chosen arbitrarily, all orthogonal to the x variables. These may be, for example, the principal components of the residuals of $\boldsymbol{y}$ after regression on $\boldsymbol{x}$. Now consider the correlation matrix of the complete set of canonical variables, the p variables $\boldsymbol{a}_i'\boldsymbol{x}$ ordered according to the values of l_i, then the corresponding values of $\boldsymbol{b}_i'\boldsymbol{y}$, then the remaining $q - p$ linear combination of the y variables. There are just $2p$ non-zero off-diagonal elements,

$$r_{i,p+i} = r_{p+i,i} = l_i^{1/2}, \quad i = 1, \ldots, p.$$

There are two main areas of application of canonical variables, in multivariate regression and classification. In multivariate regression the aim is to relate a set of random variables to another set of variables, which may or may not be random variables. This is a natural extension of the general linear model. There are obvious applications in economics, medical statistics, and many other fields. The canonical variable approach makes it possible to explain complex relationships in terms of a smaller number of pairs of variables, and, particularly if the canonical variables can be interpreted, the resulting economy should make the situation easier to interpret. Significance tests associated with canonical variables, particularly to decide how many variables to retain, are described in the Appendix.

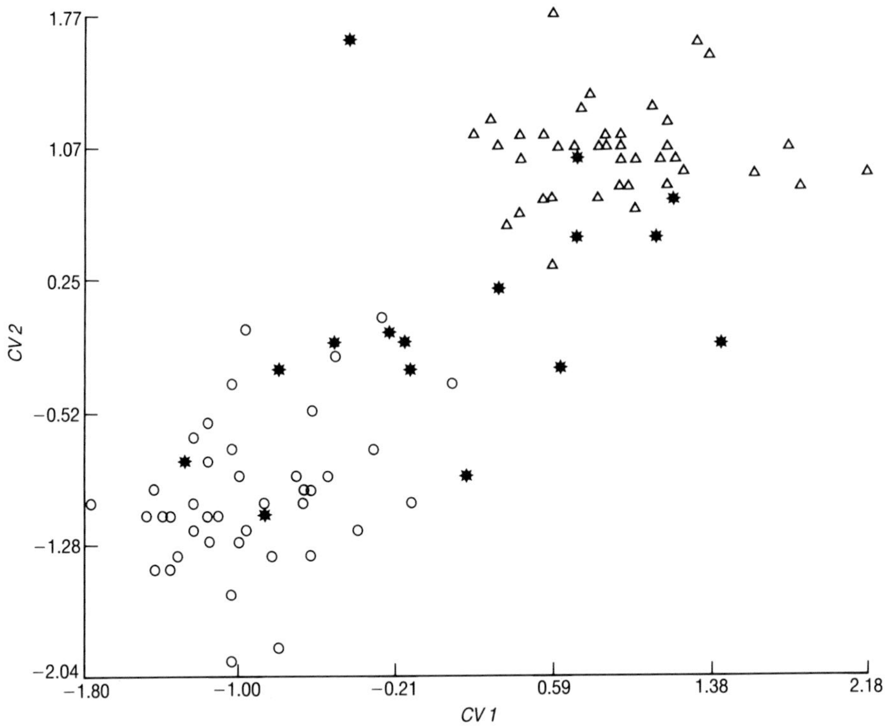

Figure 4.3 Canonical variable analysis of data on pines. Taxonomist's classification: △ *Pinus caribaea*; ○ *Pinus oocarpa*; ⋆ uncertain. CV 1 is a contrast between myrcene and β-phellandrene. CV 2 represents cone shape. Reproduced from Fernandez de la Reguera (1983).

In fact, good published instances of practical applications are surprisingly rare. Gittens (1985) gives a number of interesting ecological examples.

Example 4.3
The data of Figure 4.1 (Fernandez de la Reguera, 1983) consist of measurements on the needles, cones and resin composition of pines. Treating the cone and chemical data as two sets of variables, canonical variables can be calculated. Figure 4.3 shows the plot of the first pair of canonical variables. The abscissa represents the chemical component, the ordinate is determined by cone shape.
The contrast with Figure 4.1 is clear. The two species appear as well separated groups, and the correlation between the chemical and cone canonical variables is mainly accounted for by the difference between the two groups. There are some observations that are near the boundary between the groups, but more interestingly there are one or two typical of one species in their resin characteristics and of the other in their cones. It could be argued that these provide clearer evidence of hybridisation than intermediate cases.

The extension of canonical variables to more than two sets of variables has been discussed, particularly by Steel (1951), Horst (1965) and Kettenring (1971). A linear function is calculated for each group. With g groups of variables there are $\frac{1}{2}g(g-1)$ correlation coefficients, and some function of these correlations must be chosen as a criterion for choosing the canonical variables. Kettenring lists a number of possible criteria, all of which reduce to the canonical correlation when there are only two groups of variables.

Practical examples of the technique are uncommon; Fernandez de la Reguera *et al* (1988) used multiple-set canonical analysis on the pine data already discussed.

Canonical variables in classification

4.11 The commonest application of canonical variables is in classification problems. One set of variables defines the g groups, and the corresponding canonical variables are contrasts among the groups. Of the other set, the first canonical variable is the linear function that best discriminates among the groups, in the sense of giving the largest value to the variance ratio in an analysis of variance between and within groups. The other canonical variables are orthogonal to it, and to each other, with respect to the within-group matrix, and are ranked in decreasing order of this variance ratio. Thus, if $\boldsymbol{X}\boldsymbol{a}_i$ and $\boldsymbol{X}\boldsymbol{a}_j$ are the values of two canonical variables,

$$\boldsymbol{a}_i'\boldsymbol{W}\boldsymbol{a}_j = 0$$

where $\boldsymbol{W}$ is the within-group matrix of sums of squares and products.

There are s canonical variables, where $s = \min(p, g-1)$. If $\bar{\boldsymbol{x}}$ is a group mean in terms of the original variables, then $\bar{\boldsymbol{z}} = (z_1, \ldots, z_s)$ is its value on the canonical variates, where $z_i = \boldsymbol{a}_i'\bar{\boldsymbol{x}}$.

Standardisation is arbitrary. The coefficients may be defined so that

$$\boldsymbol{a}_i'\boldsymbol{W}\boldsymbol{a}_i = 1 \text{ or } \boldsymbol{a}_i'\boldsymbol{a}_i = 1 \text{ or } \boldsymbol{a}_i'\boldsymbol{T}\boldsymbol{a}_i = 1$$

where $\boldsymbol{T}$ is the total estimated variance–covariance matrix. If the first of these standardisations is used, then the Euclidean squared distance between two group means on the canonical variates is equal to the *Mahalanobis* squared distance

$$(\bar{\boldsymbol{z}}_i - \bar{\boldsymbol{z}}_j)'(\bar{\boldsymbol{z}}_i - \bar{\boldsymbol{z}}_j) = (\bar{\boldsymbol{x}}_i - \bar{\boldsymbol{x}}_j)\boldsymbol{W}^{-1}(\bar{\boldsymbol{x}}_i - \bar{\boldsymbol{x}}_j).$$

Standard discriminant analysis programs, such as SPSS or BMDP, routinely print plots of the first two canonical variables, showing the observations coded according to their group. These are plots that show the separation among the groups as clearly as possible in two dimensions.

The canonical variables are sometimes referred to as discriminant functions. If there are two groups, the single canonical variable is proportional to the Fisher's linear discriminant function (see Volume 2); with three or more, the canonical variables are not, of course, the discriminant functions between pairs of groups, and this usage is better avoided.

Example 4.4

A set of data published by Fauquet *et al* (1988) consists of 18 measurements (numbers of amino acid residues per molecule of coat protein) recorded for 61 viruses. These were divided into four groups according to mode of transmission; one group, however is labelled unknown. Figure 4.4 (Eslava-Gómez, 1989) shows a plot of the first two canonical variables of the variates. This figure should be contrasted with Figure 4.3, which shows the first *pair* of canonical variables, corresponding to the variates $\boldsymbol{x}$ and $\boldsymbol{y}$ respectively. Figure 4.4 shows the first two canonical variables of the $\boldsymbol{y}$ set, correlating with the contrasts between the groups defined by the dummy $\boldsymbol{x}$ variables, but by construction uncorrelated with each other.

The first canonical variable separates off the largest group, *Tobamovirus*, 39 from the others. The second separates the unclassified group (13 viruses) from *Hordeivirus*, 3 and *Tobravirus*, 6. The last two are not clearly separated in the figure; the third canonical variable is primarily a contrast between them. This pattern is to be expected when the groups are of very different sizes.

In the figure, the canonical variables show the data divided into four compact and well-separated groups—at least, when the third canonical variable is taken into account. This pattern is rather misleading; the separation is probably real enough, but the groups are not the compact and clearly defined entities suggested by the figure; quite a different view of the same data will be presented under Projection pursuit, and in fact there are clearly groupings within these groups, and not merely in the unclassified group.

This behaviour is a feature of canonical variables when the number of random variables is large and the number of items only moderate. The canonical variables display the groups they were designed to display, and figures of this sort tend to exaggerate the differences between the groups and to suppress the structure within them.

Projection pursuit

4.12 Projection pursuit is a technique for finding projections of multivariate data into spaces of lower dimension than p to give 'interesting' diagrams, in some sense to be defined. The main interest is in projections to two dimensions, to give a conventional scatter diagram. One-dimensional projections have some theoretical importance for investigating properties of different projection criteria, and projections to three or more dimensions are perfectly feasible, and may become more important as computer techniques for viewing high-dimensional data are developed, but most of the practical applications have involved two-dimensional projections.

Principal components are the oldest example of the technique. Projections are chosen to maximise the trace of the matrix of sums of squares and products. This criterion has two advantages; calculations are straightforward, and the projection to $k-1$ dimensions is simply derived from that to k. It is, however, not specifically defined to select projections with particular features of interest,

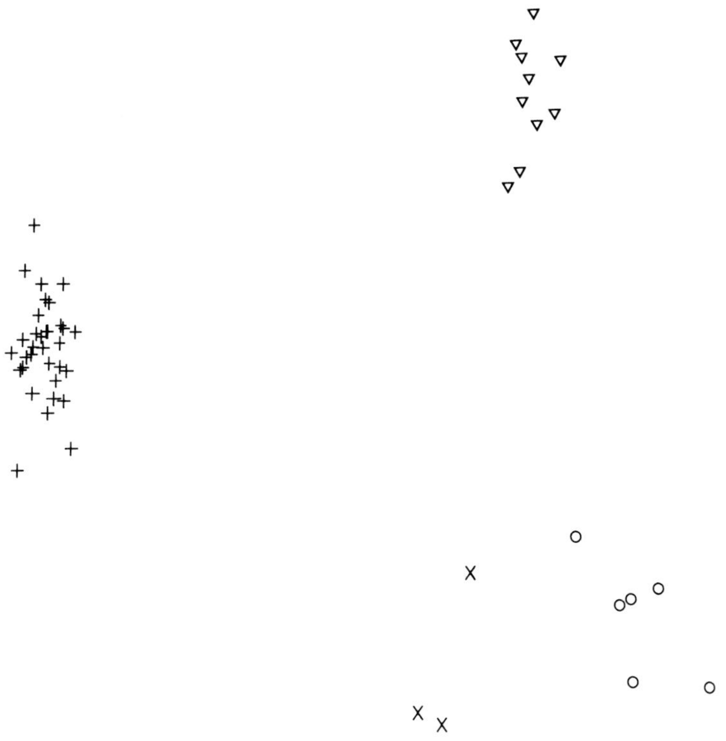

Figure 4.4 Canonical variable analysis of grouped virus data. Classification by mode of transmission: × *Hordeivirus*; ∘ *Tobravirus*; + *Tobamovirus*; ∇ unclassified. Reproduced from Eslava-Gomez (1989).

and other criteria have been shown to be more effective at revealing features such as multimodality, or non-linear relationships among variables.

The general scheme of projection pursuit is divided into steps:

(1) Choose k, the dimension of the required projection.
(2) Choose a criterion to maximise or minimise, that will, it is hoped, isolate interesting projections of the appropriate type.
(3) Evaluate the criterion for a number of projections, chosen, randomly or systematically, from the possible projections from p to k dimensions.
(4) Starting from the best, or a selection of the best, projections found in the last step, use an optimisation programme to find a local maximum or minimum.
(5) Display the chosen projections graphically.

The first step usually takes $k = 2$. If more than one value of k is to be used, it is, in general, necessary to start again for each value—principal components are exceptional.

The second step is critical, and some of the criteria that have been used will be discussed in the next section. Usually, criteria are sought that are independent of scale or location and of the choice of original variables. This implies that 'sphering' the data does not change the criterion, and often this is the first step in the calculation. The variables are linearly transformed to a new set with dispersion matrix the unit matrix. One way of doing this is to calculate principal components and then scale them to equal variance. This involves a drastic deformation of the data, and the dangers have been emphasised by Gower (1987). In particular, if there are natural clusters with their centres roughly coplanar, the transformation causes them to be elongated in the direction normal to the plane; when this happens, 'sphering' is hardly an appropriate description of the transformation.

The third step is important, because the fourth, optimisation, step is usually restricted to a neighbourhood of the starting point, and the criteria that are generally used are, as a rule, only locally smooth. It is therefore necessary to scan the complete set of projections to k dimensions, randomly or systematically, to reduce the chance of reaching a local optimum much inferior to the global optimum. Algorithms for such a scan are available; Asimov (1985) describes the Grand Tour procedure for generating a dense set of projections. Unfortunately, the number of projections needed to cover the hypersphere fairly densely, so that no direction is more than a specified angle from one in the chosen set, increases very rapidly with the dimensionality p. A table is given in Asimov (1985); roughly speaking, reasonable coverage is given by a few thousand projections for $p = 4$, but tens of thousands are needed for $p = 5$. Recent developments in graphical projections of multivariate data are discussed in Weihs and Schmidli (1990), and in the discussion and references with the paper.

The fourth step is fairly easily implemented using pseudo-Newton optimisation routines. The criterion is evaluated at a group of points around the current point, and 'pursuit' follows estimated paths of steepest ascent or descent. For most criteria, derivatives cannot be calculated algebraically, and the procedure is quite computer intensive when dimensionality is high.

Criteria for projection pursuit

4.13 The choice of criterion for projection pursuit should depend on the type of structure that is to be sought in the data. In practice, this has seldom been clearly specified. Multimodal projections, and projections showing non-linear relationships are usually regarded as interesting, while projections showing unimodal distributions with elliptical contours are not. It has often been claimed that the effectiveness of a criterion at revealing interesting projections may be related to its properties when projections are uninteresting; thus Friedman (1987) suggested that tests of k-variate normality could provide criteria for projection pursuit. This is by no means clear. A test statistic that is powerful against alternatives to an uninteresting null hypothesis does not necessarily select the most interesting projections when there is interesting structure in the data.

The first work on projection pursuit was that of Kruskal (1969, 1972). To detect clustering in the data, he proposed an *index of condensation*, based on the coefficient of variation of the inter-point distances. Results obtained with simulated data were unsatisfactory. Friedman and Tukey (1974) introduced the term projection pursuit, and were the first to develop an effective algorithm. The criterion used was complex, and great pains were taken to eliminate outliers before implementation of the algorithm. Jones and Sibson (1987) showed that it is essentially equivalent to *first order entropy*.

Friedman and Tukey applied their algorithm to a simulated data set consisting of a mixture of 15 spherical normal distributions in 14 variables, with their means approximately at the vertices of a 14-dimensional simplex. They were able to recover this structure, proceeding in stages. The algorithm typically gave bimodal projections on the line, and applying it iteratively to the parts separated in the previous stage, complete separation was eventually achieved.

Entropy indices have been widely used in projection pursuit. The index based on the entropy measure of order β, in the one-dimensional case, is

$$\sigma_x^\beta E\{f(x)\}^\beta = \sigma^\beta \int \{f(x)\}^{1+\beta} dx \tag{4.16}$$

(Yenyukov, 1988). Similarly, in k dimensions, the corresponding index may be defined. If the original p-dimensional data are sphered, so is the projection in k dimensions, and the index is

$$E\{f(\boldsymbol{x})\}^\beta = \int \{f(\boldsymbol{x})\}^{1+\beta} d\boldsymbol{x}. \tag{4.17}$$

The most important cases are $\beta \to 0$ and $\beta = 1$. The latter was used by Friedman and Tukey. The former may be written

$$E \log f(\boldsymbol{x}) = \int \log\{f(\boldsymbol{x})\} f(\boldsymbol{x}) d\boldsymbol{x}. \tag{4.18}$$

It is the Shannon–Weaver information index, with sign changed. The minimum value corresponds to the multivariate normal distribution, and maximising this information index was suggested for projection pursuit by Jones and Sibson (1987).

These indices are defined for continuous populations, and their practical use with observed data depends on smoothing each projection, or on adopting an approximation. Smoothing involves replacing $f(\boldsymbol{x})$ by a density estimate $\hat{f}(\boldsymbol{x})$, usually derived by kernel methods (see, for example, Silverman, 1986). The estimation must be carried out for every projection. This is feasible for projections onto a line, but for $k > 1$ the computations become prohibitive.

Jones and Sibson (1987) suggested maximising a moment index I_m based on the cumulants of order 3 and 4. The weights to be given to the cumulants are determined by approximating the zero-order entropy index when departures from normality are small. This leads to

$$I_m = \frac{1}{12}\left(\kappa_3^2 + \frac{1}{4}\kappa_4^2\right) \tag{4.19}$$

for $k = 1$, and

$$I_m = \frac{1}{12}\left[(\kappa_{30}^2 + 3\kappa_{21}^2 + 3\kappa_{12}^2 + \kappa_{01}^2) + \frac{1}{4}(\kappa_{40}^2 + 4\kappa_{31}^2 + 4\kappa_{13}^2 + \kappa_{04}^2)\right] \tag{4.20}$$

for $k = 2$. These definitions apply to sphered data, and the population values of the indices are zero for normal populations. The κ values, the population values of the cumulants, must in practice be replaced by the corresponding k-statistics. Maximising the indices is thus, in a sense, maximising the departure from normality. The indices, however, are not necessarily large for all interesting projections. Consider a mixture of three multivariate normal distributions with equal dispersion matrices and means equally spaced on a straight line. If the middle distribution has probability 2/3, and the others probability 1/6, the mixture has all cumulants of order 3–5 equal to zero. All projections, even when they are clearly trimodal, give zero values of the moment indices (Marriott, 1987).

Other criteria are based on measures of the distance between two distributions. Jee (1985) investigated two such measures. The L_1 difference

$$\int |f(\boldsymbol{x}) - \phi(\boldsymbol{x})|d\boldsymbol{x}$$

and the difference based on the Hellinger metric

$$\int [f^{1/2}(\boldsymbol{x}) - \phi^{1/2}(\boldsymbol{x})]^2 d\boldsymbol{x}$$

may be used in this way. Here, $\phi(\boldsymbol{x})$ represents a standard 'uninteresting' distribution—taken by Jee to be the normal distribution—while $f(\boldsymbol{x})$ corresponds to the population from which the data were drawn. Both distributions are sphered, so that the means and dispersion matrices are the same, and the projection giving the maximum difference differs most in shape from the standard (normal) distribution. Again, an approximation $\hat{f}(\boldsymbol{x})$ is needed; Jee uses a histogram.

Eslava-Gómez (1989) attempted to find criteria for projection pursuit that did not superimpose clusters, but rather, for small and comparatively simple data sets, gave a visual display of all the clusters present. She proposed two criteria.

The *polar nearest neighbour* method minimises

$$g(\theta) = \frac{1}{m}\sum_{i=1}^{m} \min\{|\theta_i - \theta_{i-1}|, |\theta_i - \theta_{i+1}|\}$$

where θ_i are the *ordered* polar angles, $\theta_0 = \theta_m$, $\theta_{m+1} = \theta_1$ and m is the total number of points, often excluding those within a certain distance of the origin.

The second criterion corresponds to maximising the mean radial distance from the centroid. Since the data have been sphered, this is equivalent to minimising the variance of the radial distance; the projection is chosen to give points as nearly as possible equidistant from the centroid.

These two criteria are simple to calculate, and in particular do not depend on smoothing the projected data. They have less tendency than most of the criteria that have been suggested to superimpose clusters, aiming to display all the clusters in moderate sized data sets. They are normally based on the first four or five principal components, because of the large number of projections needed to explore higher-dimensional data sets.

Projection pursuit and significance testing

4.14 The union-intersection tests developed by Roy (1957) involve maximising a criterion that is often associated with a particular projection of the data. Sometimes this can be done analytically, but it may involve a search of the type used in projection pursuit.

Malkovich and Afifi (1973) suggested tests of multivariate normality of union-intersection type. Univariate normality is often investigated using the measures of skewness and kurtosis

$$\beta_1 = \frac{\mu_3^2}{\mu_2^3},$$
$$\beta_2 = \frac{\mu_4}{\mu_2^2}.$$

The proposed tests were based on the maximum value of these statistics in one-dimensional projections of the data. These projections are found by numerical maximisation; the paper does not refer to projection pursuit, as the term was introduced by Friedman and Tukey (1974) a year later. Nevertheless, it can be regarded as the earliest practical application of the technique.

Malkovich and Afifi go on to derive other tests of the same type based on the union-intersection principle applied to standard tests of univariate normality. It is clearly possible to extend the same idea to other problems, such as non-parametric tests of location. Finding critical regions for such tests will involve simulation or bootstrapping, and in combination with projection pursuit the tests will become computer-intensive. Nevertheless, they are an example of an application of projection pursuit in which the criterion—the test statistic—is unambiguously fixed.

Example 4.5
Figure 4.5 shows the same virus data set that was used to illustrate canonical variables (Figure 4.4). This projection, found by polar nearest neighbour without reference to the suggested grouping, again shows clusters of observations, but they are quite different from those suggested by mode of transmission. At least, this figure suggests that the original groups are not homogeneous, though the overlap of groups of viruses with different modes of transmission should be interpreted with caution in view of the high dimensionality.

Projection pursuit regression

4.15 Projection pursuit regression was introduced by Friedman and Stuetzle (1981). Non-parametric regression methods depend essentially on local smoothing. When the number of regressor variables is high, this becomes extremely inefficient owing to the sparseness of the data. In particular, when the regressor variables are random variables, an attempt to find a mean of y in a neighbourhood of an observation $\boldsymbol{x} = (x_1, \ldots, x_p)$ is likely to be based on a

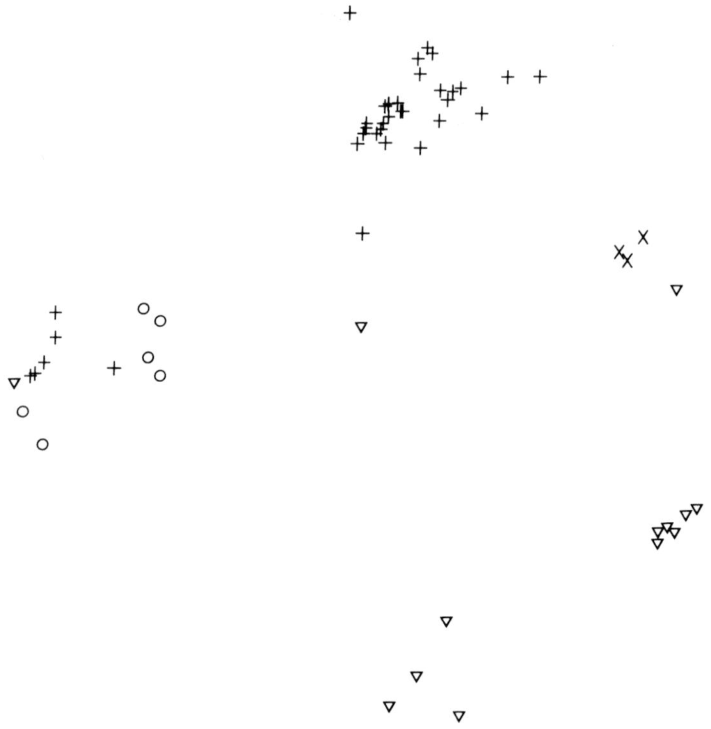

Figure 4.5 Projection pursuit (polar nearest neighbour) plot of virus data. Classification by mode of transmission: × *Hordeivirus*; ○ *Tobravirus*; + *Tobamovirus*; ∇ unclassified. Reproduced from Eslava-Gomez (1989).

very small number of points, or to involve points far enough away to induce serious bias.

Projection pursuit regression tackles this problem in a radical way. The idea is to fit y by a smooth function of a single linear function of $\boldsymbol{x}$. This linear function is chosen to optimise the fit by minimising some measure of residual variability; this is the step analogous to projection pursuit. Next, the process is repeated. The residuals from the first fit are fitted by a smooth function of another linear function, chosen as before, and the process is continued until the fit is deemed satisfactory.

Many variations have been suggested, differing in the smoothing method, the definition of the optimising criterion, and the sequence of steps, but all have two features in common.

(1) The smoothing involves just y and a single regressor variable constructed from $\boldsymbol{x}$; there is no multidimensional local averaging.

(2) The projection pursuit criterion has an unambiguous objective, to find the best fit possible with the chosen smoothing method.

The model has the form

$$y = \sum_{k=1}^{K} h_k(\boldsymbol{\alpha}_k' \boldsymbol{X}) + \epsilon. \tag{4.21}$$

Here $\boldsymbol{\alpha}_k' \boldsymbol{X}$ is a one-dimensional projection of the matrix $\boldsymbol{X}$ and h_k is a function of this variable, usually a non-parametric 'smooth'. The Friedman and Stuetzle model uses a 'figure of merit'

$$I(\boldsymbol{\alpha}) = 1 - \frac{\sum_{i=1}^{n} \epsilon_i^2}{\sum_{i=1}^{n} y_i^2} \tag{4.22}$$

as a criterion for selecting the projection $\boldsymbol{\alpha}$, where, after the first step, y and ϵ represent the residual to be fitted and the residual after the next fit respectively. The figure of merit is thus a measure of the improvement from including each successive projection in the regression. As well as a criterion for projection pursuit, it determines the stopping rule; if the best figure of merit is less than some specified value, the fit is judged adequate and the process is terminated.

This procedure can be refined, in particular by iteration. For a particular K, the initial set of projections may be modified by dropping one axis at a time and optimising again until a general optimal regression for K is achieved. Further, if the stopping rule is inappropriately chosen, the final value of K may be unreasonably high. These problems are discussed by Chen (1991), who also gives an account of the development of the subject over the past ten years.

Chen fits the projection pursuit model subject to two constraints. First, $K \leqslant p$ ensures that the number of terms in the model cannot increase indefinitely, and secondly the angle between pairs of projections is constrained to be greater than a fixed value. The choice of K and the values of $\boldsymbol{\alpha}$ are then based on a final prediction error. Chen uses a criterion based on Mallows' C_p (see Mallows, 1973) and a cubic spline smooth (Reinsch, 1967).

In conclusion, projection pursuit regression is an effective procedure for multivariate non-parametric smoothing. It is implemented in various specialised computer programs, such as Xplore (see Härdle, 1990). The main difficulty, as with principal component regression, lies in interpreting the results. Unless the vectors selected by the procedure can be simply explained, the regression is suitable only for prediction.

Projection pursuit density estimation

4.16 The problem of multivariate density estimation raises a similar set of difficulties to those encountered in non-parametric regression in high dimensions. The data are sparse, and kernel methods and nearest neighbour methods give reasonably smooth estimates only at the cost of wide bandwidth and associated bias. Further, multivariate kernel methods are far more computer intensive than the univariate technique, mainly because the multivariate fast Fourier transform is not fast in high dimensional space.

The projection pursuit density estimation method was introduced by Friedman *et al* (1984). It reduces the multidimensional problem to a sequence of univariate density estimations in directions chosen to optimise a suitably chosen criterion. The idea is to fit a standard multivariate distribution—nearly always multivariate normal—and then find the direction in which the fit is least good. The density in this projection is then estimated and compared with the marginal density of the multivariate distribution, and a new multivariate distribution is constructed by multiplying by the ratio of the two univariate distributions. This ratio is known as the *augmenting function*.

The new multivariate surface is, in fact, a density, since each profile is multiplied by a ratio of two densities. This surface is now adopted as the current model, and the next step finds the direction in which the fit to this model is least good. The process continues until the fit is judged satisfactory.

Friedman *et al* (1984) recommend a preliminary principal component analysis to eliminate any components regarded as redundant in high-dimensional data sets. Selection of directions is based on the Kullback–Leibler distance, and the comparison between marginal densities of data and model is by means of histograms derived from the data and from a Monte Carlo sample from the current model. There are clearly other possible techniques.

Figure 4.6, from this paper, shows the first stage in the process. A bivariate distribution, in fact a mixture of three bivariate normals, is being modelled. Figure 4.6a shows the histogram of the data (vertical lines) and of the projection of the simulated sample from the model—in this case, a bivariate normal distribution (marked X). Both are calculated for the first selected direction, that in which the agreement is worst. Figure 4.6b shows the ratio of the two, giving the first augmenting function. Notice the high value at the right end; the estimate is quite unreliable when both densities are low, but the effect on the next multivariate model is very small. Figure 4.6c shows the second model approximation, with the strongly bimodal projection producing ridges in the distribution, while orthogonally to this direction the conditional and marginal distributions remain bivariate normal.

Like projection pursuit regression, projection pursuit density estimation uses a criterion that corresponds to a clearly defined objective—that of maximising the discrepancy between two univariate distributions. It avoids the difficulties associated with the sparseness of high-dimensional data sets, and has been shown to work well for many artificial examples. For a review of multivariate density estimation, with examples and references to practical applications, see Izenman (1991).

Function optimisation

4.17 Many statistical problems involve optimisation, i.e. maximisation or minimisation, of a function. In multivariate problems, the functions involved are often complicated expressions involving many variables. Explicit formulation of the function in terms of the observations may be impossible, and often there will be many local maxima and minima.

Traditional algorithms are variations on the 'method of steepest descent'. A function is minimised by moving at each step along the direction in which the gradient is steepest, until an acceptable approximation to the minimum is reached. This process can actually be very inefficient when the gradients near the optimum are very different, when the minimum is the bottom of a long

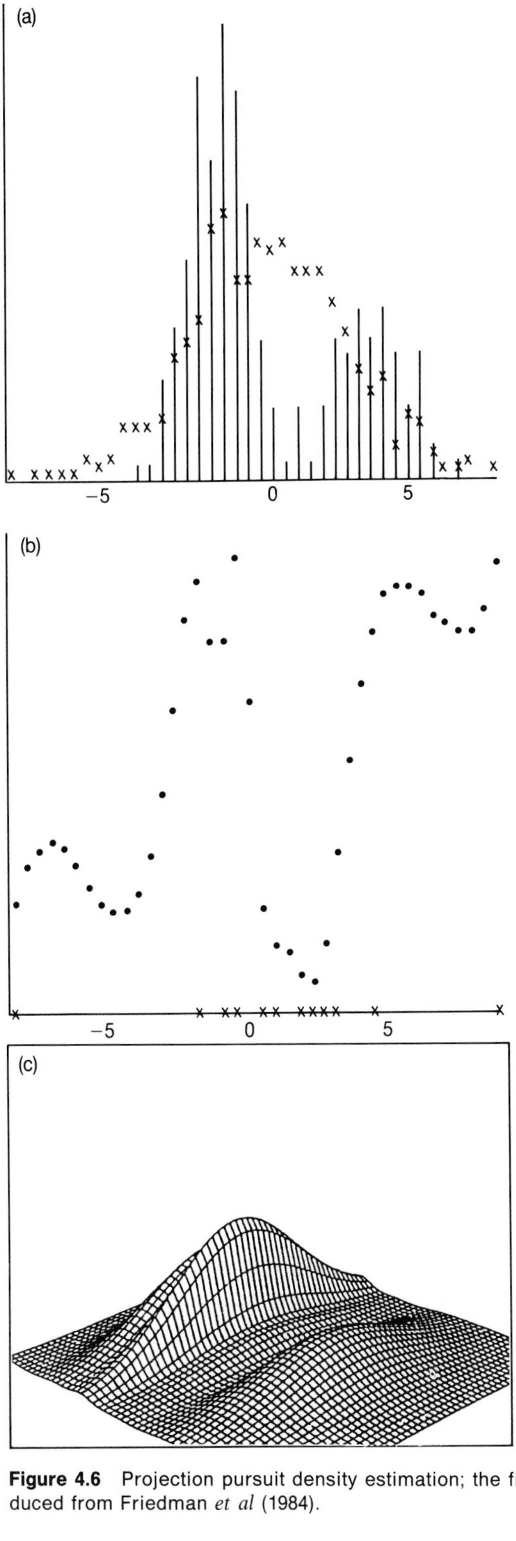

Figure 4.6 Projection pursuit density estimation; the first stage. For details, see text. Reproduced from Friedman *et al* (1984).

narrow valley, but modified versions work well. For details, see for example, Press *et al* (1989), or one of the other editions of 'Numerical Recipes'.

These methods, however, find a local minimum or maximum. The solution depends on the starting value, and in general it is necessary to try a number of different values to identify the global optimum. Quite generally, it is impossible to devise an algorithm that is certain to find such a value without assumptions about the smoothness of function to be optimised. It is clear, though, that choosing different starting values, perhaps at random, will improve the chances of success.

Recent developments in numerical methods have given much more emphasis to finding efficient algorithms with a random element specifically included. The general problem of stochastic optimisation is far too wide to be covered in any detail, but some methods are now commonly used in statistics, and three will be briefly mentioned.

- Simulated annealing is based on an analogy with the annealing process of toughening metals, glass or ceramics by slow cooling. At high temperatures, the atoms make large jumps to new positions; as cooling proceeds, the probability of movement becomes smaller, until the material assumes a more or less fixed crystalline structure. The computing method based on this model was introduced by Kirkpatrick *et al* (1983). It is related to the (deterministic) method of relaxation (Southwell, 1946).

  The numerical procedure admits of several modification. A simple algorithm to minimise $f(\boldsymbol{x})$ is:

  (1) Choose an initial guess $\boldsymbol{x}_0$, and initial parameters t_0 (temperature) and d_0 (distance).
  (2) Choose $\boldsymbol{x}_1$ at random, with $||\boldsymbol{x}_1 - \boldsymbol{x}_0|| = d$.
  (3) If $\delta = f(\boldsymbol{x}_1) - f(\boldsymbol{x}_0) \leqslant 0$, set $\boldsymbol{x} = \boldsymbol{x}_1$. If not, set $\boldsymbol{x} = \boldsymbol{x}_1$ with probability $\exp(-\delta/t)$, otherwise set $\boldsymbol{x} = \boldsymbol{x}_0$.
  This step is the essential feature of the annealing procedure. It is known as the Metropolis algorithm (Metropolis *et al*, 1953). It implies that when t is large and δ is small, there is a chance of moving to a *higher* value of $f(\boldsymbol{x})$, thus perhaps jumping out of a local minimum.
  (4) Repeat steps 2 and 3 until some convergence criterion is satisfied.
  (5) Reduce t.
  (6) Repeat steps 2 to 5 until some convergence criterion is satisfied.
  (7) Reduce d.
  (8) Repeat steps 2 to 7 until d is less than some predetermined value.

  The simulated annealing procedure has proved very successful in finding global optima in difficult optimisation problems. Statistical applications include finding maximum likelihood or maximum posterior density estimates, and it has also worked well in problems in operational research. Press *et al* (1989) give an algorithm for the Travelling Salesman problem using simulated annealing. Apart from the many possible modifications to the algorithm outlined above, the choice of initial values of temperature and distance, and the rules for changing them are important if the global optimum is to be found and the computation time is to remain reasonable.

- Neural Networks were first used for finding non-parametric linear discriminant functions in the 1950s following the work of McCulloch and Pitts (1943). The aim was to find a hyperplane that separated sets of data from two populations perfectly, or as near perfectly as possible. The method was data-based; no assumptions were made about distributions, and there was no explicit discussion of the problem of classifying *further* observations.

  The *Perceptron model* was based on simulating the way in which the nervous system recognises objects, with messages passed between successive layers of neurons. (Modern neural network models have the same idea, but the computing algorithms and the neurophysiology have diverged to some extent). Rosenblatt (1962) published the *Perceptron theorem*; this proved that, if the two data sets could be separated by a hyperplane, the perceptron model would find a plane that separated them.

  Unfortunately, the problem was by no means solved. Minsky and Papert (1969) (see also Minsky and Papert, 1988) found that the perceptron model had some unsatisfactory properties; in particular, if no separating hyperplane existed, the algorithm would not converge.

  After this, neural networks as a computing device were largely forgotten, until Rumelhart *et al* (1986) published a sound 'back propagation algorithm', that gave a method that converged to a surface giving low misclassification counts when reasonable separation was possible. Actually, the method had been independently discovered earlier, by Werbos (1974) and Parker (1982), but these papers had not reached the pattern-recognition workers.

  Since the work of Rumelhart *et al* (1986), neural network methods have been developed and modified in pattern-recognition, statistics and other computing applications; Wasserman (1989) gives a good general account. In statistics, the main application remains in discriminant analysis, though neural networks are also used in cluster analysis. These applications will be discussed in Part 2.

- Another optimisation procedure also based on a biological process is the group of techniques known as 'genetic algorithms'. Simulation of the genetic development of a population, with natural selection, was studied by von Neuman in the 1950s, and published posthumously (von Neuman, 1966).

  Consider a population of n items, each labelled with a p-variate binary string, representing alleles at p ordered sites. Suppose each individual has a 'fitness'. Select a random sample, with replacement, with probabilities proportional to fitness. This is the breeding sample—note the similarity to a bootstrap sample; see **6.18**. Now the breeding sample mates, producing n offspring, the second generation. Each new item inherits the genetic characteristics of its parents, either at random, or with added complication mimicking recombination fractions dependent on distance, mutations, and so on. This procedure is repeated until an equilibrium is reached.

  The process tends to approach maximum fitness, because of the selection at each stage. This is therefore another stochastic optimisation method. Some ingenuity is needed to devise a suitable representation of the optimisation in terms of the genetic code, and genetic algorithms have not been widely used in statistics. Michaelewicz and Janikov (1991) give a good account of the method, with examples of its use in complicated problems of constrained optimisation.

In conclusion, stochastic optimisation methods have become a major research field, with important statistical applications. They are computer intensive, and it is sometimes difficult to decide on appropriate convergence criteria. They are not readily available in standard statistical packages, but they have proved their worth in operational research and pattern recognition, and are becoming more widely used in complicated statistical problems.

Exercises

4.1 The varimax rotation (Kaiser, 1958) rotates a set of linear functions $\boldsymbol{a}'\boldsymbol{x}$ to give a new set $\boldsymbol{b}'\boldsymbol{x}$, chosen so that the variance of the squared coefficients $\text{var}(b_i^2)$ is maximised for each vector. Applied to principal components, the rotation preserves the orthogonality of the vectors and the constraint $\boldsymbol{b}'\boldsymbol{b} = 1$ holds for the new coefficients. The aim is, by giving high loadings to a small number of the original variables, to make the resulting vectors more easily interpretable.

What is the outcome if the varimax rotation is applied to the *complete* set of p principal components?

4.2 Suppose a data set is drawn from a population consisting of a mixture of two spherical p-variate normal distributions, with means $(\pm\mu, 0, \ldots, 0)$.

(a) What is the effect of standardisation, to give the correlation matrix, on the data structure?

(b) What can be said about the principal components based on the correlation matrix?

4.3 A distribution consists of a mixture of three bivariate normal distributions with centres at the vertices of an equilateral triangle. The distributions are projected on to a line to give a density $f(x)$. Show that the entropy criterion $E[\log f(x)]$ is maximised by projecting two vertices to the same point, and minimised by projecting to three equally spaced points.

5

Distance Methods and Ordination

Ordination

5.1 The techniques described in Chapter 4 are all concerned with the reduction of dimensionality of multivariate data, and all approach this objective by seeking suitable transformations of the variables. The transformations may either be explicit and linear (e.g. principal components, canonical variates) or implicit and, perhaps, more complicated (e.g. projection pursuit). However, in all cases the objective is to minimise the 'loss of information' when all the original variables are replaced by just a few of the transformed ones, and all the techniques start from a $(p \times p)$ matrix comparing every variable with every other variable. Plotting the scores of the n sample individuals on a few of the transformed variables as coordinate axes provides a useful summary of the multivariate data space, points close together indicating 'similarity' and points far apart indicating 'dissimilarity' of the corresponding individuals (subject to any distortion caused by the reduction of dimensionality). Closeness of points in the diagram is of course measured in terms of Euclidean distance, while the 'similarity' and 'dissimilarity' of individuals depends on the underlying technique for its definition. In the case of principal component analysis, for example, it is defined by Euclidean distance in the full p-dimensional space, while for canonical variate analysis it is given by the Mahalanobis distance in this space. Such a plot is termed an *ordination* of the data.

Proximity matrices

5.2 However, ordination is of interest much more widely than in just the situations mentioned above. In particular, the starting point for ordination will usually be an $(n \times n)$ matrix comparing every individual with every other individual in the sample, rather than a $(p \times p)$ matrix of inter-variable comparisons. Sometimes this is because no variables have been explicitly measured in the study, but data have been gathered directly on the inter-unit comparisons.

For example, in a now classic psychometric study, Rothkopf (1957) counted the number of occasions on which Morse code signals were judged to be the same when presented in pairs to a group of subjects; similarly, in the field of sensory studies, Chauhan *et al* (1983) discuss an experiment in which assessors were asked to rate the similarity between pairs of soft drinks. Alternatively, the raw data might be in the standard $(n \times p)$ matrix $\boldsymbol{X}$ but a measure of dissimilarity other than either Euclidean or Mahalanobis distance is felt to be appropriate when comparing the n individuals. Any of the coefficients defined in **3.24** or **3.25** might be used, and there exist many other possibilities (see, for example, Tables 2 and 3 of Gower and Legendre, 1986, plus the references therein). The classification literature abounds with instances of $(n \times n)$ dissimilarity matrices calculated from $(n \times p)$ data matrices, using a variety of measures. For some examples see Gordon (1981).

Note that in the above we have used *similarity* matrices when discussing direct assessment, but *dissimilarity* matrices when discussing calculations from raw data. However, it is immaterial to the analysis which type of matrix we start with, as the one type can always be derived from the other by means of an appropriate (monotonically decreasing) transformation. Accordingly, the term *proximity* is generally used to denote *either* a similarity *or* a dissimilarity if the distinction between them does not need to be made, and we will therefore often refer to the analysis of proximity matrices. In most practical applications, the calculation of similarity or dissimilarity between two individuals does not depend on the order in which they are presented, so the resulting proximity matrices are of necessity *symmetric*. A symmetric matrix is assumed in what follows unless explicitly stated otherwise.

Geometrical objectives and fundamentals

5.3 In this chapter we will consider ordination methods suitable for application to $(n \times n)$ proximity matrices. The basic objective is to obtain a low-dimensional pictorial representation of the n sample individuals by n points, such that the distance d_{ij} between two points i and j approximates as well as possible the proximity δ_{ij} between the corresponding individuals. Different constraints on the phrase 'as well as possible' lead to different ordination techniques, as described below. However, it is first appropriate to determine the conditions under which a satisfactory representation can be obtained, in view of the fact that the geometry in this representation must be Euclidean. We therefore start by summarising some important metric and Euclidean properties of proximity matrices.

5.4 Consider the $(n \times n)$ proximity matrix Δ, whose elements δ_{ij} give the dissimilarities between every pair of individuals in a sample of size n. Δ is said to be *metric* if the metric (i.e. triangle) inequality

$$\delta_{ij} + \delta_{ik} \geqslant \delta_{jk} \tag{5.1}$$

holds for all triplets (i, j, k). Application of this inequality first to the triplet (i, j, j) and then to the triplets $(i, j, i), (j, i, j)$ establishes that all metric dissimilarity matrices are symmetric with non-negative elements. Furthermore, if

$\delta_{ij} = 0$ then consideration of the triplets (i,k,j) and (j,k,i) yields $\delta_{ik} = \delta_{jk}$ for all k. Gower and Legendre (1986) give the following results applicable to dissimilarity matrices.

Theorem 1 If Δ is non-metric then the matrix with elements $\delta_{ij} + c$ $(i \neq j)$ is metric, where $c \geqslant max_{p,q,r} \mid \delta_{pq} + \delta_{pr} - \delta_{qr} \mid$.

Theorem 2 If Δ is metric then so are the matrices with elements:

(1) $\delta_{ij} + c^2$,
(2) $\delta_{ij}^{1/r}$, for $r \geqslant 1$,
(3) $\delta_{ij}/(\delta_{ij} + c^2)$,

where $i \neq j$ and c is any real constant.

Theorem 3 If for every triplet (i,j,k) an l can be found such that $\delta_{ij} \geqslant \delta_{lj}$ and $\delta_{ik} \geqslant \delta_{lk}$, then Δ is metric if and only if (j,k,l) is metric.

Theorem 4 Δ is metric if and only if δ_{ij} is non-negative for all pairs (i,j) and, for all triplets (i,j,k),

$$2\delta_{ij}^2\delta_{ik}^2 + 2\delta_{ij}^2\delta_{jk}^2 + 2\delta_{ik}^2\delta_{jk}^2 - \delta_{jk}^4 - \delta_{ik}^4 - \delta_{ij}^4 \geqslant 0.$$

Δ is said to be *Euclidean* if n points $P_i(i = 1, 2, \ldots, n)$ can be embedded in a Euclidean space such that the Euclidean distance between P_i and P_j is δ_{ij}. Since Euclidean distance satisfies the triangle inequality, a necessary condition for Δ to be Euclidean is that it be metric; that this is not also a sufficient condition can be seen from the following example.

Example 5.1 ; Gower and Legendre, 1986.
Suppose that $n = 4$ and that the elements of Δ are given by

$$\delta_{ii} = 0\ \forall i; \delta_{12} = \delta_{13} = \delta_{23} = 2; \delta_{14} = \delta_{24} = \delta_{34} = 1.1; \delta_{ij} = \delta_{ji}\ \forall i \neq j.$$

Establishing that Δ is metric can be done either by verifying the triangle inequality (5.1) for all triples or by application of Theorem 4. Next label the rows of Δ by P_1, P_2, P_3, P_4. Then the points P_1, P_2, P_3 form an equilateral triangle of side 2, and P_4 is equidistant (1.1 units) from each of P_1, P_2 and P_3. It is easy to see that if the configuration is to be Euclidean then the smallest distance that P_4 can be from the other vertices is when it is coplanar with them and at their centroid, giving a minimal distance of 1.15. Since this is greater than 1.1 then Δ is clearly not Euclidean.

5.5 In the light of the above, determining whether or not a Euclidean configuration $\boldsymbol{X}$ can be derived from a specified dissimilarity matrix Δ is clearly of interest. The most general result in this regard is:

Theorem 5 Δ is Euclidean if and only if the matrix $(\boldsymbol{I} - \mathbf{1}\boldsymbol{s}')\boldsymbol{\Gamma}(\boldsymbol{I} - \boldsymbol{s}\mathbf{1}')$ is positive semi-definite, where $\boldsymbol{\Gamma}$ is the matrix with elements $-\frac{1}{2}\delta_{ij}^2$, $\boldsymbol{I}$ is the unit matrix, $\mathbf{1}$ is a vector of n ones, and $\boldsymbol{s}$ is an n-element vector that satisfies $\boldsymbol{s}'\mathbf{1} = 1$. Furthermore, the derived configuration $\boldsymbol{X}$ can always be centred in such a way that $\boldsymbol{s}'\boldsymbol{X} = 0$ is also satisfied. Gower (1982) gives a discussion and proof of this theorem; the special cases $\boldsymbol{s} = \frac{1}{n}\mathbf{1}$ with centring at the origin, and $\boldsymbol{s} = \boldsymbol{e}_i$ (a vector having 1 in its ith position and zeros elsewhere) with centring at the ith point, were first proved by Schoenberg (1935). The first of these centrings is the usual one, and this special case of the theorem is proved in most standard multivariate texts (e.g. Mardia *et al*, 1979; Seber, 1984). Gower (1984) shows that if the result holds for any one choice of $\boldsymbol{s}$ then it holds for every valid choice of $\boldsymbol{s}$.

An equivalent statement to Theorem 5 is that $\boldsymbol{\Delta}$ is Euclidean if and only if $\boldsymbol{x}'\boldsymbol{\Gamma}\boldsymbol{x} \geqslant 0$ for all vectors $\boldsymbol{x}$ such that $\boldsymbol{x}'\mathbf{1} = 0$. There are two results giving simple monotonic transformations that carry general dissimilarity matrices into Euclidean distance matrices. Lingoes (1971) establishes a lower bound on h for the matrix with elements $(\delta_{ij}^2 + h)^{1/2}$ to be Euclidean, while Cailliez (1983) establishes a corresponding bound on k for the matrix with elements $\delta_{ij} + k$ to be Euclidean. Finally, if interest focuses on similarity rather than dissimilarity matrices, then Gower and Legendre (1986) give the following result.

Theorem 6 If $\boldsymbol{S}$ is a positive semi-definite similarity matrix with elements $0 \leqslant s_{ij} \leqslant 1$ and $s_{ii} = 1$, then the dissimilarity matrix with elements $\delta_{ij} = (1 - s_{ij})^{1/2}$ is Euclidean.

Metric scaling

5.6 We now turn to the pictorial representation of proximity matrices. First suppose that the matrix $\boldsymbol{\Delta}$ is Euclidean. Then there exists a configuration of n points such that the distance d_{ij} between points i and j equals the dissimilarity δ_{ij} between the corresponding individuals. This configuration can be determined as follows. Let its dimensionality be k, so that the coordinates of the points can be written as the rows of an $(n \times k)$ matrix $\boldsymbol{X}$. Thus $d_{rs}^2 = \sum_{j=1}^k (x_{rj} - x_{sj})^2$. Now if we write $\boldsymbol{Q} = \boldsymbol{X}\boldsymbol{X}'$, and if $\boldsymbol{Q}$ has (i, j)th element q_{ij}, then

$$q_{rs} = \sum_{j=1}^{k} x_{rj}x_{sj}, \tag{5.2}$$

so that

$$d_{rs}^2 = q_{rr} + q_{ss} - 2q_{rs}. \tag{5.3}$$

Hence, given $\boldsymbol{X}$, we can readily find all the d_{ij}^2. We require to do the reverse operation, i.e. given all the d_{ij}^2 to find $\boldsymbol{X}$. To obtain a unique solution we must impose a location constraint, and the most convenient one is to place the centre of gravity of the points, $\bar{\boldsymbol{x}}$, at the origin. Thus $\mathbf{1}'\boldsymbol{X} = \mathbf{0}$. Now if we write $\boldsymbol{D}$ for the matrix with elements d_{ij}^2 and $\boldsymbol{E} = \text{diag}(q_{11}, \ldots, q_{nn})$, the diagonal matrix containing the diagonal elements of $\boldsymbol{Q}$, then the matrix form of (5.3) is

$$\boldsymbol{D} = \boldsymbol{E}\mathbf{1}\mathbf{1}' + \mathbf{1}\mathbf{1}'\boldsymbol{E} - 2\boldsymbol{X}\boldsymbol{X}'. \tag{5.4}$$

Hence $(\boldsymbol{I}-\boldsymbol{1}\boldsymbol{1}'/n)\boldsymbol{D}(\boldsymbol{I}-\boldsymbol{1}\boldsymbol{1}'/n) = -2\boldsymbol{X}\boldsymbol{X}' = -2\boldsymbol{Q}$. Thus given the matrix $\boldsymbol{\Delta}$ of dissimilarities, this shows that the matrix $\boldsymbol{Q}$ can be generated as $\boldsymbol{Q} = (\boldsymbol{I}-\boldsymbol{1}\boldsymbol{1}'/n)\boldsymbol{\Gamma}(\boldsymbol{I}-\boldsymbol{1}\boldsymbol{1}'/n)$ where the (i,j)th entry of $\boldsymbol{\Gamma}$ is $-\frac{1}{2}\delta_{ij}^2$. Since $\boldsymbol{\Delta}$ is Euclidean, then by Theorem 5 $\boldsymbol{Q}$ must be positive semi-definite. It is also symmetric, so using the spectral decomposition theorem we can write $\boldsymbol{Q} = \boldsymbol{T}\boldsymbol{\Lambda}\boldsymbol{T}'$ where $\boldsymbol{\Lambda} = \text{diag}(\lambda_1, \ldots, \lambda_k)$, the diagonal matrix of eigenvalues of $\boldsymbol{Q}$, and $\boldsymbol{T}$ is the matrix whose columns are the eigenvectors of $\boldsymbol{Q}$. Positive semi-definiteness of $\boldsymbol{Q}$ ensures that $\lambda_i \geqslant 0\ \forall i$, so that we can obtain $\boldsymbol{\Lambda}^{\frac{1}{2}} = \text{diag}(\lambda_1^{\frac{1}{2}}, \ldots, \lambda_k^{\frac{1}{2}})$. Hence $\boldsymbol{Q} = \boldsymbol{T}\boldsymbol{\Lambda}^{\frac{1}{2}}\boldsymbol{\Lambda}^{\frac{1}{2}}\boldsymbol{T}' = \boldsymbol{X}\boldsymbol{X}'$ where $\boldsymbol{X} = \boldsymbol{T}\boldsymbol{\Lambda}^{\frac{1}{2}}$. This matrix $\boldsymbol{X}$ thus provides a set of coordinates (the *principal coordinates*) yielding the required d_{ij}^2.

5.7 Given an $(n \times n)$ Euclidean matrix of dissimilarities $\boldsymbol{\Delta} = (\delta_{ij})$ between every pair of entities in a sample, the above development thus shows that we can find a geometrical representation of the n entities by n points in the following manner.

(1) Form the matrix $\boldsymbol{\Gamma}$ with (i,j)th element $\gamma_{ij} = -\frac{1}{2}\delta_{ij}^2$.
(2) Subtract from each element of $\boldsymbol{\Gamma}$ the means of the row and column in which it is located, and add to it the mean of all elements of $\boldsymbol{\Gamma}$. Denote the resulting matrix by $\boldsymbol{\Phi}$.
(3) Find the eigenvalues $\lambda_1 \geqslant \lambda_2 \geqslant \ldots \geqslant \lambda_n = 0$ and corresponding eigenvectors $\boldsymbol{v}_i$ $(i = 1, \ldots, n)$ of $\boldsymbol{\Phi}$. The dimensionality of the representation is given by the number of non-zero eigenvalues.
(4) Normalise the eigenvectors so that $\boldsymbol{v}_i'\boldsymbol{v}_i = \lambda_i\ \forall i$. The coordinates of the n points on the ith axis of the Euclidean representation are given by the elements of $\boldsymbol{v}_i$.

Algebraic reconstruction of a configuration from its interpoint distances dates back to Young and Householder (1938). The main theoretical and substantive foundations are attributable to Torgerson (1952 and 1958), while Gower (1966a) developed the above method under the name *principal coordinate analysis.* It is now perhaps more commonly referred to as *classical scaling.* In its most general form it would allow weighting of the n points in the fitting procedure, and centring the configuration at the weighted average (i.e. *barycentre*) $\boldsymbol{s}$ of the points. If the weights attached to the points are $w_1, \ldots, w_n$ and $\boldsymbol{D}_w$ is the diagonal matrix containing these weights, then the steps of the classical scaling procedure are modified as follows.

(1) Form the matrix $\boldsymbol{\Gamma}$ as before.
(2) Obtain $\boldsymbol{\Phi}$ as $(\boldsymbol{I}-\boldsymbol{1}\boldsymbol{s}')\boldsymbol{\Gamma}(\boldsymbol{I}-\boldsymbol{s}\boldsymbol{1}')$.
(3) Find the eigenvalues $\lambda_1, \ldots, \lambda_n$ and corresponding eigenvectors $\boldsymbol{v}_i$ of $\boldsymbol{D}_w^{1/2}\boldsymbol{\Phi}\boldsymbol{D}_w^{1/2}$.
(4) Normalise the eigenvectors so that $\boldsymbol{v}_i'\boldsymbol{v}_i = \lambda_i\ \forall i$. The coordinates of the n points on the ith axis of the Euclidean representation are given by the elements of $\boldsymbol{D}_w^{-1/2}\boldsymbol{v}_i$.

5.8 Exact Euclidean representation of n entities by points can require up to $n-1$ dimensions. Interest therefore focuses on finding suitable low-dimensional configurations in which the between-point distances *approximate* as well as possible the inter-entity dissimilarities, and one possible approach is to find the best projection of the $(n-1)$-dimensional configuration into a k-dimensional subspace. Gower's solution, as given in **5.7**, is optimal in this respect because it is referred to its principal axes, and so arguments similar to those for principal component analysis in Chapter 4 establish that the best k-dimensional representation is given by the eigenvectors corresponding to the k largest eigenvalues of $\boldsymbol{\Phi}$. It can be shown easily (e.g. see Mardia *et al*, 1979 p406) that projecting a configuration reduces interpoint distances, i.e. $d_{ij}^2 \leqslant \delta_{ij}^2 \ \forall i, j$, where d_{ij} is the distance between points i, j in the projection, and that this k-dimensional representation is 'best' in the sense that it is the projection minimising the measure of discrepancy

$$\psi = \sum_{i=1}^{n} \sum_{j=1}^{n} (\delta_{ij}^2 - d_{ij}^2). \tag{5.5}$$

Furthermore, for this representation $\psi = 2n(\lambda_{k+1} + \ldots + \lambda_n)$, so that a measure of 'goodness-of-fit' of the k-dimensional configuration to the original set of dissimilarities is the principal component 'per cent trace' measure $\alpha_{1,k} = (\sum_{i=1}^{k} \lambda_i / \sum_{i=1}^{n} \lambda_i) \times 100\%$. The evident resemblance between principal component analysis and classical scaling becomes a formal duality under certain circumstances. If $\boldsymbol{X}$ is an $(n \times p)$ data matrix, and if the $(n \times n)$ dissimilarity matrix $\boldsymbol{\Delta}$ has as its (i, j)th element the Euclidean distance between the ith and jth rows of $\boldsymbol{X}$, then the principal component scores calculated from the covariance matrix of the data coincide with the coordinates of the scaling procedure (Gower, 1966a). Also, if the rows of $\boldsymbol{X}$ are partitioned into g groups (e.g. when the data comprise samples from g populations) and the $(g \times g)$ matrix $\boldsymbol{\Delta}$ has as its (i, j)th element the Mahalanobis distance between the ith and jth groups, then the canonical variate scores (**4.11**) calculated using the *unweighted* between-group covariance matrix coincide with the coordinates of the scaling procedure (Gower, 1966b).

5.9 It can happen that the matrix $\boldsymbol{\Delta}$ in a particular case is not Euclidean. Then the matrix $\boldsymbol{\Phi}$ constructed in the course of the scaling process will not be positive semi-definite and hence some of the eigenvalues λ_i will be negative. Coordinates of points on the corresponding axes will thus be imaginary, and a Euclidean representation of the entities does not exist in this case. There has been some work on finding the positive semi-definite matrix closest to a matrix with negative eigenvalues; see, for example, Schwerteman and Allen (1981) or Hong and Yang (1991). Such matrix approximation will enable approximate Euclidean representations to be obtained in the usual way. Alternatively, it is possible to obtain an approximate representation by employing merely those eigenvectors corresponding to the positive eigenvalues. This representation will be adequate if all negative eigenvalues are small in absolute value, but will clearly become poorer as the absolute sizes of the negative eigenvalues increase.

Mardia (1978) has discussed optimality properties of the classical scaling procedure in the non-Euclidean case. In particular, he has shown that if $\hat{\boldsymbol{\Phi}} = \sum_{i=1}^{k} \lambda_i \mathbf{v}_i \mathbf{v}_i'$ then the k-dimensional solution provided by classical scaling minimises the discrepancy measure $\psi' = \mathrm{tr}(\boldsymbol{\Phi} - \hat{\boldsymbol{\Phi}})^2$. This is a special case of the Eckart–Young (1936) theorem; to remove the distortion caused by the negative eigenvalues, the goodness-of-fit measure can be modified to Eckart and Young's criterion $\alpha_{1,k} = (\sum_{i=1}^{k} \lambda_i / \sum_{i=1}^{n} \mid \lambda_i \mid) \times 100\%$. An alternative measure proposed by Mardia is $\alpha_{2,k} = (\sum_{i=1}^{k} \lambda_i^2 / \sum_{i=1}^{n} \lambda_i^2) \times 100\%$.

Robustness of classical scaling was also studied by Mardia (1978) and by Sibson (1979). The method has been shown to be robust against a variety of perturbations to the δ_{ij}. Furthermore, Sibson's perturbation analysis has yielded a number of useful approximate distributional results, as well as some auxiliary techniques for choice of dimensionality and correction of bias.

5.10 Classical scaling is just one way of representing objects by points in space such that inter-point distances approximate inter-object proximity as well as possible; it is an orthogonal projection method in which the phrase 'as well as possible' means that the measure of discrepancy ψ (or ψ') is minimised. However, many other representations of objects by points are possible if the restriction to orthogonal projections is relaxed or if a different measure of discrepancy is optimised. For example, Sammon (1969) looked for a representation in k dimensions by minimising the discrepancy measure

$$\psi'' = \sum_{i=1}^{n} \sum_{j=1}^{n} (\delta_{ij} - d_{ij})^2. \tag{5.6}$$

Exact algebraic solution is no longer possible in such cases, and recourse must be made to numerical methods. A starting configuration must be specified in the chosen number of dimensions k, and the discrepancy measure is then viewed as a function of nk variables (the coordinates of the points) to be minimised by a standard method such as steepest descent (**4.17**). The classical scaling solution in k dimensions generally provides a good initial configuration, and if a configuration is subsequently required in, say, $k + 1$ dimensions, then the whole process must be repeated *ab initio*. In general, the 'optimum' dimensionality for representing the data can be determined by considering a scree plot (see item 5 in **4.6**) of the minimum values of ψ'' over a range of values of k.

More generally, to smooth the fitting process and at the same time to optimise location and scale aspects, the distances d_{ij} can be regressed on the proximities δ_{ij} at the end of each iteration of the numerical optimisation procedure. This produces a set of 'estimated' distances, often called *disparities*,

$$\hat{d}_{ij} = a + b\delta_{ij}, \tag{5.7}$$

and the residual sum of squares from this regression provides yet another discrepancy measure. For comparability across different situations this residual sum of squares should be normalised by its 'size' $\sum_i \sum_j d_{ij}^2$, yielding (Kruskal,

Table 5.1 Road distances in miles between seven English towns

Bristol	0						
Cardiff	47	0					
Dover	210	245	0				
Exeter	84	121	250	0			
Hull	231	251	266	305	0		
Leeds	220	240	271	294	61	0	
London	120	155	80	200	218	199	0
	Bristol	Cardiff	Dover	Exeter	Hull	Leeds	London

1964a,b) the standardised residual sum of squares defined by

$$\text{STRESS} = \left[\sum_i \sum_j (d_{ij} - \hat{d}_{ij})^2 \Big/ \sum_i \sum_j d_{ij}^2\right]^{\frac{1}{2}} . \tag{5.8}$$

Takane *et al* (1977) used alternating least squares in place of steepest descent for the minimisation, and advocated replacing d_{ij} and $\hat{d}_{ij}$ by their squares. This yields the discrepancy measure

$$\text{SSTRESS} = \left[\sum_i \sum_j (d_{ij}^2 - \hat{d}_{ij}^2)^2 \Big/ \sum_i \sum_j d_{ij}^4\right]^{\frac{1}{2}} . \tag{5.9}$$

Normalisation ensures that STRESS and SSTRESS always take values between 0 and 1; an optimised value below about 0.1 is usually considered to be indicative of a good representation of objects by configuration points.

Since the goodness-of-fit measures are all based on direct numerical comparison of dissimilarities and distances, and disparities are obtained by metric regression methods, the derivation of a configuration by optimisation of any of these criteria is usually referred to as *metric scaling.*

Example 5.2

The Automobile Association of Great Britain (AA) issues a handbook every two years for its members. In this handbook there is a matrix of road distances (in miles) between every pair out of a list of major towns in England, Scotland and Wales. A small extract from this matrix is shown in Table 5.1. The full matrix was subjected to a metric scaling, minimising STRESS using the alternating least squares approach as implemented in the ALSCAL procedure of the SAS computer package, and the resulting two-dimensional configuration is shown in Fig. 5.1. The value of STRESS for this configuration was 0.067, so it can be considered to be a 'good' representation of the original distances. The picture is indeed a recognisable reconstruction of the map of Great Britain, but there are a few evident distortions. For example, the places in Scotland are squashed into the centre of the configuration, while in the south Exeter is positioned incorrectly above Barnstaple. However, a small amount of distortion is to be expected as the distances in the AA matrix are not 'crow-fly' distances

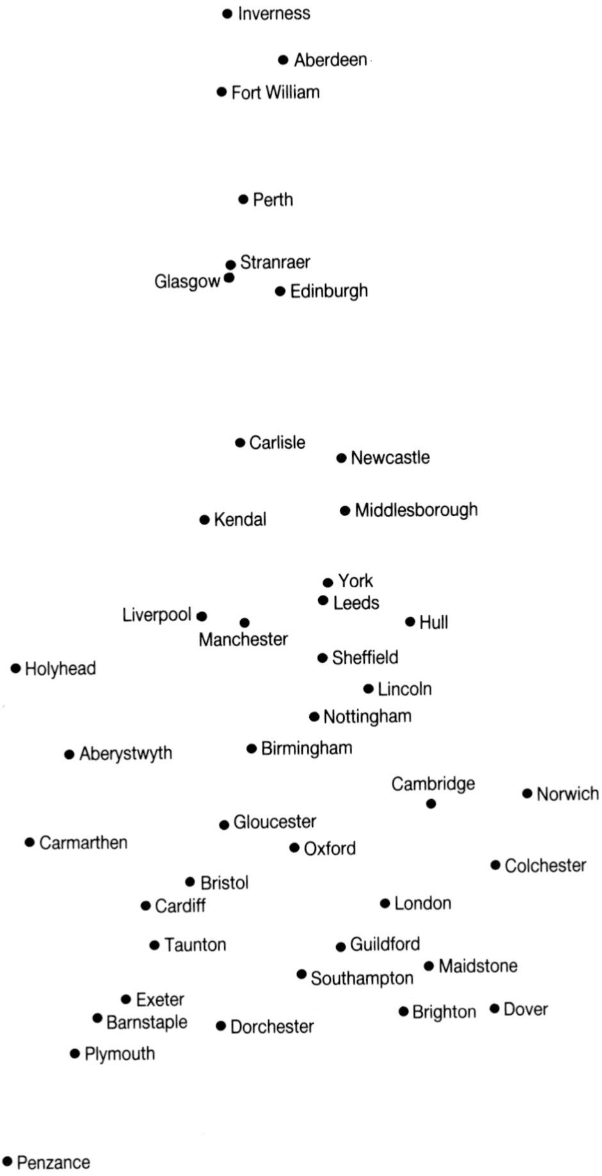

Figure 5.1 Metric scaling reconstruction of the map of Great Britain from a matrix of road distances between pairs of towns

but road distances, and moreover, they are not even the shortest road distances but those obtained when travelling between the towns along 'AA recommended routes'. It is thus evident that the recovered configuration is indeed a good one, and that metric scaling can represent inter-object dissimilarities by configurations of points both accurately and usefully.

5.11 Whenever approximate configurations are derived in a reduced dimensionality, there is a danger of misrepresentation of points relative to each other. It is therefore prudent, when examining a scaling plot, to check that such distortion has not occurred. A simple check in the case of classical scaling is provided by calculating the squared 'residuals' for each point, $r_i^2 = \sum_{j=k+1}^{n-1} v_{ij}^2$. These are the squared distances through which the points have been displaced in the projection from $n-1$ to k dimensions, so points that have large r_i^2 values warrant further inspection.

Another useful device, applicable to the results of any scaling, is to superimpose on the recovered configuration the *minimum spanning tree* calculated from the original dissimilarities δ_{ij}. The minimum spanning tree is a concept from graph theory. For a comprehensive discussion of this topic see, e.g., Harary (1969); the relevant features in the present context are as follows. Any configuration resulting from application of multidimensional scaling can be treated as a *graph*, in which the points representing the observations are the *nodes* and lines connecting pairs of points are the *edges*. The *length* of the edge joining points i and j is defined to be the dissimilarity δ_{ij}. A *spanning tree* of the graph is a set of edges which provides a unique path between every pair of nodes, and the *minimum* spanning tree is the one whose total length is the least of all possible spanning trees. The idea is to give a direct visual impression of each individual's 'nearest neighbours', as these will in general be the individuals connected to it by edges of the tree. Since 'similar' individuals should thus be joined by edges of the tree, nearby points on the plot that *aren't* joined by edges indicate possible areas of distortion (where points more distant in $n-1$ dimensions have been represented as lying close together in k dimensions).

Minimum spanning trees are also important in Cluster Analysis, and will therefore be considered again in Volume 2.

Example 5.3

Corbet *et al* (1970) report a study of the water vole, genus *Arvicola.* The study was set up to investigate the hypothesis that two distinct species, *Arvicola terrestris* and *Arvicola sapidus*, were present in the British Isles. Information on the presence or absence of thirteen characteristics was obtained from about 300 vole skulls subdivided into fourteen groups; there were six British groups (Surrey, Shropshire, Yorkshire, Perthshire, Aberdeen and Eilean Gamhna), five *terrestris* groups from mainland Europe (Germany, Norway, Alps, Yugoslavia and Pyrenees I), and three *sapidus* groups from mainland Europe (North Spain, South Spain and Pyrenees II). Sample sizes ranged from 11 to 50 in each group. The percentage incidences $x_1, \ldots, x_{13}$ were first subjected to an angular transformation $y_i = \sin^{-1}(1 - 2x_i/100)$, and then the dissimilarity between every pair of groups was calculated as the square root of the bias-corrected squared Euclidean distance calculated from the y_i. The correction for bias involved subtracting $(1/n_1 + 1/n_2)$ from the squared Euclidean distances between groups of n_1 and n_2 voles respectively; this introduced two very small negative squared dissimilarities, but negligible distortion was caused by simply taking their absolute values.

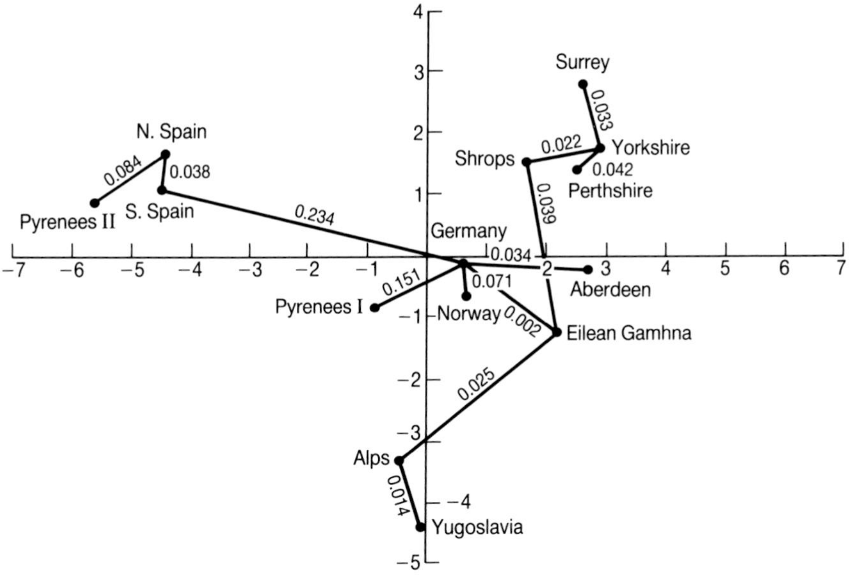

Figure 5.2 Two-dimensional classical scaling representation of voles data. Reproduced with permission from Corbet *et al* (1970).

Classical scaling was performed on the final dissimilarity matrix, and the resulting 2-dimensional configuration is shown in Fig. 5.2. Over eighty per cent of the trace was accounted for by these two dimensions, so the representation should be accurate. However, in case any distortion has been introduced in projecting from the original thirteen dimensions into just two, the minimum spanning tree is superimposed on the configuration; the correct dissimilarity values are attached to the branches of this tree. It seems that the configuration in general is an accurate one, but the point corresponding to Eilean Gamhna has been displaced a little; the dissimilarities put it closest to Germany, while on the plot it appears to be nearer to Aberdeen. However, this is only a very minor distortion and the overall picture enabled a clear conclusion to be drawn. All the British groups form a tight cluster which is aligned with the mainland *terrestris* populations and far distant from the *sapidus* populations. The latter, moreover, form a well-separated cluster of their own. There is thus no evidence in favour of the hypothesis that both *terrestris* and *sapidus* populations are present in Britain.

Non-metric scaling

5.12 The methods described above assume that we have available a set of numerical proximities δ_{ij} between every pair of individuals in a sample, and we wish to construct a configuration of points representing the individuals such that inter-point distances match the inter-individual proximities as closely as possible. However, application of these methods will not be appropriate under the following circumstances.

(1) Exact numerical proximities are not available, but only their rank order. This situation arises frequently in such areas as sensory assessment or psychology. For example, if asked to compare the tastes of different brands of chocolate, or the quality of different concert pianists, most people would be unable to ascribe numerical values to the δ_{ij} but might be prepared to settle on an ordering

$$\delta_{i_1 j_1} < \delta_{i_2 j_2} < \ldots < \delta_{i_M j_M}, \tag{5.10}$$

where $M = \frac{1}{2}n(n-1)$ and the i_k, j_k are distinct integers in the set $\{1, 2, \ldots, n\}$. Such an ordering quantifies the perceived *relative* strengths of the pairwise proximities.

(2) Numerical proximities *are* available, but the quality of the measuring process is such that only an ordering such as (5.10) is trustworthy.

(3) Implicit in the metric scaling methods is the assumption that there is a 'true' configuration in k dimensions, and that in this configuration the inter-point distances satisfy

$$d_{ij} = \delta_{ij} + \epsilon_{ij} \tag{5.11}$$

where the ϵ_{ij} represent measurement errors. In some situations it may be more realistic to seek a configuration in which

$$d_{ij} = f(\delta_{ij} + \epsilon_{ij}) \tag{5.12}$$

for some arbitrary monotone function f.

For any of these situations, the only information that we can use when seeking a configuration to reconstruct the δ_{ij} is the *rank order* of the d_{ij}. The seminal papers on this topic are those by Shepard (1962a,b), but Shepard's solution was adapted by Kruskal (1964a,b) into the form that is best known today. His procedure was essentially the one already described in **5.10** for metric scaling, but with the metric constraint (5.7) replaced by the non-metric one

$$\delta_{ij} < \delta_{rs} \Rightarrow \hat{d}_{ij} \leqslant \hat{d}_{rs} \; \forall i, j, r, s. \tag{5.13}$$

A *monotone* regression (Barlow *et al*, 1972) is thus required in each cycle of the iterative procedure to minimise STRESS, and Kruskal gives the computational details for embedding this monotone regression into the steepest descent algorithm. The adjective *non-metric* is used to distinguish this solution from the previous ones, but it should be understood that the term non-metric relates to the nature of the (minimal) data requirements and not to the properties of the constructed space.

The Shepard–Kruskal solution is invariant under translation, rotation and uniform dilation of the constructed configuration. Sibson (1979) demonstrated that it is insensitive to errors in the δ_{ij} at the lower end of the range, but can be upset if the ordering of the δ_{ij} is disturbed at the upper end. Missing values are readily accommodated, by omitting the missing dissimilarities in

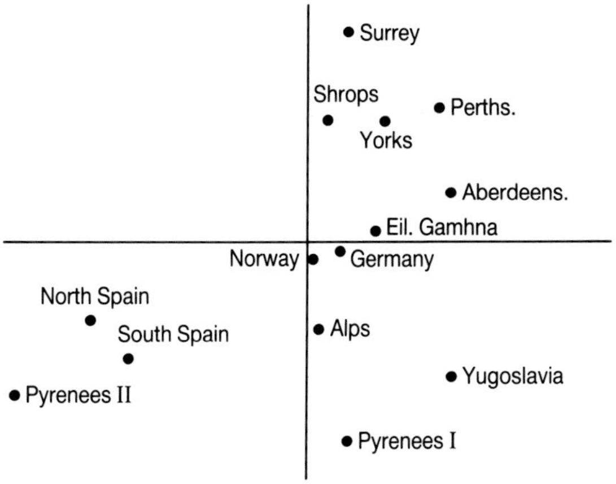

Figure 5.3 Non-metric scaling configuration for *Arvicola* data. Reproduced with permission from Krzanowski (1988a).

the ordering (5.10) and deleting the corresponding terms from (5.8); providing that not too many values are missing the method still works well. Likewise, ties among the dissimilarities can be handled readily, in one of several possible ways. The constraint given by (5.13) is called the *primary* treatment of ties; if $\delta_{ij} = \delta_{rs}$ then no constraint is made on $\hat{d}_{ij}$ and $\hat{d}_{rs}$. A stronger requirement, called the *secondary* treatment of ties, is given by

$$\delta_{ij} \leqslant \delta_{rs} \Rightarrow \hat{d}_{ij} \leqslant \hat{d}_{rs} \ \forall i, j, r, s. \tag{5.14}$$

This constraint has the property that $\delta_{ij} = \delta_{rs} \Rightarrow \hat{d}_{ij} = \hat{d}_{rs}$. Kruskal (1964a,b) discusses implementation of both methods of treating ties.

For further discussion of the Shepard–Kruskal method see Lingoes and Roskam (1973), Kruskal (1977), Kruskal and Wish (1978), Carroll and Arabie (1980) and De Leeuw and Heiser (1980). Numerous Monte Carlo studies of the properties of the method have been published. One topic extensively studied in this way is the choice of starting configurations for the iterative process, in particular whether random or rationally chosen configurations should be used; for the arguments from each viewpoint see Arabie (1978) and Spence and Young (1978). Shepard (1966), Young (1970) and Sibson (1972) have considered the extent to which metric information can be recovered using non-metric methods. Various alternative non-metric scaling methods have been proposed, most notably by Guttman (1968), Johnson (1973) and Borg and Lingoes (1980). Young and Null (1978) have extended the methodology to cope with nominal level of data, while Takane *et al* (1977) have subsumed all possible levels of measurement within a single computational procedure which optimises SSTRESS using alternating least squares. This procedure also allows individual differences to be catered for (see **5.13**); it is available in a number of commercial software packages (e.g. the ALSCAL option within SAS, already mentioned in Example 5.2).

Example 5.4
Returning to the *Arvicola* data of Example 5.3, let us suppose that the dissimilarities calculated there are only deemed to be trustworthy up to their rank order. A non-metric scaling, minimising STRESS, yielded the two-dimensional solution given in Fig. 5.3. It can be seen that there is a high degree of resemblance between this configuration and that of the metric scaling in Fig. 5.2. Disregarding small local fluctuations, the only group of voles that appears to have changed position significantly is that of Pyrenees I. However, the STRESS value of this configuration was 0.125, so a more accurate representation might be sought in three dimensions before drawing any conclusions.

Example 5.5
Manly (1986, p134) gives a dissimilarity matrix between fifteen Congressmen from New Jersey in the United States House of Representatives. The data come from Romesburg (1984, p155), and the dissimilarities are simply the numbers of times that the pairs of Congressmen voted differently on nineteen environmental bills. In calculating the dissimilarities, the possible categories for each bill were taken to be 'for', 'against' and 'abstain' (so that two Congressmen voted 'similarly' if they both abstained for a particular bill). Manly reports the results of a non-metric scaling of this dissimilarity matrix. STRESS values for 2-, 3- and 4-dimensional configurations were 0.134, 0.089 and 0.065 respectively, so a 3-dimensional configuration gives a good representation of the relationships among the Congressmen and the fourth dimension provides negligible extra improvement.
Conducting a classical scaling on these data yields eigenvalues 497.76, 146.18, 102.91, 76.88, 55.12, 24.74, 8.01, 6.17, 2.36, 0.00, −2.03, −15.21, −18.69, −20.40, −33.99. We thus note the presence of some negative eigenvalues, showing that the dissimilarity matrix is not Euclidean. However, these negative eigenvalues are all small in absolute terms relative to the first three, so the distortion in fitting a Euclidean representation should not be great. For 3-dimensional fitting, the discrepancy measures of **5.9** are $\alpha_{1,3} = 73.91$ and $\alpha_{2,3} = 96.12$ so a 3-dimensional classical scaling representation should also be a good one. Table 5.2 shows the coordinates of the points representing the Congressmen in this solution, and also the coordinates of Manly's non-metric scaling solution for comparison. The Congressmen are grouped in the table by party allegiance, R denoting Republican and D denoting Democrat. When due allowance is made for the different scales of the two solutions, it is evident that there is very little difference between the two configurations. Formal methods of comparing two such representations will be discussed later in this chapter, but for the present we accept the equivalence of the two solutions and focus on just one of them. Fig. 5.4 shows the first two dimensions of Manly's solution, with the value for the third dimension given next to each point of the configuration.
Manly discusses interpretation of this configuration. Since all Democrats fall on the left-hand side of the figure and all Republicans except Rinaldo on the right, the first dimension represents party allegiance. The second dimension is not so obviously interpreted, and requires deeper consid-

Table 5.2 Coordinates of configurations of 15 Congressmen obtained by non-metric and by classical scaling; non-metric coordinates taken from Manly (1986), with permission

	Non-metric solution			*Classical solution*		
	Dimension			*Dimension*		
Congressmen	1	2	3	1	2	3
Hunt (R)	2.25	0.15	0.53	9.16	0.02	2.48
Sandman (R)	1.74	2.06	0.64	8.37	7.68	2.51
Frelinghuysen (R)	1.47	-0.83	-1.23	5.34	-2.89	-4.38
Forsythe (R)	0.81	-0.93	-0.43	3.71	-3.50	-1.24
Widnall (R)	2.25	-0.28	-0.46	8.44	-0.83	-3.66
Rinaldo (R)	-1.27	-0.18	-0.27	-6.03	-0.72	-1.32
Maraziti (R)	1.20	-1.20	0.97	4.76	-4.64	4.38
Howard (D)	-1.37	-0.01	0.84	-5.63	-0.27	2.95
Thompson (D)	-0.85	1.42	-0.45	-2.75	6.55	-2.82
Roe (D)	-1.40	-0.01	0.60	-5.69	-0.22	2.50
Helstoski (D)	-1.50	0.22	-0.18	-6.53	-0.06	0.15
Rodino (D)	-1.09	-0.19	0.10	-4.42	-0.02	1.03
Minish (D)	-1.13	-0.21	-0.24	-4.89	-0.79	-0.90
Daniels (D)	-0.12	-0.16	0.52	-0.21	-0.43	1.29
Patten (D)	-0.99	0.14	-0.94	-3.63	0.11	-2.99

eration of the original data. When these are studied, it turns out that Sandman and Thompson (at the top of the diagram) abstained from a large proportion of the votes – Sandman nine times and Thompson six times – while Congressmen near the bottom of the diagram voted most of the time. Thus dimension 2 reflects abstention from voting. While dimension 3 must also represent some systematic differences in voting patterns between the Congressmen, no simple or obvious interpretation has been found for it. Nevertheless, the analysis has produced a useful summary of the data regarding voting of Congressmen on environmental issues.

A special case of multidimensional scaling occurs when there is a one-dimensional ordering among the objects being scaled, and the objective of the analysis is to recover this ordering. For example, Kendall (1971) discusses the analysis of the Munsingen-Rain incidence matrix in which the occurrences of seventy types of artefact are given for each of fifty-nine excavated tombs. Tombs laid down close together in time would be expected to have plenty of artefacts in common, while tombs laid down at well-separated periods of time would have few artefacts in common. One possible way of *seriating* the tombs, i.e. arranging them in temporal order, would thus be to calculate a dissimilarity between every pair of tombs based on the number of common types of artefact found in each, and then to conduct a multidimensional scaling on the resulting dissimilarity matrix. In theory, displaying the first two dimensions of this scaling should reveal a linear ordering of tombs as defined by their temporal order. However, Kendall found on doing this that the tombs were arranged along a curve that resembled a horse's shoe. The explanation for this is that

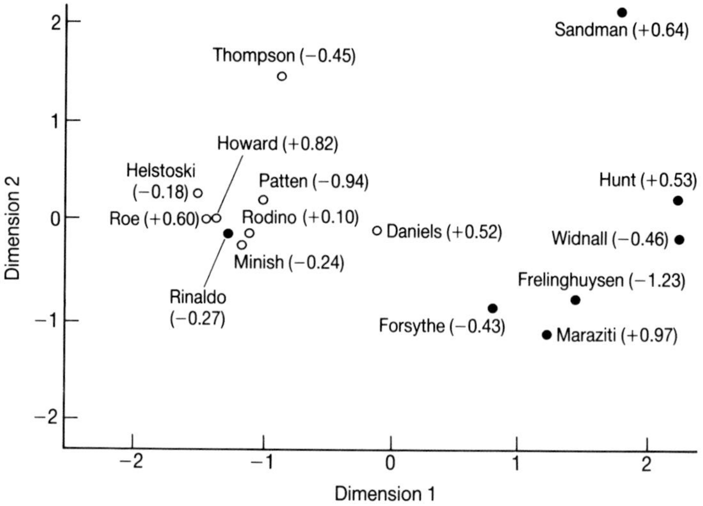

Figure 5.4 Non-metric scaling configuration of Congressmen. Open circles indicate Democrats, closed circles indicate Republicans. The coordinate on the third dimension is indicated in parentheses for each point. Reproduced with permission from Manly (1986).

tombs close together in time have accurately determined dissimilarities, but the dissimilarities become less accurate the further apart in time that the tombs are. Indeed, once the time interval exceeds some threshold, it is likely that two tombs will have no artefacts in common in which case any such pair of tombs will have the same dissimilarity value irrespective of their actual temporal separation. Thus large dissimilarities tend to be underestimates of their true values, causing the ends of the linear arrangement of tombs to be bent towards each other into a curve. This phenomenon is observed quite widely whenever there is an underlying one-dimensional structure to the data, and has thus been termed the *horseshoe effect*. A range of examples exhibiting this effect may be found in Gifi (1990).

Individual differences

5.13 All the methods described above are appropriate for analysing a single proximity matrix. In many applications, particularly in such areas as psychology or sensory studies, we might be presented with a *series* of proximity matrices for analysis. For example, in a comparison of a set of soft drinks, each member of a panel of tasters may provide a matrix of dissimilarities between pairs of drinks; in market research, individuals in different parts of the country may be asked to compare various competing products on the market; and, in a psychological experiment, subjects in different age groups may be asked to judge the similarities between various pairs of stimuli. While the primary focus in all of these cases is on the *objects* being compared, it is also recognised that there are likely to be systematic differences between the *individuals* doing the comparisons. Thus not only are we interested in a pictorial representation of the overall relationships between the objects, but we might also wish to quantify the differences between the individuals and perhaps represent these differences pictorially. Such an analysis is usually termed *three-way*, or *individual difference*, scaling.

Early contributions towards a solution were provided by Tucker and Messick (1963), Ross (1966), Cliff (1968), McGee (1968) and Horan (1969); for a brief overview of this work see Mead (1992). However, the first widely implemented approach was the one due to Carroll and Chang (1970). Their premise was that there exists an underlying space, the 'group stimulus' space, in which the objects are uniquely representable by points, and that systematic differences arise between individuals because they perceive this space in different ways. In particular, there is a fixed set of reference axes in the space such that all differences between individuals can be explained by assuming that different individuals attach differential 'weights' to these axes. In other words, each individual identifies the same underlying sources of variation among the objects but the individuals differ in the relative importance they attach to each of these sources.

Suppose that there are k individuals, each of whom has provided an $(n \times n)$ matrix of dissimilarities $\boldsymbol{\Delta}_i = (\delta_{irs})$ for $i = 1, \ldots, k$ and $r, s = 1, \ldots, n$. Writing $\boldsymbol{Q}_i = (\boldsymbol{I}-\mathbf{1}\mathbf{1}'/\mathbf{n})\boldsymbol{\Gamma}_i(\boldsymbol{I}-\mathbf{1}\mathbf{1}'/\mathbf{n})$ where the (r,s)th entry of $\boldsymbol{\Gamma}_i$ is $-\frac{1}{2}\delta_{irs}^2$, then the classical scaling procedure of **5.7** yields a p-dimensional configuration of points with coordinates $\boldsymbol{Y}_i = (y_{iuv})$ for $i = 1, \ldots, k$, $u = 1, \ldots, n$ and $v = 1, \ldots, p$ satisfying $\boldsymbol{Q}_i = \boldsymbol{Y}_i\boldsymbol{Y}_i'$. Carroll and Chang's model then postulates a set of group stimulus coordinates x_{uv} for $u = 1, \ldots, n$ and $v = 1, \ldots, p$, and a set of weights w_{iv} for $i = 1, \ldots, k$ and $v = 1, \ldots, p$, such that $y_{iuv} = x_{uv}\sqrt{w_{iv}}$ for all u, v. Writing $\boldsymbol{W}_i^{1/2} = \text{diag}(\sqrt{w_{i1}}, \ldots, \sqrt{w_{ip}})$ and $\boldsymbol{X} = (x_{uv})$, this is equivalent to $\boldsymbol{Y}_i = \boldsymbol{X}\boldsymbol{W}_i^{1/2}$ and hence to $\boldsymbol{Q}_i = \boldsymbol{X}\boldsymbol{W}_i\boldsymbol{X}'$.

The problem is thus to find, for given input dissimilarities $\boldsymbol{\Delta}_i$ and specified dimensionality p, the group stimulus coordinates $\boldsymbol{X}$ and the individual subject weights $\boldsymbol{W}_i$ such that $\boldsymbol{X}\boldsymbol{W}_i\boldsymbol{X}'$ approximates as closely as possible the derived $\boldsymbol{Q}_i$. In terms of the matrix elements, this is equivalent to finding x_{uv} and w_{iv} such that

$$q_{irs} = \sum_{t=1}^{p} w_{it}x_{rt}x_{st} + \epsilon_{irs}, \tag{5.15}$$

where ϵ_{irs} is a small 'error'. This is a generalisation of the two-way problem treated by Eckart and Young (1936). The full three-way specification is to seek values a_{it}, b_{rt} and c_{st} such that a set of known values z_{irs} can be approximated in the form

$$z_{irs} = \sum_{t=1}^{p} a_{it}b_{rt}c_{st} + \epsilon_{irs}. \tag{5.16}$$

An alternating least squares solution proceeds as follows. Set the b_{rt} and c_{st} to arbitrary initial values, and find the values of a_{it} minimising

$$V = \sum_i \sum_r \sum_s \left(z_{irs} - \sum_{t=1}^{p} a_{it}b_{rt}c_{st} \right)^2 .$$

Retaining these values of a_{it} and the original values of c_{st}, next find the values of b_{rt} minimising V. Finally, for these computed values of a_{it} and b_{rt}, find the values of c_{st} minimising V. These three minimisations form one cycle of the iterative scheme. Continue cycling using current values of a_{it}, b_{rt} and c_{st} until there is negligible change in these values between successive cycles. The individual differences model is the special case of this procedure with $z_{irs} = q_{irs}$, $a_{it} = w_{it}$, and $b_{rt} = c_{rt} = x_{rt}$. Thus *two* minimisations with respect to the x_{rt} take place in each cycle, and it is customary to retain the second one of the pair for carrying forward. Also, to give each individual equal weight in the analysis, the matrices $\boldsymbol{Q}_i$ are normalised at the outset so that $\sum_r \sum_s q_{irs}^2 = 1$ for each i.

The above analysis was given the acronym INDSCAL by Carroll and Chang. Note that it is essentially a metric technique, but it has the feature common to earlier non-metric solutions that the whole fitting process has to be repeated whenever a solution in a different dimensionality is sought. Carroll and Chang (1970) also briefly considered a quasi non-metric version of this technique, but with limited success. Bloxom (1974) suggested an alternative method for fitting the Carroll and Chang model, but the most comprehensive generalisation to date has been provided by Takane *et al* (1977) who show how data at any of the four levels of measurement (nominal, ordinal, interval or ratio) can be handled within the single framework.

Equation (5.16) is a particular form of the *trilinear* model, a generalisation to three-way data of the familiar *bilinear* model for two-way data that is exemplified by the singular value decomposition of a matrix (**4.1**). There has been much interest in trilinear and even more general (*multilinear*) models in recent years. A good summary of developments can be found in the review paper by Leurgans and Ross (1992), and in the discussion that follows it.

Example 5.6

Chauhan *et al* (1983) report various investigations into the similarities between seven commercially available soft drinks, as perceived by a panel of ten assessors. The seven drinks were

(1) Hunts Dry Ginger Ale,
(2) Schweppes Dry Ginger Ale,
(3) Hunts American Ginger Ale,
(4) Schweppes American Ginger Ale,
(5) Idris Ginger Beer,
(6) Corona Lemonade,
(7) Corona Limeade.

In one of the investigations, the panel members were asked to assess each drink by means of *descriptive profiling*, i.e. by giving each drink a score on a prescribed set of descriptors relating to flavour, taste, appearance etc. In this case there were 32 descriptors, each descriptor was scored for intensity on a 0–5 category scale, and each panel member provided two replicate assessments (on two separate tasting occasions). The experiment thus yielded twenty (7×32) data matrices. Each of these matrices was converted to a (7×7) dissimilarity matrix among the soft drinks by finding the Euclidean distances of the raw data, and the resulting set of

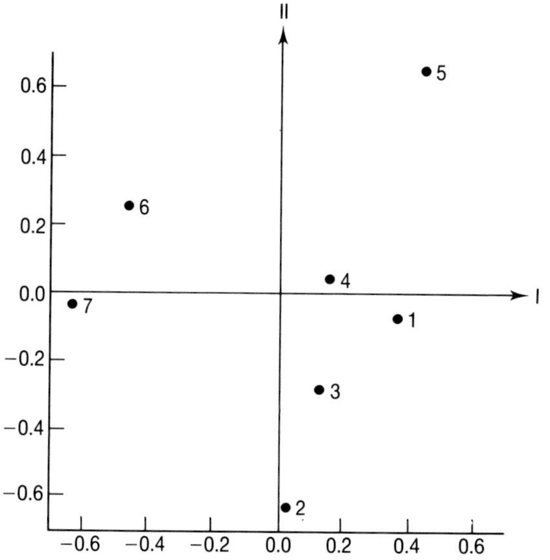

Figure 5.5 Two-dimensional configuration of the INDSCAL group stimulus space derived from 20 matrices of dissimilarities among seven soft drinks. Reproduced from Chauhan *et al* (1983).

twenty dissimilarity matrices was subjected to individual scaling analysis by invoking the INDSCAL option of the software package MDS(X). (Note that the ALSCAL procedure in SAS also offers the same option). The INDSCAL solutions in 2-, 3- and 4-dimensions accounted for 47%, 59% and 69% respectively of the variance among the dissimilarity matrices. The two-dimensional group stimulus space is shown in Fig. 5.5; coordinates in the third dimension are 0.5 for points 1 and 2, 0.0 for points 5, 6 and 7, −0.4 for point 3, and −0.5 for point 4. Thus the seven drinks are primarily differentiated into two distinct groups, the citrus-flavoured drinks falling in one group and the ginger drinks in the other. Among the latter, the Ginger Beer is perceived as being unique, with the two Dry Ginger Ales being differentiated from the two American Ginger Ales when the third dimension is taken into account. However, the distance between drinks 3 and 4 is smaller than that between 1 and 2, indicating less distinction between the two varieties of American Ginger than between the two Dry Gingers. Also, the American Gingers appear to be closer to the citrus drinks than do the Dry Gingers. The first axis of the configuration distinguishes citrus from ginger, while the second and third axes differentiate among the gingers.

To investigate differences among the assessors, the most instructive approach is to plot the derived axis weights w_{it} against each other. There will be one such weight for each axis for each dissimilarity matrix. Plotting the weights on axis one against their counterparts on axis two for the soft drinks comparison yields the twenty points of Fig. 5.6. Assessors are numbered 1 to 10, and the two replicates for each assessor are labelled *a* and *b*. The weights indicate by how much each assessor stretches or

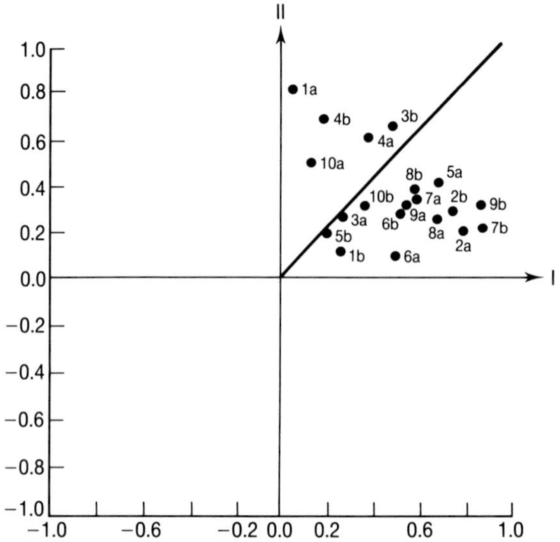

Figure 5.6 Plot of individual weights for the first two dimensions of the INDSCAL analysis of 20 matrices of dissimilarities among seven soft drinks. Reproduced from Chauhan *et al* (1983).

shrinks a particular axis in order to arrive at his/her view of the stimuli. Thus points above the 45 degree line in the diagram correspond to those assessments that place more weight on axis two (i.e. the 'ginger taste') than to axis one (i.e. the 'citrus versus ginger' contrast), and vice-versa for the points below this line. Also, the distance of a point from the origin provides a rough 'goodness-of-fit' measure, indicating how well the INDSCAL solution recovers that individual's set of dissimilarities. Fig. 5.6 shows that there are considerable individual differences among the assessors in their judgements of the drinks. Assessors 2, 4, 6, 8 and 9 show good agreement between the two replicate assessments, in contrast to assessors 1, 3, 5, 7 and 10 whose replicate assessments vary substantially.

5.14 All the foregoing methods are purely descriptive. They do not incorporate any estimation of variability of points on a diagram, so that any inferences drawn from such diagrams must be informal ones. In a series of papers, Ramsay (1977, 1978, 1982) has addressed this issue by postulating distributional models for the observed dissimilarities. This approach leads on to the use of maximum likelihood methods in multidimensional scaling, which in turn allows the possibility of estimating standard errors of observations; the construction of confidence or credibility regions round points on derived configurations; the testing of points for significant separation; and the testing of the extent to which some other relationship between subsets of points is satisfied. Ramsay's methods focus on metric scaling; Takane (1981) has applied maximum likelihood ideas to dissimilarity data measured on rating scales, while Takane and Carroll (1981) and Brady (1985) have extended the concepts to non-metric multidimensional scaling.

An alternative approach to the estimation of variability in general is via a data resampling procedure such as jack-knifing or bootstrapping (Efron and Gong, 1983). Jack-knifing operates by successively omitting either single individuals or groups of individuals from the data and recomputing the statistics of interest on each omission, thereby generating artificial replicates from their sampling distributions. Bootstrapping generates such artificial replicates by sampling individuals with replacement from the existing data. Either of these techniques is thus ideally suited to the INDSCAL situation; Weinberg *et al* (1984) have discussed the calculation of confidence intervals in individual scaling by these means. In the absence of replicate observations in the data it is less obvious how these methods can be used; De Leeuw and Meulman (1986) provide an interesting possibility by deleting one *stimulus* at a time, and then combining the resulting configurations by a least squares matching method. This idea can be used for stability analysis of *any* multidimensional scaling.

5.15 A tacit assumption in all the methods discussed above, as mentioned at the outset in **5.2**, is that the proximity matrix presented for analysis is symmetric. This will be so for the vast majority of practical applications, but nevertheless situations do arise in which there is asymmetry of similarities or dissimilarities; examples can be found in diallel-cross experiments, immigration/emigration statistics, food preference studies, and confusion matrices. In all these cases we may be faced with an $(n \times n)$ proximity matrix Δ the elements δ_{ij} of which are such that $\delta_{ij} \neq \delta_{ji}$ for some, or all, i, j.

One way of tackling such a matrix is to view the rows and columns as corresponding to *different* entities, and to seek a pictorial representation containing $2n$ points, n labelled $i, j, k, \ldots$ for the row entities and n labelled $I, J, K, \ldots$ for the column entities, such that δ_{ij} is approximated by the distance between points i and J for all elements of Δ. A symmetric Δ would give rise to a collapsed configuration in which points i and I coincide, as do j and J, k and K, and so on. The further points i and I are from each other in the configuration, the more asymmetry is there in the proximities involving the ith stimulus. The general approach to construction of such a configuration is through *multidimensional unfolding*; see Schönemann (1970). However, this is a general technique which can be applied to *any* $(m \times n)$ matrix of quantitative elements. Asymmetric square proximity matrices can more profitably be viewed as the central $(n \times n)$ block of the lower triangle of a $(2n \times 2n)$ proximity matrix, for which the 'top' and 'side' $n \times n$ lower triangles are 'missing'. Most multidimensional scaling programs, such as ALSCAL previously mentioned, can handle missing values. A suitable configuration can therefore be obtained by providing the expanded proximity matrix as input to such a program.

Constantine and Gower (1978) proposed an alternative approach. They noted that any square matrix Δ can be written in the form $\boldsymbol{M} + \boldsymbol{N}$, where $\boldsymbol{M} = \frac{1}{2}(\Delta + \Delta')$ is symmetric and $\boldsymbol{N} = \frac{1}{2}(\Delta - \Delta')$ is skew-symmetric. They therefore suggested that graphical representation of Δ can be accomplished by constructing *two* configurations: one picture would be a multidimensional scaling of the symmetric component $\boldsymbol{M}$ while the second would be a representation of the skew-symmetric component $\boldsymbol{N}$. The latter is obtained from the canonical decomposition

$$N = \sum_{i=1}^{[n/2]} \lambda_i(\boldsymbol{u}_i\boldsymbol{v}_i' - \boldsymbol{v}_i\boldsymbol{u}_i'), \tag{5.17}$$

where $[n/2]$ denotes the greatest integer less than or equal to $n/2$ and the $\lambda_i, \boldsymbol{u}_i, \boldsymbol{v}_i$ are obtained from the spectral decomposition of the symmetric matrix $\boldsymbol{NN}'$, which produces pairs of equal eigenvalues λ_i^2 with associated pairs of eigenvectors $\boldsymbol{u}_i, \boldsymbol{v}_i$. Constantine and Gower (1978) show that if λ_1 is the largest eigenvalue, then the configuration of n points with coordinates (u_{1j}, v_{1j}) for $j = 1, \ldots, n$ is the best two-dimensional representation of the skew-symmetric component. They also discuss fully the interpretation of such diagrams.

Example 5.7

Chauhan *et al* (1983) report a second experiment involving the same ten assessors and the same seven soft drinks as previously discussed in Example 5.6. This time all possible pairs of drinks were presented in turn to each assessor, and the assessors were asked to rate (directly) the dissimilarity of each pair for flavour in the mouth. The experiment was repeated a second time, providing two replicates of the direct assessments for each panellist to go with the two replicates of the descriptive profiling assessments described in Example 5.6. Averaging each set of twenty dissimilarity matrices produced a single dissimilarity matrix for direct assessment and a single matrix for descriptive profiling, and interest then centred on comparing these two matrices.

To do this, the lower triangle of the first was replaced by the upper triangle of the second to yield a single asymmetric dissimilarity matrix, the descriptive profiling assessments being in the lower triangle and the direct assessments being in the upper triangle. This asymmetric matrix was then subjected to a multidimensional scaling as described above. The seven row labels (i.e. the drinks as assessed by descriptive profiling) and the seven column labels (i.e. the same drinks treated by direct assessment) were considered to be fourteen different entities. The central (7×7) square portion of the resulting (14×14) lower triangular dissimilarity matrix was taken to be this asymmetric matrix, and the two remaining (7×7) lower triangles were assigned missing values. Presenting this (14×14) matrix for non-metric scaling yielding the two-dimensional configuration shown in Fig. 5.7. Open circles denote the position of a drink assessed by descriptive profiling, solid circles the position as determined by direct assessment.

It is evident that that the overall pattern of the configuration is similar to that of the group stimulus space of Fig. 5.5 (after suitable rotation): three separate groups of drinks with the Ginger Beer being unique amongst the seven drinks. With the exceptions of points representing drinks 1 and 5, the two points for each of the other five drinks are fairly close together, indicating that the two methods of assessment are equivalent for these latter five drinks. Reasons for differences between the two methods of assessment in the case of drinks 1 and 5 were left for further investigation.

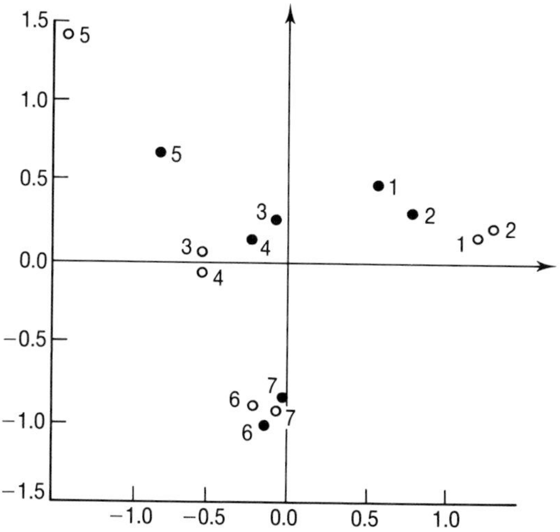

Figure 5.7 Two-dimensional configuration of similarities between seven soft drinks as assessed by two different methods: solid circles denote direct assessment, open circles denote descriptive profiling. Reproduced from Chauhan *et al* (1983).

Contingency tables

5.16 Contingency tables are frequently encountered in many areas of research (e.g. sociology, education, psychology, marketing). A typical analysis involves the Pearson chi-square statistic, which is used to determine whether there is evidence of any significant association, or dependence, between rows and columns of the table (see, e.g, Stuart and Ord, 1991). Equivalently, we say that a significant chi-square indicates a departure from row or column homogeneity, the homogeneity hypothesis being the same as the hypothesis of row-column independence. If the test is significant, then it is of interest to ascertain the specific nature of the heterogeneity in the table. One way of doing this is by investigating various partitions of the rows and columns and their associated subtables (Goodman, 1964; Gabriel, 1966; Hirotsu, 1983). An alternative approach is to expose a more continuous form of structure in the contingency table as a whole, either by formal modelling (Goodman, 1985) or by graphical displays (Greenacre, 1988a). We concentrate here on the latter approach, showing first how the ideas of multidimensional scaling developed earlier can be used to advantage and then demonstrating their equivalence with the more formal methodology of correspondence analysis.

5.17 Consider a two-way contingency table having I rows and J columns. Let the entry in the ith row and jth column be n_{ij}, and write $\boldsymbol{N}$ for the $I \times J$ matrix with entries n_{ij}, $i = 1, \ldots, I; j = 1, \ldots, J$. Denoting the row and column totals of $\boldsymbol{N}$ by $n_{i.}$ and $n_{.j}$ respectively, and the grand total of all entries by n, we can define the marginal relative frequencies by $r_i = n_{i.}/n$ for the rows $(i = 1, \ldots, I)$ and $c_j = n_{.j}/n$ for the columns $(j = 1, \ldots, J)$. Then the Pearson chi-square statistic for testing the null hypothesis of no row-column association is

$$X^2 = \sum_{i=1}^{I}\sum_{j=1}^{J}[n(n_{ij} - n_{i.}n_{.j}/n)^2/n_{i.}n_{.j}]. \tag{5.18}$$

If we set $\boldsymbol{P}= (p_{ij}) = (n_{ij}/n) = \frac{1}{n}\boldsymbol{N}$, then this statistic can be rewritten as

$$X^2 = n\sum_{i=1}^{I}\sum_{j=1}^{J}[(p_{ij} - r_i c_j)^2/(r_i c_j)]. \tag{5.19}$$

The quantity $t = X^2/n$ is the coefficient of association known as Pearson's mean-square contingency (Greenacre, 1988a); it is now more usually called the *total inertia* of the contingency table. Homogeneity in the table is therefore characterised by 'small' values of t, heterogeneity by 'large' values of t. But the total inertia can be re-expressed as

$$t = \sum_{i=1}^{I} r_i \sum_{j=1}^{J}[(p_{ij}/r_i - c_j)^2/c_j], \tag{5.20}$$

where the second summation is a weighted squared Euclidean distance between the vector of relative frequencies for the ith row [i.e. the jth *row profile* $(p_{i1}/r_i, \ldots, p_{iJ}/r_i)$] and the average row profile $\boldsymbol{c} = (c_1, \ldots, c_J)$, the weights being the inverses of the elements c_j of this average row profile. This weighted squared Euclidean distance is known as the *chi-square distance* between the ith row profile and the average row profile. The total inertia is a further weighted combination of the I chi-square distances, the weights this time being given by the elements r_i. Thus it can be seen that homogeneity in the table arises when all I row profiles are 'close' to the average row profile, and heterogeneity arises when some or all row profiles are 'far' from the average row profile, the distances being gauged by the chi-square metric. The former case is equivalent to all the row profiles being close to each other, the latter to some or all of them being far apart. A graphical exploration of heterogeneity can thus be effected by applying classical scaling (**5.7**) to the square roots of the chi-square distances between every pair of row profiles. The above discussion suggests that the generalised form of classical scaling described in **5.7** is the appropriate one, with the barycentre $\boldsymbol{s}$ set to be the average row profile $\boldsymbol{c}$ and the weights w_j given by the inverses of the elements c_j of this average row profile. To obtain the chi-square distance between row profiles i and k, we simply replace c_j by p_{kj}/r_k in the numerator of the second sum in (5.20):

$$d^2_{ik(r)} = \sum_{j=1}^{J}[(p_{ij}/r_i - p_{kj}/r_k)^2/c_j]. \tag{5.21}$$

5.18 The above analysis has been in terms of the row profiles, and the investigation of heterogeneity in the table thus involves plotting row profiles as points to see which rows cause departures from the independence hypothesis. In a symmetric fashion, however, we can equivalently decompose the total inertia of the table column-wise. Here we use the jth *column profile* $(p_{1j}/c_j, \ldots, p_{Ij}/c_j)$ and the average column profile $\boldsymbol{r} = (r_1, \ldots, r_I)$, so that the total inertia is

Table 5.3 Eye and hair colour data for Caithness schoolchildren

Eye colour	Fair	Red	Hair colour Medium	Dark	Black	Total
Light	688	116	584	188	4	1580
Blue	326	38	241	110	3	718
Medium	343	84	909	412	26	1774
Dark	98	48	403	681	85	1315
Total	1455	286	2137	1391	118	5387

Table 5.4 Row profiles for Caithness schoolchildren

	Fair	Red	Medium	Dark	Black
Light	0.435	0.073	0.370	0.119	0.003
Blue	0.454	0.053	0.336	0.153	0.004
Medium	0.193	0.047	0.512	0.232	0.015
Dark	0.075	0.037	0.306	0.518	0.065
Average	0.270	0.053	0.397	0.258	0.022

written as the weighted average of chi-square distances between the column profiles and their average:

$$t = \sum_{j=1}^{J} c_j \sum_{i=1}^{I} [(p_{ij}/c_j - r_i)^2/r_i]. \tag{5.22}$$

The chi-square distance between column profiles j and k is thus

$$d^2_{jk(c)} = \sum_{i=1}^{I} [(p_{ij}/c_j - p_{ik}/c_k)^2/r_i]. \tag{5.23}$$

Heterogeneity in the table can thus be investigated also by plotting column profiles as points to see which columns cause departures from the independence hypothesis. Here the average column profile and its elements replace the average row profile and its elements in the barycentre and weights of the classical scaling procedure. It is immaterial which representation is used, as the two configurations are merely the graphical depiction of the two ways of viewing departures from independence: either as variation among the row proportions or as variation among the column proportions in the table.

Example 5.8
Table 5.3 shows a 4 × 5 contingency table of 5387 schoolchildren from Caithness in Scotland, classified according to the colours of their hair and eyes. These data have been analysed previously by Fisher (1940), Maung (1941), Goodman (1981), Hill (1982), and Greenacre (1984); we use them here to illustrate the ideas outlined above. The null hypothesis of no association between eye and hair colour is clearly untenable, confirmed

Table 5.5 Column profiles for Caithness schoolchildren

	Fair	Red	Medium	Dark	Black	Average
Light	0.473	0.406	0.273	0.135	0.034	0.293
Blue	0.224	0.133	0.113	0.079	0.025	0.133
Medium	0.236	0.294	0.425	0.296	0.220	0.329
Dark	0.067	0.168	0.189	0.490	0.720	0.244

Table 5.6 Chi-square distances between row profiles for Caithness schoolchildren

Light	0.0			
Blue	0.0168	0.0		
Medium	0.3376	0.3602	0.0	
Dark	1.3103	1.2224	0.5914	0.0
	Light	Blue	Medium	Dark

by a Pearson chi-square statistic value $X^2 = 1240.04$ on 12 degrees of freedom. We can therefore investigate sources of heterogeneity by the above methods. First we calculate the row and column profiles; these are given in Tables 5.4 and 5.5, along with their average profiles. Chi-square distances computed from these data are given in Tables 5.6 and 5.7 respectively. We then conduct weighted classical scaling on each distance matrix. The barycentre for the 'eye colour' scaling is given by the vector (0.293, 0.133, 0.329, 0.244) from Table 5.5, with weights obtained from the row profiles of Table 5.4, while the barycentre for the 'hair colour' scaling is the vector (0.270, 0.053, 0.397, 0.258, 0.022) of Table 5.4 and the weights are obtained from the column profiles of Table 5.5. The non-zero eigenvalues are the same for each of the weighted scalings, in this case being 0.1992, 0.0301 and 0.0009. Thus two dimensions account for 99.6 per cent of differences among the row or column profiles, and the two-dimensional configurations that are obtained are displayed in Figs. 5.8 and 5.9. In the case of eye colour, it can be seen that the profiles for 'light' and 'blue' are very similar, but the other two profiles are very different from them and from each other, while in the case of hair colour we find a steady trend among the five profiles.

Table 5.7 Chi-square distances between column profiles for Caithness schoolchildren

Fair	0.0				
Red	0.1294	0.0			
Medium	0.3981	0.1171	0.0		
Dark	1.2879	0.6952	0.4954	0.0	
Black	2.7004	1.8245	1.5386	0.2922	0.0
	Fair	Red	Medium	Dark	Black

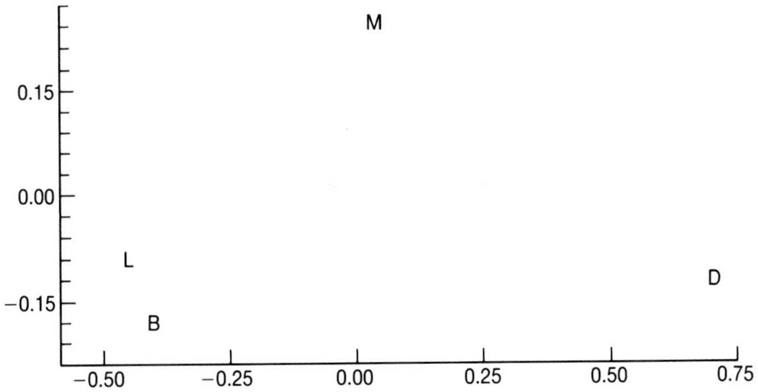

Figure 5.8 Two-dimensional configuration of eye-colour profiles for Caithness schoolchildren.

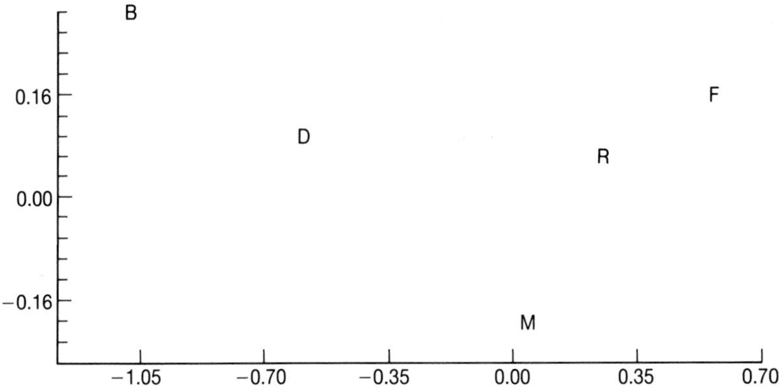

Figure 5.9 Two-dimensional configuration of hair-colour profiles for Caithness schoolchildren.

Correspondence analysis

5.19 The above development has shown how classical scaling can be used to investigate the contingency table $\boldsymbol{N}$ graphically. The objective is to display the categories of the classifying variables of the table as points, such that the Euclidean distance between two points is equal to the chi-square distance between the corresponding categories. One picture is obtained for the row categories and another one for the column categories, while the principal axis representation of classical scaling ensures that plotting the points on the first k axes provides the best k-dimensional approximation to the true configuration in each case.

Precisely the same solution can be obtained much more directly, as follows. Let the matrix $\boldsymbol{P}$ and the vectors $\boldsymbol{r}$ and $\boldsymbol{c}$ be as defined in **5.17** (so that $\boldsymbol{r} = \boldsymbol{P1}$ and $\boldsymbol{c} = \boldsymbol{P}'\boldsymbol{1}$), and set $\boldsymbol{D}_r = \text{diag}(\boldsymbol{r})$, $\boldsymbol{D}_c = \text{diag}(\boldsymbol{c})$, and $\boldsymbol{E} = \boldsymbol{D}_r^{-1/2}(\boldsymbol{P} - \boldsymbol{rc}')\boldsymbol{D}_c^{-1/2}$. Thus the elements of the matrix $\boldsymbol{E}$ are proportional to the standardised Pearsonian residuals for the contingency table $\boldsymbol{N}$, i.e. the signed square roots

Table 5.8 Pearsonian residuals and two-dimensional correspondence analysis for Caithness schoolchildren

			Hair				
Eyes	Fair	Red	Med.	Dark	Black	f_1	f_2
Light	0.1723	0.0478	-0.0233	-0.1484	-0.0709	-0.441	-0.088
Blue	0.1292	-0.0003	-0.0354	-0.0755	-0.0437	-0.400	-0.165
Med.	-0.0847	-0.0143	0.1054	-0.0293	-0.0281	0.034	0.245
Dark	-0.1859	-0.0356	-0.0708	0.2525	0.1427	0.702	-0.134
g_1	0.544	0.233	0.042	-0.589	-1.094		
g_2	0.174	0.048	-0.208	0.104	0.286		

of the terms making up the chi-square statistic X^2. Obtain the singular value decomposition of $\boldsymbol{E}$, i.e. $\boldsymbol{E} = \boldsymbol{UDV}'$ where $\boldsymbol{D}$ is the diagonal matrix containing the square roots of the non-zero eigenvalues of either $\boldsymbol{E}'\boldsymbol{E}$ or $\boldsymbol{EE}'$ (ranked in descending order) and $\boldsymbol{U}$, $\boldsymbol{V}$ are orthogonal matrices whose columns are the corresponding eigenvectors (normalised to have unit sums of squared elements) of $\boldsymbol{EE}'$ and $\boldsymbol{E}'\boldsymbol{E}$ respectively. Then the coordinates of the row profiles of the table are given by the rows $\boldsymbol{f}_i$ of $\boldsymbol{F} = \boldsymbol{D}_r^{-1/2}\boldsymbol{UD}$ while the coordinates of the column profiles are given by the rows $\boldsymbol{g}_i$ of $\boldsymbol{G} = \boldsymbol{D}_c^{-1/2}\boldsymbol{VD}$. The pairs of row and column coordinates $\boldsymbol{f}_i, \boldsymbol{g}_i$ are thus elements in the orthogonal decomposition of the residuals from the independence model in decreasing order of importance.

This approach is termed the *correspondence analysis* of the table $\boldsymbol{N}$. The centroids of the two sets of coordinates are at zero, and the scores $\boldsymbol{f}_i$ (for $i = 1, \ldots, p = \text{rank}[\boldsymbol{N}]$) are uncorrelated, as also are the scores $\boldsymbol{g}_i$. However, the two sets of scores are linked to each other by the formulae $\boldsymbol{G} = \boldsymbol{D}_c^{-1}\boldsymbol{P}'\boldsymbol{FD}^{-1}$ and $\boldsymbol{F} = \boldsymbol{D}_r^{-1}\boldsymbol{PGD}^{-1}$. The elements $d_1, \ldots, d_p$ of $\boldsymbol{D}$ are known as the *principal inertias* of the two configurations, and their squares d_i^2 are used in place of the λ_i in the goodness-of-fit measure $\alpha_{1,k}$ of **5.8** for the k-dimensional correspondence analysis solution. The two configurations are often superimposed to provide a compact representation of the whole system. Note, however, that there is no direct distance relation between a point representing a row profile and one representing a column profile, so such a superposition of diagrams must be interpreted with caution. If a pictorial representation relating row and column profiles is required, then biplots (**4.9**) should be used, see Example 4.2.

Example 5.9

Table 5.8 shows the matrix $\boldsymbol{E}$ for the Caithness schoolchildren. Singular value decomposition of this matrix yields the non-zero principal inertias 0.1992, 0.0301 and 0.0009. Thus the goodness-of-fit measure $\alpha_{1,2}$ is 99.99%, indicating excellent fit in two dimensions. The coordinates $\boldsymbol{f}_1, \boldsymbol{f}_2, \boldsymbol{g}_1, \boldsymbol{g}_2$ in the two-dimensional representations of the row and column profiles obtained from the singular value decomposition of $\boldsymbol{E}$ are also given in Table 5.8, and these coordinates recover the configurations of Figs. 5.8 and 5.9 exactly.

5.20 Various alternative approaches to the analysis of an $I \times J$ contingency table have been proposed over the years, having seemingly different objectives to those of correspondence analysis. For example, in *reciprocal averaging* (Hill, 1973), we seek to assign numerical scores to the categories of the row and column classifications. This generates two 'continuous' variables, x and y say, whose bivariate frequency distribution is given by the contingency table $\boldsymbol{N}$. The objective of reciprocal averaging is to allocate the scores in such a way as to maximise the correlation between x and y. *Dual scaling* (Nishisato, 1980) also seeks to construct two such continuous variables x and y, but the bivariate frequency distribution that arises is viewed this time from the perspective of two-way analysis of variance. The objective is to find scores such that the values 'within rows' should be as similar as possible while those 'between rows' are as different as possible. Yet a third variation on the same theme is the simultaneous linear regressions approach of Lingoes (1968), who seeks the scores in such a way that the regressions of y on x and of x on y are simultaneously as optimal as possible. Greenacre (1984) outlines the algebra for each of these approaches and demonstrates in fact that they are all equivalent to the correspondence analysis of **5.19** above, while Greenacre (1993) presents a practical view of all aspects of the technique. We will see the extension of these ideas to more general nonlinear multivariate methodology in Chapter 8.

Note that correspondence analysis has been presented here as a method for analysing contingency tables, in which the entries are counts of independent events. This is the only situation in which inferential arguments are possible, but the technique has also been widely used (particularly by French statisticians) as a data-analytic method for other types of data. This usage can be justified if the chi-squared distance (**5.17**) is a reasonable dissimilarity measure for the data in hand. An exposition of this approach to data analysis may be found, for example, in Jambu (1991).

Indicator matrices and higher-order tables

5.21 An $I \times J$ contingency table with grand total of its entries n is a summary of observations made on n individuals. Each of these n observations can be thought of as a vector that indicates which of the I row categories and which of the J column categories is exhibited by a given individual. Such a vector will have $I + J$ elements, the first I corresponding to the row categories and the remaining J corresponding to the column categories, with ones in the two positions corresponding to the occupied categories and zeros everywhere else. Thus the contingency table $\boldsymbol{N}$ can be expanded to an $n \times (I + J)$ matrix $\boldsymbol{Z}$, each row of which is such an indicator vector for one of the n individuals; i.e. $\boldsymbol{Z}$ contains n_{ij} rows with a one in the ith and $(I + j)$th columns and zeros elsewhere ($i = 1, \ldots, I; j = 1, \ldots, J$). The matrix $\boldsymbol{Z}$ is called the *indicator matrix* of the contingency table. It represents the data matrix from which the table was formed (apart from permutations of its rows).

Greenacre (1984) shows that correspondence analysis of $\boldsymbol{Z}$ is closely related to that of the contingency table itself, and also that the latter is equivalent to a canonical correlation analysis (**4.10**) between the first I and remaining

J columns of $\boldsymbol{Z}$. However, the main use of the indicator matrix is in the analysis of higher-order contingency tables. Suppose, for example, that $\boldsymbol{N}$ is an $(I \times J \times K \times L)$ contingency table formed from cross-classification of four factors. Then the matrix $\boldsymbol{Z}$ has dimension $n \times (I + J + K + L)$, and each row contains four ones with the remaining elements all being zero. The symmetric matrix $\boldsymbol{Z}'\boldsymbol{Z}$, often called the *Burt* matrix, gives the elements of pairwise marginal tables formed from $\boldsymbol{N}$. A simple correspondence analysis of this matrix is called a *multiple correspondence analysis* of $\boldsymbol{N}$; it is equivalent to a decomposition of the residuals from a main-effects model for the contingency table.

Full details of multiple correspondence analysis are given by Greenacre (1984) , while Van der Heiden *et al* (1989) show how the concept of decomposing residuals allows correspondence analysis to be linked with more complex log-linear models in the analysis of contingency tables. Greenacre (1988b) extends the methodology to cope with correspondence analysis of multivariate categorical data. More generally, Heiser (1987) considers least absolute residuals in place of least squares as a criterion of fit, while Pack and Jolliffe (1992) and Kim (1992) investigate diagnostics for influential observations in correspondence analysis.

Procrustes analysis

5.22 Various techniques have now been described for producing a configuration of points representing multivariate observations, starting either from a data matrix of objects by variables or from a proximity matrix between objects. The opportunity thus exists for generating different geometrical represention of a single set of individuals. Two different configurations will be obtained, for example, if two different techniques (such as metric and non-metric scaling) are applied to the same proximity matrix, or if a single technique is used but on two different proximity matrices derived from the same data matrix (by employing two different dissimilarity measures). Gower (1971b) lists other ways in which the situation can arise. In all such cases, it is of interest to quantify the difference between the two configurations, as this will provide a means of comparing the two multivariate techniques, or the two dissimilarity measures, for the given set of data. But since the two representations are of the same multivariate observations, each point of one configuration corresponds directly to a single point of the other configuration, so the difference between the two configurations can be measured by aggregating in some way the differences between their corresponding points. Moreover, any configuration is defined purely in terms of the internal relationships among its points, and is not affected either by its position or its orientation in space. Consequently, the two configurations should be matched as closely as possible by translation, rotation and reflection of one configuration relative to the other before the difference between them is determined. 'Closeness of matching' can also be measured in various ways, but standard statistical practice and intuitive geometrical concepts suggest that we should use the criterion of least squares. Mathematically, therefore, the problem is stated as follows: given two p-dimensional configurations of n points, with coordinates $(\boldsymbol{x}_1, \dots, \boldsymbol{x}_n)$ and $(\boldsymbol{y}_1, \dots, \boldsymbol{y}_n)$ respectively, we wish to find the transformation $z_i = Ay_i + b$ for $i = 1, \ldots, n$ and orthogonal A such that

$$M^2 = \sum_{i=1}^{n} \| x_i - z_i \| \qquad (5.24)$$

is minimised, where $\| x \| = x'x$. The minimum value M_0^2 is then a measure of the difference between the two configurations.

5.23 To find this minimum value, we need to find the minimising translation b and rotation/reflection A of the second configuration relative to the first. It is easy to see that, from their nature, these two operations can be conducted separately. Considering the translation first, simple algebra shows that $\sum_{i=1}^{n} \| x_i - z_i \|$ is equal to $\sum_{i=1}^{n} \| x_i - \bar{x} \| + \sum_{i=1}^{n} \| z_i - \bar{z} \| + n(\bar{x} - \bar{z})^2$. This expression is clearly minimised when $\bar{x} = \bar{z}$, so $b = \bar{x} - \bar{y}$. Thus the required translation is obtained by superimposing the centroids of the two configurations, and this can be achieved most easily by mean-centring each one at the outset.

Assuming therefore that the configurations are both centred at the origin, their coordinates can be written as the rows of the matrices $X = (x_1 - \bar{x}, \ldots, x_n - \bar{x})'$ and $Y = (y_1 - \bar{y}, \ldots, y_n - \bar{y})'$. Equation (5.24) thus reduces to

$$\begin{aligned} M^2 &= \sum_{i=1}^{n} \| x_i - Ay_i \| && (5.25) \\ &= \operatorname{tr}[(X - YA)(X - YA)'] && (5.26) \\ &= \operatorname{tr}(XX') + \operatorname{tr}(YY') - 2\operatorname{tr}(X'YA) && (5.27) \end{aligned}$$

where A is orthogonal. Thus minimising M^2 with respect to rotation and reflection is equivalent to maximising $\operatorname{tr}(X'YA)$ with respect to A, subject to the $p(p+1)/2$ constraints on its elements given by $AA' = I$. Let $\frac{1}{2}\Lambda$ be a $(p \times p)$ symmetric matrix for these constraints, so that we need to maximise

$$V = \operatorname{tr}[Y'XA - \tfrac{1}{2}\Lambda(AA' - I)]. \qquad (5.28)$$

Differentiating this expression directly and equating the derivatives to zero, we find that A must satisfy

$$Y'X = \Lambda A. \qquad (5.29)$$

Let the singular value decomposition of $Y'X$ be given by VDU', where V and U are orthogonal $(p \times p)$ matrices and D is a diagonal matrix of non-negative elements. Thus, remembering that Λ is symmetric and that A is orthogonal, we deduce from (5.29) that

$$\Lambda^2 = Y'XA'AX'Y = Y'XX'Y = (VDU')(UDV'). \qquad (5.30)$$

Thus we can take $\Lambda = VDV'$. Substituting for $Y'X$ and Λ into (5.29) shows that the minimising rotation/reflection is given by $A = VU'$; this is known as the *Procrustes rotation* for comparison of the two configurations, and the 'best' rotation of Y relative to X is given by YA. Further substitution for $X'Y$ and A into (5.27) gives the measure of difference between the two configurations as

$$M_0^2 = \operatorname{tr}(XX') + \operatorname{tr}(YY') - 2\operatorname{tr}(UDU').$$

This has the alternative expressions

$$M_0^2 = \mathrm{tr}(\boldsymbol{XX}') + \mathrm{tr}(\boldsymbol{YY}') - 2\mathrm{tr}\boldsymbol{D}$$

(using the fact that $\mathrm{tr}(\boldsymbol{AB}) = \mathrm{tr}(\boldsymbol{BA})$), or

$$M_0^2 = \mathrm{tr}(\boldsymbol{XX}') + \mathrm{tr}(\boldsymbol{YY}') - 2\mathrm{tr}(\boldsymbol{X}'\boldsymbol{YY}'\boldsymbol{X})^{1/2}$$

(on noting that $\boldsymbol{X}'\boldsymbol{YY}'\boldsymbol{X} = \boldsymbol{UD}^2\boldsymbol{U}'$ from the singular value decomposition above), or

$$M_0^2 = \mathrm{tr}(\boldsymbol{X}'\boldsymbol{X}) + \mathrm{tr}(\boldsymbol{Y}'\boldsymbol{Y}) - 2\mathrm{tr}[(\boldsymbol{X}'\boldsymbol{X})^{1/2}(\boldsymbol{Y}'\boldsymbol{Y})(\boldsymbol{X}'\boldsymbol{X})^{1/2}]$$

(on using $\mathrm{tr}(\boldsymbol{AB}) = \mathrm{tr}(\boldsymbol{BA})$ in each term of the previous expression). The first form is the best for computation, the second was first given (in the context of factor analysis) by Green (1952) while the third involves only the inner product matrices $\boldsymbol{X}'\boldsymbol{X}$ and $\boldsymbol{Y}'\boldsymbol{Y}$ so may be useful in certain cases. The statistic M_0^2 is also known as the *Procrustes statistic* for comparison of the two configurations. Commutability of matrices under the trace operation shows immediately that the same value of M_0^2 results whether $\boldsymbol{Y}$ is fitted to $\boldsymbol{X}$ or vice-versa.

5.24 Two problems are likely to occur with the above procedure as regards direct practical application. The first is that the two configurations for comparison may not have the same dimensionalities. Suppose that $\boldsymbol{X}$ is $(n \times p)$ as before, but that $\boldsymbol{Y}$ is $(n \times k)$ where $k < p$. This problem is overcome most commonly by appending $p - k$ columns of zeros to $\boldsymbol{Y}$, thereby 'filling it out' to be $(n \times p)$, and then applying the above procedure directly. By doing this we are essentially treating the first k axes of the $\boldsymbol{X}$ configuration as coincident with those of the $\boldsymbol{Y}$ configuration, and taking the latter configuration as lying in this k-dimensional subspace of the former. Rather than expanding the k-dimensional configuration to p dimensions, however, it may be felt more appropriate to collapse the p-dimensional one to k. Here we would want first to project $\boldsymbol{X}$ into the subspace of $\boldsymbol{Y}$ before applying the above procedure to the two configurations in this subspace, or equivalently to seek a $(p \times k)$ matrix $\boldsymbol{B}$ such that $\boldsymbol{XB}$ best fits $\boldsymbol{Y}$. Other variations may arise in special circumstances.

The second problem occurs when the scales of the two configurations are different. One way of dealing with this problem is to extend the above procedure to include uniform stretching or shrinking (i.e. *dilation*) along with translation and rotation/reflection in the fitting process. Thus we now seek a scale constant c as well as an orthogonal matrix $\boldsymbol{A}$ and a vector $\boldsymbol{b}$, the transformation in (5.24) becoming $\boldsymbol{z}_i = c\boldsymbol{A}\boldsymbol{y}_i + \boldsymbol{b}$ for $i = 1, \ldots, n$. The translation $\boldsymbol{b}$ is once again taken care of by ensuring that $\boldsymbol{X}$ and $\boldsymbol{Y}$ are both mean-centred. Proceeding as before, we now wish to minimise

$$M^2 = \mathrm{tr}(\boldsymbol{XX}') + c^2\mathrm{tr}(\boldsymbol{YY}') - 2c\mathrm{tr}(\boldsymbol{X}'\boldsymbol{YA}) \qquad (5.31)$$

with respect to c and orthogonal $\boldsymbol{A}$. For fixed $c > 0$, maximisation with respect to $\boldsymbol{A}$ gives the same solution as previously so that

$$M^2 = \mathrm{tr}(\boldsymbol{XX}') + c^2\mathrm{tr}(\boldsymbol{YY}') - 2c\mathrm{tr}[(\boldsymbol{Y}'\boldsymbol{YX}'\boldsymbol{Y})^{1/2}]. \qquad (5.32)$$

Differentiation with respect to c then yields the minimising value as

$$c = \mathrm{tr}[(\boldsymbol{Y}'\boldsymbol{YX}'\boldsymbol{Y})^{1/2}]/\mathrm{tr}[\boldsymbol{YY}'], \qquad (5.33)$$

and back substitution yields

$$M_0^2 = \text{tr}[XX'] - \text{tr}[(Y'YX'Y)^{1/2}]/\text{tr}[YY']. \quad (5.34)$$

However, M_0^2 is now no longer symmetric in X and Y, so that if dilation is permitted then optimal fitting of Y to X yields a different solution from optimal fitting of X to Y. This is clearly an unsatisfactory feature. Instead of including dilation in the process, therefore, Gower (1971b) suggests initial standardisation of the configurations so that $\text{tr}(XX') = \text{tr}(YY') = 1$, followed by the rotation step only.

5.25 The name 'Procrustes analysis' was first coined by Hurley and Cattell (1962) in the context of factor analysis, where interest often centres on matching a set of factor loadings, either to a previously obtained set or to some hypothesised 'target' set. In this context the technique can be traced back to Mosier (1939); other principal references are Green (1952), Cliff (1966), Schönemann (1966, 1968), Gruvaeus (1970), and Schönemann and Carroll (1970). Its use in multidimensional scaling and other ordination methods was initiated by Gower (1971b). Goodall (1991), in the course of a study on Procrustes methods in the analysis of shape (see **4.3** and also Volume 2), introduces the idea of weighted Procrustes analysis. Here the objective is to minimise

$$M_0^2 = \text{tr}[W(X - YA)(X - YA)'], \quad (5.35)$$

where W is a matrix of weights, and the centring of the two configurations has been made with respect to suitably weighted means (i.e. barycentres). Goodall draws connections between this analysis and regression methods. Note that if W is a diagonal matrix with elements $w_1, \ldots, w_n$, then interpretation of M_0^2 is as a weighted sum of squares with the ith points of the two configurations receiving weight w_i. This case can be handled by multiplying each row of the centred X and Y by $\sqrt{w_i}$, and then using ordinary Procrustes analysis. Further theoretical results are given by Ten Berge (1977), who establishes existence of Procrustes rotations, and Sibson (1978), who shows that M_0^2 is a metric (but not Euclidean). Alternative statistics for the comparison of multivariate configurations have been suggested by Robert and Escoufier (1976) and Siegel and Benson (1982). Verboon and Heiser (1992) consider alternative loss criteria for least squares Procrustes analysis, based on (i) the Huber function and (ii) the biweight function, in order to provide a method that is resistant to outliers.

Example 5.10

Table 5.9 gives measurements of various blood groups on seven Indian tribes, for each of the characters *ABO*, *Rh* and *MN* (Sanghvi, 1966). The data are in the form of multinomial proportions for each character, there being four multinomial categories for *ABO*, seven for *Rh* and two for *MN*. To investigate the relationships among the tribes for any such character, we require a measure of distance between two multinomial populations. Bhattacharyya (1946) defined such a distance D_c by

$$D_c^2 = [\cos^{-1} \sum_{k=1}^{m} \sqrt{(p_{1k}p_{2k})}]^2, \quad (5.36)$$

Table 5.9 Blood group measurements on seven Indian tribes for the characters *ABO, Rh* and *MN*, from Sanghvi (1966).

		Tribes						
Char.	Cat.	Koli	Bhil	Dubla	Naika	Dhanka	Dhodia	Gamit
ABO	A_1	.114	.203	.151	.181	.166	.253	.274
	A_2	.016	.008	.017	.018	.018	.010	.010
	B	.208	.257	.254	.211	.234	.127	.147
	O	.662	.532	.579	.590	.583	.610	.569
Rh	R_1	.652	.673	.671	.751	.769	.793	.760
	R_2	.060	.013	.071	.069	.050	.070	.059
	R_0	.049	.121	.101	.088	.099	.062	.110
	R_z	.004	.023	.000	.004	.003	.003	.000
	r	.234	.133	.128	.088	.080	.072	.036
	r'	.000	.000	.029	.000	.000	.000	.004
	r''	.000	.037	.000	.000	.000	.000	.000
MN	M	.636	.585	.604	.494	.552	.448	.537
	N	.364	.415	.396	.506	.448	.552	.463

if there are m multinomial categories and p_{1k}, p_{2k} are the proportions in category k of the two populations. D_c was also shown by Edwards and Cavalli-Sforza (1964) to be the arc along the great circle joining two points representing the populations, when the sample space is transformed into $(\frac{1}{2})^m$ of the surface of the unit hyperspere in m dimensions by means of the angular transformation $\theta = \sin^{-1}\sqrt{p}$. This being a curved space, it is of interest to find a projection into a Euclidean space together with an associated distance between the populations. Edwards (1971) defined the optimal projection required to achieve a Euclidean representation to be the orthomorphic zenithal projection, also called the *stereographic* projection. He showed that the Euclidean distance between the two populations under stereographic projection is given by

$$D_e^2 = \frac{8[1 - \sum_{k=1}^m \sqrt{(p_{1k}p_{2k})}]}{[1 + \sum_{k=1}^m \sqrt{(p_{1k}/m)}][1 + \sum_{k=1}^m \sqrt{(p_{2k}/m)}]}. \tag{5.37}$$

A much simpler procedure would be to ignore the curved nature of the population space and to use the the straightforward Euclidean distance

$$D_x^2 = \sum_{k=1}^m (p_{1k} - p_{2k})^2, \tag{5.38}$$

but it is unclear how good an approximation this would provide. To investigate the two approximations D_e^2 and D_x^2 to D_c^2, Krzanowski (1971) used Procrustes methods on the data in Table 5.9. For each of the three characters *ABO*, *Rh* and *MN* separately, he first obtained the three (7×7) matrices of distances between the tribes using in turn each of the three distances given above. He then derived 7-point configurations from each of these distance matrices by means of classical scaling. Thus

Table 5.10 M_0^2 values between three distance measures, as obtained from data on three characters for seven Indian tribes; values in each cell are for characters *ABO*, *Rh* and *MN*, in that order reading downwards

D_e	0.00012 0.00054 0.00030	
D_x	0.02530 0.26472 0.00049	0.02479 0.25460 0.00006
	D_c	D_e

for each character there were three distinct configurations depicting the seven tribes, one configuration corresponding to each distance measure. Pairwise matching of these three configurations were then conducted by Procrustes analysis for each character, and the resultant M_0^2 values are given in Table 5.10. We note that the M_0^2 values between D_e and D_c are always very small. This indicates a very good fit between the coordinates obtained from Bhattacharyya's measure and those from the measure after stereographic projection, across all characters. Using the fact that M_0^2 is a metric, we can now treat Table 5.10 as providing three distance matrices, one for each character, between the three measures D_c, D_e and D_x. Classical scaling of each of these three matrices produced the pictures shown in Fig. 5.10. Points representing D_c and D_e are always in close proximity, indicating that the stereographic projection gives a consistently good approximation to the original curved space (noting that for three points and Euclidean space, only two dimensions are needed for exact representation). The simple distance D_x approximates D_c poorly when extreme values are present [as for *Rh*, shown in (ii)], but well when all values lie near the centre of the population space [as for *MN*, shown in (iii)].

5.26 Krzanowski (1987a) uses Procrustes analysis as an essential component in a procedure for selecting variables to preserve the structure of a given multivariate data set. The basic idea is as follows. Suppose that $\boldsymbol{X}$ is an $(n \times p)$ data matrix whose effective structure is embodied in the $(n \times k)$ matrix of principal component scores $\boldsymbol{Y}$, and the m 'most important' variables in determining this structure are sought. There are $\frac{p!}{m!(p-m)!}$ subsets of m variables to be considered. Let $[j]$ be the jth such subset (with respect to any chosen ordering) ; denote by $\boldsymbol{X}_{[j]}$ the $(n \times m)$ data matrix using these variables and by $\boldsymbol{Y}_{[j]}$ the $(n \times k)$ matrix of principal component scores computed from $\boldsymbol{X}_{[j]}$. The extent to which subset $[j]$ has 'lost' the original structure in the data is then measured by $M_{0,[j]}^2$, the Procrustes statistic obtained from comparison of $\boldsymbol{Y}_{[j]}$ with $\boldsymbol{Y}$; the 'best' subset is the one with minimum $M_{0,[j]}^2$. An 'all subset' search may be computationally prohibitive, so Krzanowski (1987a) also discusses a backward elimination implementation of this procedure. Krzanowski (1993a)

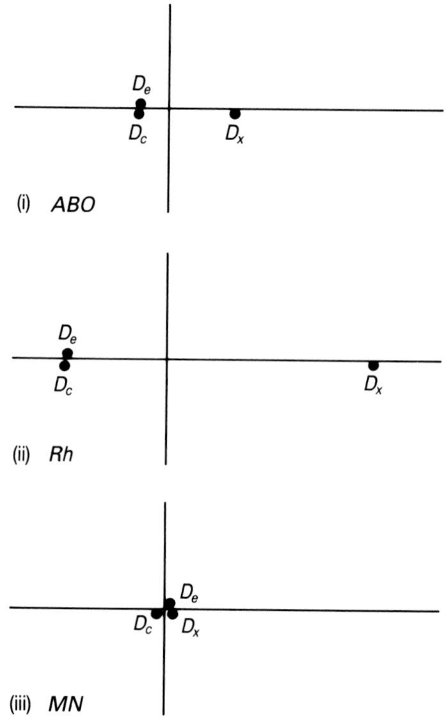

Figure 5.10 First two principal axes for comparison of D_e, D_c and D_x. Reproduced with permission from Krzanowski (1971).

extends the same idea to incidence matrices via correspondence analysis, which requires a weighted Procrustes analysis in place of an ordinary one.

5.27 All the above theory and application of Procrustes methodology is purely descriptive in nature. What it lacks is any guideline as to the amount of sampling variability to be expected in the statistic M_0^2, so that objective decisions can be made in given circumstances about distinctness of two matched configurations. No exact distributional results for M_0^2 have yet been obtained, however, and we have to be content with some asymptotic approximations. Davis (1978) showed that the asymptotic distribution in the case of two independent sets of Mahalanobis D^2 distances, obtained from the same p-variate normal population (equal numbers of samples, equal sample sizes), is approximated by a multiple of the chi-square distribution. Sibson (1979) considered perturbations of a configuration. More specifically, he assumed that $\boldsymbol{X}$ is a centred $(n \times p)$ matrix of full rank p, that $\boldsymbol{Y}$ is a perturbed value of $\boldsymbol{X}$ given by $\boldsymbol{Y} = \boldsymbol{X} + \epsilon\boldsymbol{Z} + O(\epsilon^2)$, and that the elements of $\boldsymbol{Z}$ are i.i.d. $N(0, 1)$. Under these circumstances, he showed that M_0^2 is distributed as $\epsilon^2\chi^2_{[np-\frac{1}{2}p(p+1)]} + O(\epsilon^3)$ for matching under translation and rotation/reflection. If dilation is also permitted, then the distribution is the same except that one degree of freedom is lost in the chi square. Langron and Collins (1985) extended this result to the case of comparison of two perturbations of the same configuration, i.e. they considered the case of matching $\boldsymbol{X}_1 = \boldsymbol{X}+\epsilon\boldsymbol{Z}_1+O(\epsilon^2)$ and $\boldsymbol{X}_2 = \boldsymbol{X}+\epsilon\boldsymbol{Z}_2+O(\epsilon^2)$ where the elements of both $\boldsymbol{Z}_1, \boldsymbol{Z}_2$ are i.i.d. $N(0,1)$. They showed that in this case M_0^2 is distributed as $2\epsilon^2\chi^2_{[np-\frac{1}{2}p(p+1)]} + O(\epsilon^3)$ for matching under translation and rotation/reflection with, again, one degree of freedom lost when dilation is included. This result enabled them to partition M_0^2 into terms corresponding to each of the separate operations of translation, rotation/reflection and dilation, and to summarise them in an analysis of variance that has the usual F tests of significance for each operation.

Generalised Procrustes analysis

5.28 Suppose now that there are m p-dimensional configurations, the coordinates for the ith being given by the rows of $\boldsymbol{X}_i$ for $i = 1, \ldots, m$, and that we wish to compare these configurations. Example 5.10 shows one way of doing this, namely by pairwise Procrustes analysis of the configurations followed by multidimensional scaling of the resulting matrix of M_0^2 values. A more direct approach would be to find *simultaneous* translations, rotations, reflections and scalings of the m configurations into positions of best fit with respect to each other. Simultaneous 'closeness' of all m configurations would then be measured by the resulting goodness of fit value, and this value could be interpreted by inspecting the m matched configurations. Again, various goodness of fit criteria are possible, but if the measure adopted is the residual sum of squares between each point of each configuration and the corresponding point of the average (or 'consensus') configuration then we obtain a generalisation of the above Procrustes methodology. This is known as *generalised Procrustes analysis (GPA)*. The idea was first considered by Kristof and Wingersky (1971), but it was put into its currently adopted framework by Gower (1975) while Ten Berge (1977) provided some improvements to the algorithm which guarantee convergence of the iterative procedure. Summaries of the method are given by Langron and Collins (1985) and Goodall (1991); the following brief description essentially draws on the former.

5.29 The goodness of fit measure can be written most conveniently as

$$M_G^2 = \operatorname{tr}\left[\sum_{i=1}^{m}(\boldsymbol{Z}_i - \boldsymbol{Z}^*)(\boldsymbol{Z}_i - \boldsymbol{Z}^*)'\right], \tag{5.39}$$

where the $\boldsymbol{Z}_i$ are the configurations $\boldsymbol{X}_i$ after any appropriate translations, rotations, reflections and scalings $(i = 1, \ldots, m)$ while $\boldsymbol{Z}^* = \frac{1}{m}\sum_{i=1}^{m}\boldsymbol{Z}_i$ is the consensus of these transformed configurations. GPA thus seeks the various transformations that minimise M_G^2.

Optimum matching of configurations under translation is again achieved by ensuring that the $\boldsymbol{X}_i$ have a common origin, which will be the case if they are all initially mean-centred. We therefore assume that this has been done.

Matching under rotation and reflection is achieved by the series of transformations $Z_i = X_i A_i$, where

$$A_i = X^* X_i'(X_i X^{*\prime} X^* X_i')^{-1/2} \tag{5.40}$$

for $i = 1, \ldots, n$ and $X^* = \frac{1}{m}\sum_{i=1}^{m} X_i$. However, as the consensus configuration changes with each individual transformation, the process is an iterative one. Clearly, also, the final solution is arbitrary up to orthogonal transformations of X^*; a unique solution is obtained by referring X^* to its principal axis representation.

GPA under the above operations in the case $m = 2$ is equivalent to ordinary Procrustes analysis (Gower, 1975). However, if we additionally wish to include dilations among the permitted transformations then standard theory does not generalise to m configurations as the consensus contracts to the origin. This problem is obviated by imposing an additional constraint. Ten Berge (1977) shows that if the constraint

$$\sum_{i=1}^{m} s_i^2 \mathrm{tr}(X_i X_i') = \sum_{i=1}^{m} \mathrm{tr}(X_i X_i') \tag{5.41}$$

is imposed, then the optimum scaling factors s_i are given by

$$s_i = \left[\frac{\sum_{i=1}^{m} \mathrm{tr}(X_i X_i')}{\mathrm{tr}(X_i X_i')}\right] p_{1i} \tag{5.42}$$

where $p_1' = (p_{11}, \ldots, p_{1m})$ is the eigenvector corresponding to the largest eigenvalue of the matrix Φ whose (i, j)th element is given by

$$\phi_{ij} = (\mathrm{tr}[X_i X_j'])(\mathrm{tr}[X_i X_i'])^{-1/2}(\mathrm{tr}[X_j X_j'])^{-1/2}. \tag{5.43}$$

Furthermore, the A_i given by equation (5.40) remain unchanged by a rescaling of the X_i, so the order of rotation/reflection and dilation is unimportant.

5.30 Peay (1988) considers a variation of the goodness of fit measure M_G^2, by optimising the matching of the m configurations in a reduced number of dimensions. This is motivated by the fact that displaying the outcome of a GPA can generally only be done in two or three dimensions. Langron and Collins (1985) extend Sibson's (1979) perturbation analysis to GPA. They show that if $X_i = XR_i + \epsilon Z_i + O(\epsilon^2)$ for $i = 1, \ldots, m$, where X_i is an $(n \times p)$ matrix of observations, R_i is an orthogonal $(p \times p)$ matrix, X is an $(n \times p)$ 'true' configuration, and Z_i is an $(n \times p)$ matrix of errors whose elements are i.i.d. $N(0, 1)$, then the minimised value of M_G^2 is distributed as $\epsilon^2 \chi^2_{[m-1][np-\frac{1}{2}p(p+1)]} + O(\epsilon^3)$ for matching under rotation and reflection. If dilations are also included in the matching, then a further $m - 1$ degrees of freedom are lost in the chi-square. These results enable the analysis of variance breakdown of ordinary Procrustes analysis to be extended to GPA.

All the foregoing theory has assumed that the X_i all have the same dimensions $(n \times p)$. If X_i is $(n \times p_i)$ where the p_i are not all equal, the simplest procedure is to set $p = \max(p_1, \ldots, p_m)$ and then to 'fill out' each X_i to have dimension $(n \times p)$ by appending a suitable number of columns of zeros.

Example 5.11

Generalised Procrustes analysis has become a popular technique in food

Table 5.11 Key to meat products investigated by GPA

1.	Sausage	10.	Minced Beef	18.	Roast Chicken
2.	Luncheon Meat	11.	Steak	19.	Duck
3.	Paté	12.	Corned Beef	20.	Roast Turkey
4.	Liver	13.	Veal	21.	Chicken Casserole
5.	Salami	14.	Pork Chops	22.	Lamb Chops
6.	Black Pudding	15.	Bacon	23.	Roast Lamb
7.	Tongue	16.	Pork Pies	24.	Beefburgers
8.	Roast Beef	17.	Ham	25.	Rabbit
9.	Stewed Beef				

research for the analysis of sensory data, where it is used for comparing the differences and agreements between the views of several assessors regarding the properties of the same (food) substances. Gains *et al* (1988) report the results of an investigation in which twenty-eight assessors were asked to compare the twenty-five meat products listed in Table 5.11. The investigation was done using *free-choice profiling*, in which each assessor devises his or her own list of features on which to score each product. Thus if assessor i chooses p_i features, then the data matrix $\boldsymbol{X}_i$ for that assessor will be $(25 \times p_i)$ for $i = 1, \ldots, 28$. For further discussion of free-choice profiling, see e.g. Williams and Langron, 1984; in the present case p_i ranged between 11 and 36. A major objective of the study was to investigate the perceived similarities and differences between the twenty-five products, and this can best be achieved by obtaining the consensus configuration derived from GPA of the twenty-eight data matrices $\boldsymbol{X}_i$. Since the p_i varied between assessors, and since the maximum p_i was 36, each $\boldsymbol{X}_i$ was first 'filled out' to be (25×36) by appending an appropriate number of columns of zeros. The first two principal axes of the resulting consensus configuration are shown in Fig. 5.11. Groupings of products, e.g. 13 (Veal) 19 (Duck) and 25 (Rabbit), indicate those products perceived to be very similar in general, while well separated products, e.g. 7 (Tongue) and 10 (Minced Beef), indicate those products perceived to be rather different from each other.

This analysis takes all the information generated by each assessor. However, it can be argued that when an assessor devises a list of features in the free-choice profiling procedure, many of the chosen features will be inter-correlated, perhaps highly so, and the essential information provided by each assessor has dimensionality considerably smaller than the chosen p_i. To test this assertion Gains *et al* subjected each of the twenty-eight $\boldsymbol{X}_i$ separately to the variable selection procedure described in **5.26** above, choosing just the 'best' four features for each assessor. The resulting twenty-eight (25×4) matrices were then subjected to GPA, and the first two principal axes of the consensus configuration are shown in Fig. 5.12. It can be seen that the relationships among the meat products are virtually indistinguishable from the previous patterns, indicating that the comparison of the products can be done adequately on just four features for each assessor. The assessor who chose thirty-six features was thus being grossly over conscientious!

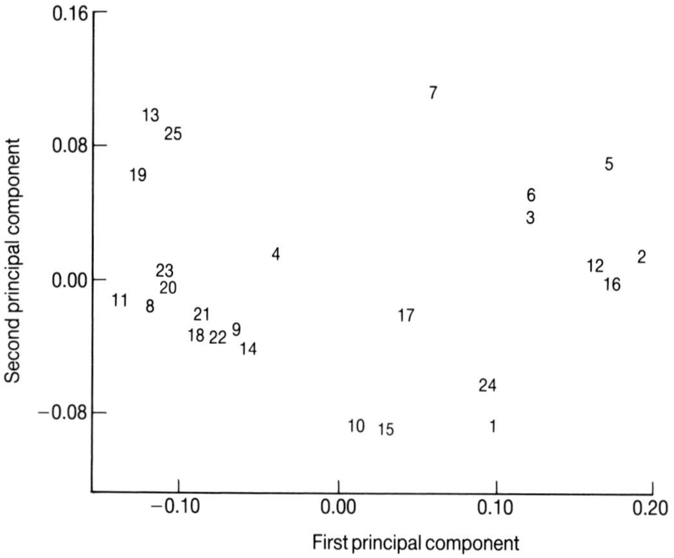

Figure 5.11 Plot of the 25 meats from Table 5.11 on the first two principal axes of the consensus configuration derived from GPA of the full data set. Reproduced with permission from Gains *et al* (1988).

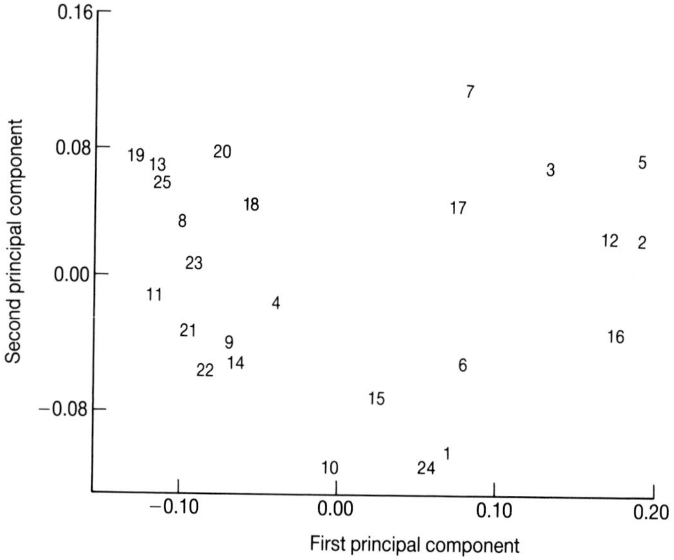

Figure 5.12 Plot of the 25 meats from Table 5.11 on the first two principal axes of the consensus configuration derived from GPA of the reduced data set. Reproduced with permission from Gains *et al* (1988).

Exercises

5.1 Show that the Jaccard dissimilarity coefficient defined in **3.25** is not Euclidean.
Hint. Set up the following counterexample. Suppose that four units have $3+q$ variables observed on them such that the first q variables have value 1 on all four units, variable $q+1$ has value 1 for the first unit and 0 for the others, variable $q+2$ has value 1 for the second unit and zero for the others, and variable $q+2$ has value 1 for the third unit and 0 for the others. Calculate the inter-unit dissimilarities and use Example 5.1.

(Gower and Legendre, 1986)

5.2 If $\boldsymbol{S}$ is positive semi-definite, show that $s_{ii} + s_{jj} - 2s_{ij} > 0$ and that the distance d_{ij} defined by $d_{ij}^2 = s_{ii} + s_{jj} - 2s_{ij}$ satisfies the triangle inequality.

5.3 If $\boldsymbol{D}$ is a dissimilarity matrix with elements d_{ij} and $\boldsymbol{\Delta}$ is the matrix with elements $-\frac{1}{2}d_{ij}^2$, show that the matrix with elements $(d_{ij}^2 + h)^{1/2}$ is Euclidean when $h \geqslant -\lambda_n$, the smallest eigenvalue of

$$\boldsymbol{\Delta}_1 = (\boldsymbol{I}-\mathbf{11}'/\mathbf{n})\boldsymbol{\Delta}(\boldsymbol{I}-\mathbf{11}'/\mathbf{n}).$$

(Lingoes, 1971)

5.4 If $\boldsymbol{D}, \boldsymbol{\Delta}$ and $\boldsymbol{\Delta}_1$ are as defined in exercise 5.3, and $\boldsymbol{\Delta}_2$ is defined as $\boldsymbol{\Delta}_1$ but for elements $-\frac{1}{2}d_{ij}$ rather than $-\frac{1}{2}d_{ij}^2$, show that the matrix with elements $d_{ij} + k$ is Euclidean when $k \geqslant \mu_n$, the largest eigenvalue of

$$\begin{pmatrix} \mathbf{0} & 2\boldsymbol{\Delta}_1 \\ -\boldsymbol{I} & 2\boldsymbol{\Delta}_2 \end{pmatrix}.$$

(Cailliez, 1983)

5.5 Prove Theorem 5 for the special case $\boldsymbol{s} = \frac{1}{n}\mathbf{1}$.

(Seber, 1984, p236)

5.6 Suppose that the dissimilarity matrix $\boldsymbol{D}$ is obtained by calculating Euclidean distances (**3.24**) between all pairs of rows of the $(n \times p)$ data matrix $\boldsymbol{Y}$. Show that the principal coordinates in k dimensions obtained from classical scaling of $\boldsymbol{D}$ are given by the centred scores of the n objects on the first k principal components of $\boldsymbol{Y}$.

(Gower, 1966a; Mardia *et al*, 1979, p405)

5.7 Suppose that the $(n \times k)$ matrix $\boldsymbol{X}$ gives the principal coordinates in k dimensions derived from an $(n \times n)$ Euclidean matrix $\boldsymbol{D}$, and suppose that $d_{i,n+1}$ for $i = 1, \ldots, n$ give the Euclidean distances from a new, $(n+1)$th, point to each of the n existing points. We wish to position the new point optimally in this configuration. Let d_i^2 be the square of the distance of the ith point from the centroid of the configuration for $i = 1, \ldots, n$, so that d_i^2 is the ith diagonal element of $\boldsymbol{XX}'$. Show that the coordinates giving the optimal position of the new point on the k dimensions of the configuration are given by the elements of the vector $\frac{1}{2}(\boldsymbol{X}'\boldsymbol{X})^{-1}\ \boldsymbol{X}'\boldsymbol{d}$, where $\boldsymbol{d}' = (d_1^2 - d_{1,n+1}^2, \ldots, d_n^2 - d_{n,n+1}^2)$.

(Gower, 1968)

5.8 Consider the first term of equation (5.17), i.e. $\lambda(\boldsymbol{uv}' - \boldsymbol{vu}')$ where λ is the largest eigenvalue, of multiplicity 2, and $\boldsymbol{u}, \boldsymbol{v}$ are the corresponding eigenvectors of $\boldsymbol{NN}' = -\boldsymbol{N}^2$ for skew-symmetric $(n \times n)$ matrix $\boldsymbol{N}$. By plotting the vectors $\boldsymbol{u}, \boldsymbol{v}$ as n points relative to two orthogonal axes we obtain a two-dimensional configuration. Discuss the interpretation of this configuration in representing an asymmetric dissimilarity matrix graphically.

(Constantine and Gower, 1978)

5.9 In correspondence analysis of the matrix $\boldsymbol{N}$, prove that the two sets of scores $\boldsymbol{f}_i$ and $\boldsymbol{g}_i$ are linked by the formulae $\boldsymbol{G} = \boldsymbol{D}_c^{-1}\boldsymbol{P}'\boldsymbol{F}\boldsymbol{D}^{-1}$ and $\boldsymbol{F} = \boldsymbol{D}_r^{-1}\boldsymbol{P}\boldsymbol{G}\boldsymbol{D}^{-1}$, where all quantities are defined in **5.19**.

(Greenacre, 1984 pp. 88–89)

5.10 Suppose that a correspondence matrix $\boldsymbol{P}$ (cf **5.17**) has the block structure

$$\begin{pmatrix} \boldsymbol{P}_1 & \boldsymbol{0} \\ \boldsymbol{0} & \boldsymbol{P}_2 \end{pmatrix}$$

where $\boldsymbol{P}$ is $(I \times J)$, $\boldsymbol{P}_1$ is $(I_1 \times J_1)$ and $\boldsymbol{P}_2$ is $(I_2 \times J_2)$ with $I = I_1 + I_2$ and $J = J_1 + J_2$. The sum of the elements of $\boldsymbol{P}$ is 1 by definition; let the sums of the elements of $\boldsymbol{P}_1$ and $\boldsymbol{P}_2$ be t_1 and t_2 respectively, and let $(\boldsymbol{F}_1, \boldsymbol{G}_1, \boldsymbol{D}_1)$,$(\boldsymbol{F}_2, \boldsymbol{G}_2, \boldsymbol{D}_2)$ denote the results of correspondence analyses of $\boldsymbol{P}_1$, $\boldsymbol{P}_2$ respectively (cf **5.19**). Show that the largest non-trivial principal inertia in the correspondence analysis of $\boldsymbol{P}$ is 1, and that the other principal inertias are those of $\boldsymbol{D}_1$ and $\boldsymbol{D}_2$ arranged in descending order.

(Greenacre, 1984 pp. 123–125)

5.11 Let $\boldsymbol{A}$ be a square matrix, and $\boldsymbol{P}$ an orthogonal matrix of the same size. Write $\boldsymbol{M}^{1/2}$ for the unique positive semi-definite symmetric square root of a positive semi-definite symmetric matrix $\boldsymbol{M}$. Show that $\text{tr}(\boldsymbol{P}'\boldsymbol{A}) \geqslant \text{tr}(\boldsymbol{A}'\boldsymbol{A})^{1/2}$, with equality if and only if $\boldsymbol{P}$ satisfies $\boldsymbol{P}'\boldsymbol{A} = (\boldsymbol{A}'\boldsymbol{A})^{1/2}$.
Hint : use the singular value decomposition of $\boldsymbol{A}$.

(Sibson, 1978)

5.12 Show that M_0 (**5.23**) is not a Euclidean metric.
Hint : set up the following counterexample. Let W, X, Y, Z be four four-point configurations in one-dimensional space having point coordinates : $W = (-3, -1, 1, 3); X = (-3, 1, -1, 3); Y = (-1, -3, 3, 1); Z = (1, -3, 3, -1)$. Obtain all pairwise M_0 values and show that they are not Euclidean distances.

(Sibson, 1978)

6

Inference: Estimation and Hypothesis Testing

6.1 *Statistical Inference* is the use of sample data to make statements about the population (possibly hypothetical) from which the sample has been taken. The general principles remain the same whether the data are univariate or multivariate; they will be governed by the type of inference required and by the philosophy of inference adopted.

The chief distinction as regards type of inference is between *parametric* and *non-parametric* inference. In the former, a specific distributional form is assumed for each population of interest so that the process of inference reduces to the making of statements about the parameters of these distributions. In the latter, by contrast, the emphasis is on developing methods that are appropriate for populations having any one member of a whole class of distributional forms. Parametric methods are usually more powerful than their non-parametric counterparts when the distributional assumptions are met, but the non-parametric methods compensate for this by their less restrictive assumptions and hence broader applicability. However, some parametric methods can tolerate quite substantial departures from assumptions without much deterioration in performance; such methods are said to be *robust* to these departures. Whichever approach is adopted, the inferential framework is determined by the philosophy of inference that is held. Here the two chief contenders are *frequentist* and *Bayesian* inference, although a number of alternative frameworks can also be identified (e.g. decision theory, likelihood, empirical Bayes). Frequentist interpretation of results is in terms of probabilities of observed outcomes, and is made against the background of (hypothetical) repeated sampling from the given populations, while Bayesian interpretation requires the assignment of subjective probabilities to parameter values and subsequent weighing of evidence as provided by these probabilities. A full account of the general principles embodied in frequentist inference may be found in Stuart and Ord (1991), while those of Bayesian inference are discussed by O'Hagan (1994).

6.2 In this chapter we survey the main results available for drawing inferences about unstructured multivariate populations, the case of structured populations being deferred to the next chapter. The overwhelming majority of methods for multivariate inference are parametric methods, based on the assumption that samples have been taken from multivariate normal distributions. Reasons for this include the derivation of such methods as generalisations of the corresponding univariate procedures, the use of the multivariate central limit theorem to justify the assumption of multivariate normality, the robustness of many of the methods to moderate departures from normality, and the tractability of the mathematics associated with the multivariate normal distribution (which ensured that relatively simple analytical expressions could be derived and used in the early days of the subject when computation was more difficult than today). The following account reflects this imbalance, although more recent emphasis on computer-based inference is also surveyed. One area that is not included, however, is that of analytical non-parametric multivariate inference, since this would lead to a lengthy cataloguing of relatively infrequently used individual test statistics; the interested reader is referred instead to the book by Puri and Sen (1971).

Point estimation

6.3 Following the above discussion, we assume that the data vectors $\boldsymbol{x}_1, \boldsymbol{x}_2, \ldots, \boldsymbol{x}_n$ form a random sample from a multivariate normal population which has mean $\boldsymbol{\mu}$ and dispersion matrix $\boldsymbol{\Sigma}$. The likelihood $L(\boldsymbol{\mu}, \boldsymbol{\Sigma})$ of the sample is thus given by

$$\log L(\boldsymbol{\mu}, \Sigma) = -\frac{np}{2}\log(2\pi|\Sigma|) - \frac{1}{2}\sum_{i=1}^{n}[(\boldsymbol{x}_i - \boldsymbol{\mu})'\Sigma^{-1}(\boldsymbol{x}_i - \boldsymbol{\mu})], \qquad (6.1)$$

and this expression is maximised at the values $\hat{\boldsymbol{\mu}} = \bar{\boldsymbol{x}}$ and $\hat{\boldsymbol{\Sigma}} = \frac{1}{n}\boldsymbol{A} = \frac{1}{n}\sum_{i=1}^{n}(\boldsymbol{x}_i - \bar{\boldsymbol{x}})(\boldsymbol{x}_i - \bar{\boldsymbol{x}})'$ (see **3.20**). These are thus the maximum likelihood estimates of $\boldsymbol{\mu}$ and $\boldsymbol{\Sigma}$. From **2.7** and **A.3** we see that the sampling distributions of $\hat{\boldsymbol{\mu}}$ and $n\hat{\boldsymbol{\Sigma}}$ are $N(\boldsymbol{\mu}, \frac{1}{n}\Sigma)$ and $W(n-1, \Sigma)$ respectively. Thus $\hat{\boldsymbol{\mu}}$ is an unbiased estimate of $\boldsymbol{\mu}$, but $\hat{\boldsymbol{\Sigma}}$ is a biased estimate of Σ; the appropriate unbiased estimate is $\frac{n}{n-1}\hat{\boldsymbol{\Sigma}} = \frac{1}{n-1}\boldsymbol{A} = \boldsymbol{S}$.

6.4 The multivariate normal distribution serves as a model for most situations involving continuous vector variables, so that in the frequentist approach to inference $\bar{\boldsymbol{x}}$ and either $\frac{1}{n}\boldsymbol{A}$ or $\frac{1}{n-1}\boldsymbol{A}$ are nearly always used to estimate the mean and dispersion matrix of the parent population. If contamination by presence of outliers is suspected, then one of the robust estimates described in **3.22** should be used instead. More recently, there has been some interest in theory associated with elliptical distributions (**2.11–2.14**). These distributions share many of the features of the multivariate normal (which is itself a member of this class of distributions), but they include distributions which have heavier tails than the multivariate normal. Samples from the elliptic class of distributions are thus more likely to include outlying values, and this class therefore provides a useful probability model for real situations. Fang and Zhang (1990) show that if $\boldsymbol{x}_1, \boldsymbol{x}_2, \ldots, \boldsymbol{x}_n$ form a random sample from an elliptic distribution which has mean $\boldsymbol{\mu}$ and dispersion matrix $\boldsymbol{\Sigma}$, i.e. if the density function of each p-element vector $\boldsymbol{x}$ has the form

$$f(\boldsymbol{x}) = |\boldsymbol{\Sigma}|^{-\frac{1}{2}}\psi[(\boldsymbol{x}-\boldsymbol{\mu})'\boldsymbol{\Sigma}^{-1}(\boldsymbol{x}-\boldsymbol{\mu})] \tag{6.2}$$

for some function $\psi(.)$, then the maximum likelihood estimates of $\boldsymbol{\mu}$ and $\boldsymbol{\Sigma}$ are $\bar{\boldsymbol{x}}$ and $\lambda_0\boldsymbol{A}$, where λ_0 is the maximum of the function $\phi(\lambda) = \lambda^{-np/2}\psi(p/\lambda)$.

Example 6.1
Suppose that $\boldsymbol{x}_1, \boldsymbol{x}_2, \ldots, \boldsymbol{x}_n$ is a random sample from a $N(\boldsymbol{\mu},\boldsymbol{\Sigma})$ distribution. Then $\psi(z) = (2\pi)^{-p/2}\exp(-z/2)$, so that $\phi(\lambda) = \lambda^{-np/2}(2\pi)^{-p/2}\exp(-p/2\lambda)$. Thus $\frac{\partial\psi}{\partial\lambda} = \frac{p}{2\lambda}(\frac{1}{\lambda} - n)\psi$, from which it readily follows that $\lambda_0 = 1/n$. This yields the maximum likelihood estimator $\hat{\boldsymbol{\Sigma}} = \frac{1}{n}\boldsymbol{A}$ as previously derived.

6.5 Maximum likelihood estimation can be employed for any multivariate density function $f(\boldsymbol{x}, \boldsymbol{\theta})$, providing that the likelihood can be written down analytically and maximised with respect to the unknown parameter(s). The approach breaks down either if the distributions become intractable or if the likelihood cannot be written down explicitly (e.g. for implicit stochastic models). Diggle and Gratton (1984) have proposed Monte Carlo methods for such situations. Given a set of observations $\boldsymbol{x}_1, \boldsymbol{x}_2, \ldots, \boldsymbol{x}_n$ and a model involving the parameter $\boldsymbol{\theta}$, the proposal is to simulate an independent random sample $\boldsymbol{y}_1, \boldsymbol{y}_2, \ldots, \boldsymbol{y}_m$ for suitably large m (say 200) at each value $\boldsymbol{\theta}_i$ over a mesh of values, use a kernel method to estimate the density $f(\boldsymbol{x}, \boldsymbol{\theta})$ for each $\boldsymbol{x}_j$ at each $\boldsymbol{\theta}_i$, obtain the set of estimated log-likelihoods $L^*(\boldsymbol{\theta}_i) = \sum_{j=1}^{m}\log f(\boldsymbol{x}_j, \boldsymbol{\theta}_i)$, and then find the value $\boldsymbol{\theta}^*$ maximising $L^*(\boldsymbol{\theta}_i)$. Full details are given by Diggle and Gratton (1984), and a recent application of this idea has been presented by Crowder (1994).

6.6 Moving from the frequentist approach, it is possible to adopt either a Bayesian approach, or a decision theoretic approach, or a mixture of the two approaches to point estimation problems.

In the pure Bayesian approach we are required to provide a prior distribution $\pi(\boldsymbol{\theta})$ for the unknown parameter vector $\boldsymbol{\theta}$. Multiplying this prior distribution by the likelihood of the sample yields the posterior distribution $\pi(\boldsymbol{\theta}|\boldsymbol{x}_1, \boldsymbol{x}_2, \ldots, \boldsymbol{x}_n)$, and the Bayesian point estimate of $\boldsymbol{\theta}$ is then given by a summary measure of this posterior distribution. The most commonly used summary measure is the mode, as this represents the 'most likely' value of $\boldsymbol{\theta}$ given the sample data, but the mean of the posterior distribution is also often used. If the prior is locally flat, the posterior mode and the maximum likelihood estimator will almost coincide.

In the pure decision theoretic approach we are required to provide a loss function $l(\boldsymbol{\theta}, \boldsymbol{T})$ that represents the loss incurred to the statistician when $\boldsymbol{\theta}$ is estimated by $\boldsymbol{T}$. Averaging the loss over the distribution of the data produces the risk function $R(\boldsymbol{\theta}, \boldsymbol{T}) = E[l(\boldsymbol{\theta}, \boldsymbol{T})]$, the expected loss when $\boldsymbol{\theta}$ is estimated by $\boldsymbol{T}$. In decision theoretic terms, an estimator $\boldsymbol{T}_1$ is better than an estimator $\boldsymbol{T}_2$ if $R(\boldsymbol{\theta}, \boldsymbol{T}_1) \leqslant R(\boldsymbol{\theta}, \boldsymbol{T}_2)$ for all $\boldsymbol{\theta}$ with $R(\boldsymbol{\theta}, \boldsymbol{T}_1) < R(\boldsymbol{\theta}, \boldsymbol{T}_2)$ for at least one $\boldsymbol{\theta}$.

An estimator is said to be *admissible* if no other estimator is better than it in this sense, and the goal of decision theory is to find such an estimator. An estimator that is not admissible is said to be *inadmissible.*

In a mixture of both Bayesian and decision theoretic approaches we are required to specify *both* a prior distribution *and* a loss function as outlined above. Calculation of the risk function and the posterior distribution proceeds as before, but the final stage is to take the expectation of the risk function with respect to the posterior distribution. This produces the average risk, and the optimum estimator is the one that minimises this average risk. For certain types of loss function this procedure results in the optimum estimator emerging as a summary measure of the posterior distribution, and both the mean and mode of this distribution can be justified as optimal estimators with respect to particular loss functions: the quadratic loss function gives the posterior mean, while a zero-one loss function gives the posterior mode. In addition, absolute error loss yields the posterior median as the optimal estimator.

6.7 It can be recognised readily that optimum estimators will vary according to the choices of loss function and prior distribution. Also, analytical results will not necessarily exist for arbitrary choices of these functions or for sampling from arbitrary populations, and recourse in a particular situation may have to be made either to numerical methods or to Monte Carlo techniques such as Gibbs sampling (see **6.12** below). However, considerable analytical work has been done in the case of sampling from a multivariate normal distribution, and a brief summary now follows.

Consider first the pure decision theoretic approach. The seminal result in this area is due to Stein (1956), who showed that in sampling from a $N_p(\boldsymbol{\mu}, \Sigma)$ distribution the maximum likelihood estimator $\bar{\boldsymbol{x}}$ is inadmissible as an estimator of $\boldsymbol{\mu}$ under quadratic loss when $p \geqslant 3$. Using the loss function $(\boldsymbol{T} - \boldsymbol{\mu})'\Sigma^{-1}(\boldsymbol{T} - \boldsymbol{\mu})$, James and Stein (1961) showed that a better estimator is given by

$$\boldsymbol{t} = (1 - \frac{\alpha}{n\bar{\boldsymbol{x}}'\boldsymbol{A}^{-1}\bar{\boldsymbol{x}}})\bar{\boldsymbol{x}} \qquad (6.3)$$

where $\alpha = (p-2)/(n-p-2)$. Many subsequent papers have addressed the admissibility question for estimation of $\boldsymbol{\mu}$, and have investigated the use of different loss functions to find estimators (see Muirhead, 1982 p128, Seber, 1984 p62, and Fang and Zhang, 1990 p144, for a comprehensive list of references; also Stigler, 1990, for discussion and simple proofs of results). Similar studies have been conducted for estimation of Σ. Here the results are quite complicated, but it can be shown that the unbiased estimate $\boldsymbol{S}$ does have smallest risk under certain loss functions (Muirhead, 1982 p129). Despite the radical findings of James and Stein, therefore, the fact that different estimators are in general obtained with different loss functions and different underlying populations has led most statisticians to fall back on the traditional maximum likelihood, unbiased or robust estimates of $\boldsymbol{\mu}$ and Σ in practical applications.

Turning to the Bayesian approach, it is necessary to specify prior distributions for the unknown parameters. Assume again that we are sampling from a $N_p(\boldsymbol{\mu}, \Sigma)$ distribution. If we have no prior knowledge concerning $\boldsymbol{\mu}$ and Σ then a suitable choice of prior distribution (Press, 1972a p167) is

$$\pi(\boldsymbol{\mu}, \boldsymbol{\Sigma}) \propto |\boldsymbol{\Sigma}|^{-(p+1)/2}. \tag{6.4}$$

Combining this with the joint distribution of $\bar{\boldsymbol{x}}$ and $\boldsymbol{A}$ yields the posterior distribution

$$\pi(\boldsymbol{\mu}, \boldsymbol{\Sigma} \mid \bar{\boldsymbol{x}}, \boldsymbol{A}) \propto |\boldsymbol{\Sigma}|^{-(n+p+1)/2} \exp\{-\tfrac{1}{2}\mathrm{tr}\boldsymbol{\Sigma}^{-1}[\boldsymbol{A} + n(\bar{\boldsymbol{x}} - \boldsymbol{\mu})(\bar{\boldsymbol{x}} - \boldsymbol{\mu})']\}. \tag{6.5}$$

For fixed $\boldsymbol{\mu}$ this function can be recognised as proportional to the density (in $\boldsymbol{\Sigma}$) of an inverted Wishart distribution (see equation (A.23) in the Appendix), while for fixed $\boldsymbol{\Sigma}$ it is proportional to a multivariate normal density (in $\boldsymbol{\mu}$). Using the normalising constant of the inverted Wishart distribution and simplifying, we thus find that the marginal posterior distribution of $\boldsymbol{\mu}$ has the multivariate t-distribution

$$\pi(\boldsymbol{\mu} \mid \bar{\boldsymbol{x}}, \boldsymbol{A}) \propto [1 + n(\boldsymbol{\mu} - \bar{\boldsymbol{x}})'\boldsymbol{A}^{-1}(\boldsymbol{\mu} - \bar{\boldsymbol{x}})]^{-n/2}, \tag{6.6}$$

while integrating the joint posterior distribution with respect to $\boldsymbol{\mu}$ shows that the marginal posterior distribution of $\boldsymbol{\Sigma}$ has the inverted Wishart distribution given in (A.23) but with $\boldsymbol{A}$ replacing $\boldsymbol{U}$ and $(n-1)$ replacing n. The mean of the former distribution is just $\bar{\boldsymbol{x}}$, and this is also the mode of this distribution. Bayesian estimation of $\boldsymbol{\mu}$ under prior uncertainty thus coincides with maximum likelihood estimation. On the other hand, the mean of the latter distribution is $\frac{1}{n-p-2}\boldsymbol{A}$, which is a different estimator of $\boldsymbol{\Sigma}$ from either the maximum likelihood or the unbiased frequentist estimators.

Once there is prior knowledge available about the parameters $\boldsymbol{\mu}$ and $\boldsymbol{\Sigma}$, many more possibilities exist because a number of different prior distributions can usually be chosen to represent this knowledge and each will give rise to different parameter estimates. However, once the actual prior distribution has been chosen then the stages in the inference process are as before. For further work on Bayesian estimation of the parameters of a multivariate normal distribution, see Evans (1965), Chen (1979), Dickey *et al* (1985) and Leonard and Hsu (1992).

Example 6.2
Press (1972a p168) suggests using the 'natural conjugate' prior

$$\pi(\boldsymbol{\mu}, \boldsymbol{\Sigma}) \propto |\boldsymbol{\Sigma}|^{-(m+1)/2} \exp\{-\tfrac{1}{2}[\mathrm{tr}\boldsymbol{\Sigma}^{-1}\boldsymbol{G} + (\boldsymbol{\mu} - \boldsymbol{\phi})'\boldsymbol{\Sigma}^{-1}(\boldsymbol{\mu} - \boldsymbol{\phi})]\} \tag{6.7}$$

where $\boldsymbol{\phi}, \boldsymbol{G}$ and $m > 2p - 1$ are parameters. Working through all the same stages as above (for details see Press, *op. cit.*) we find that the means of the respective marginal posterior distributions, and hence a set of Bayes estimators of $\boldsymbol{\mu}$ and $\boldsymbol{\Sigma}$, are given by

$$(\boldsymbol{\phi} + n\bar{\boldsymbol{x}})/(1+n)$$

and

$$\{n\boldsymbol{A} + \boldsymbol{G} + n(\bar{\boldsymbol{x}} - \boldsymbol{\phi})(\bar{\boldsymbol{x}} - \boldsymbol{\phi})'/(1+n)\}/(n+m-2p-2).$$

Note that both of these expressions are weighted averages of prior estimators and sample-based estimators; the larger the sample size n, the greater is the role of the sample-based estimator.

6.8 We see from the preceding section that a Bayesian point estimate of a parameter requires evaluation of the marginal posterior density of that parameter. Derivation of the analytical results given above for samples from a multivariate normal distribution was eased by two specific features: the fact that we chose prior distributions which yielded tractable expressions for the joint posterior distribution of the parameters, and the fact that the marginal density of each parameter of interest could be obtained analytically by a single integral. Had we chosen an arbitrary prior distribution other than the natural conjugate prior of Example 6.2, the situation might have been much more complicated. Similarly, once we move away from the case of sampling from a multivariate normal distribution, we are liable to encounter severe problems with the implementation of the (conceptually straightforward) Bayesian approach. Typically, posterior distributions will end up as complicated analytical expressions; we may only know the kernel of the posterior density and not the normalising constant (which requires another multivariate integral for its evaluation); and we generally cannot compute marginal posterior densities and moments in terms of exact closed form explicit expressions. For these reasons, much effort has been directed towards approximation methods, numerical methods, and computer based methods for the evaluation of marginal posterior distributions.

6.9 The simplest of the approximation methods is a Bayesian version of the central limit theorem, which provides a very general large-sample result. Suppose that $\boldsymbol{x}_1, \ldots, \boldsymbol{x}_n$ is a set of observations with joint density $f(\boldsymbol{x}_1, \ldots, \boldsymbol{x}_n | \boldsymbol{\theta})$, where $\boldsymbol{\theta}$ is a k-element unknown parameter with prior density $\pi(\boldsymbol{\theta})$. Let $\hat{\boldsymbol{\theta}}$ be the maximum likelihood estimator of $\boldsymbol{\theta}$, and write ω_{ij} for $-\frac{\partial^2}{\partial\theta_i \partial\theta_j} \log f(\boldsymbol{x}_1, \ldots, \boldsymbol{x}_n | \boldsymbol{\theta})$ evaluated at $\boldsymbol{\theta} = \hat{\boldsymbol{\theta}}$. The contribution of any prior distribution for $\boldsymbol{\theta}$ is swamped in large samples by the data so that, under suitable regularity conditions, the limiting posterior distribution $\pi(\boldsymbol{\theta} | \boldsymbol{x}_1, \ldots, \boldsymbol{x}_n)$ is multivariate normal with mean $\hat{\boldsymbol{\theta}}$ and dispersion matrix $\boldsymbol{\Omega}^{-1}$ where $\boldsymbol{\Omega} = (\omega_{ij})$. A proof of this result is given by Le Cam (1956), a heuristic discussion by Lindley (1965), and some detailed consideration of the required regularity conditions by Heyde and Johnstone (1979). The result effectively arises from a Taylor series expansion of the log-likelihood function about $\hat{\boldsymbol{\theta}}$.

Being essentially a large-sample approximation to the likelihood function, the above result may be adequate for some cases involving small or medium samples, but in general alternative methods must be found when sample sizes are not large. The sticking point in the practical implementation of Bayesian methodology in such cases is in the evaluation of integrals of the general form

$$I = \frac{\int u(\boldsymbol{\theta})\, L(\boldsymbol{\theta}, \boldsymbol{x})\, \pi(\boldsymbol{\theta})\, d\boldsymbol{\theta}}{\int L(\boldsymbol{\theta}, \boldsymbol{x})\, \pi(\boldsymbol{\theta})\, d\boldsymbol{\theta}}, \tag{6.8}$$

where $L(\boldsymbol{\theta}, \boldsymbol{x})$ is the likelihood of the sample, $\pi(\boldsymbol{\theta})$ is the prior distribution of $\boldsymbol{\theta}$ and the integral in the denominator provides the normalising constant in the posterior distribution of $\boldsymbol{\theta}$. The expression I encompasses a range of moments of the posterior distribution, depending on the function $u(\boldsymbol{\theta})$, and marginal posterior densities can also be expressed as a variant of such ratio of integrals

(Press, 1982 p73). Lindley (1980) has developed specific expansions to order n^{-1} for such ratios of integrals, yielding an approximation to I in terms of the maximum likelihood estimate $\hat{\boldsymbol{\theta}}$ and of the elements ω_{ij} of $\boldsymbol{\Omega}$. Tierney and Kadane (1986), on the other hand, prefer to apply the Laplace method for evaluating integrals (De Bruijn, 1961), separately to both numerator and denominator of I. Setting

$$M(\boldsymbol{\theta}) = n^{-1}[\log L(\boldsymbol{\theta}, \mathbf{x}) + \log \pi(\boldsymbol{\theta})]$$

and

$$N(\boldsymbol{\theta}) = n^{-1}[\log u(\boldsymbol{\theta}) + \log L(\boldsymbol{\theta}, \mathbf{x}) + \log \pi(\boldsymbol{\theta})],$$

then the numerator and denominator of I are given by $\int \exp[nN(\boldsymbol{\theta})]\,d\boldsymbol{\theta}$ and $\int \exp[nM(\boldsymbol{\theta})]\,d\boldsymbol{\theta}$ respectively. Taylor series expansions of the functions $N(\boldsymbol{\theta})$ and $M(\boldsymbol{\theta})$ about their maximising values $\boldsymbol{\theta}^*$, $\boldsymbol{\theta}^{**}$, plus multivariate normal approximation for the distributions of these maximising values, produces

$$I \approx \left(\frac{|\boldsymbol{\Sigma}^*|}{|\boldsymbol{\Sigma}^{**}|}\right)^{1/2} \exp\{n[N(\boldsymbol{\theta}^*) - M(\boldsymbol{\theta}^{**})]\}$$

where $\boldsymbol{\Sigma}^*$, $\boldsymbol{\Sigma}^{**}$ are minus the inverse Hessians of $N(\boldsymbol{\theta})$ and $M(\boldsymbol{\theta})$ evaluated at $\boldsymbol{\theta}^*$ and $\boldsymbol{\theta}^{**}$ respectively. Some further refinements are given by Tierney *et al* (1989).

6.10 An alternative approach is to evaluate I by numerical integration, and a description of quadrature techniques may be found, for example, in Cohen *et al* (1973). Attention has more recently turned to development of efficient methods based on Gaussian quadrature; for work in this area see Naylor and Smith (1982,1983), Smith and Naylor (1984), Smith *et al* (1985) and Smith (1991).

Implementation of these methods needs a certain amount of numerical analytic expertise, however, and they also become more problematic as the number of parameters (and hence order of integration) increases. Growing interest in high-dimensional applications such as image analysis, neural networks and expert systems has led to the development of conceptually simple and easily implemented (but often computer intensive) Monte Carlo sampling methods. The earliest of these methods is *importance sampling*. This is based on the observation that if f and g are two density functions, then

$$\int f(x)\,dx = \int [f(x)/g(x)]g(x)\,dx = E[f(x)/g(x)]$$

where the expectation is with respect to g. Thus a Monte Carlo method of integration consists of generating a sample from this distribution, and using the mean of the values of the ratio f/g as an estimate of $\int f(x)\,dx$. Now equation (6.8) can be written as

$$I = \int u(\boldsymbol{\theta})w(\boldsymbol{\theta})\,d\boldsymbol{\theta}, \tag{6.9}$$

where

$$w(\boldsymbol{\theta}) = \frac{L(\boldsymbol{\theta}, \mathbf{x})\,\pi(\boldsymbol{\theta})}{\int L(\boldsymbol{\theta}, \mathbf{x})\,\pi(\boldsymbol{\theta})\,d\boldsymbol{\theta}}. \tag{6.10}$$

Suppose that we can choose an *importance function* $g(\boldsymbol{\theta})$ from which samples can be drawn. Then if we generate M values $\boldsymbol{\theta}_1, \ldots, \boldsymbol{\theta}_M$ from $g(\boldsymbol{\theta})$, we can estimate I of (6.9) by the weighted average $\sum_{i=1}^{M} w_i u(\boldsymbol{\theta}_i)$ where the weights are given by

$$w_i = \frac{L(\boldsymbol{\theta}_i, \boldsymbol{x})\, \pi(\boldsymbol{\theta}_i)/g(\boldsymbol{\theta}_i)}{\sum_{m=1}^{M} L(\boldsymbol{\theta}_m, \boldsymbol{x})\, \pi(\boldsymbol{\theta}_m)/g(\boldsymbol{\theta}_m)}. \tag{6.11}$$

The effectiveness of this approach clearly rests on suitable choice of $g(\boldsymbol{\theta})$. Although in principle any density function can be used, variance considerations suggest that g be chosen to be 'similar' to f. Some general aspects regarding this choice, as well as possible strategies for implementation of the scheme, may be found in Press (1989) and Smith (1991), while some further particular ideas on importance sampling are given by Geweke (1988 and 1989).

6.11 In practice, however, directly generating samples from an arbitrary high-dimensional joint distribution may not be possible. Recent developments have therefore centred on indirect approaches, using Markov chain Monte Carlo methods. Suppose that we wish to generate a sample from $g(\boldsymbol{\theta})$, and we can construct a Markov chain which is straightforward to simulate from and the equilibrium distribution of which is $g(\boldsymbol{\theta})$. If we then run the chain for a long time, simulated values of the chain can be used as a basis for summarising features of $g(\boldsymbol{\theta})$ of interest. Construction of the transition probabilities in an appropriate Markov chain was first made possible by means of the Metropolis–Hastings algorithm (Metropolis *et al*, 1953; Hastings, 1970), and two particular methods that have subsequently evolved are *substitution sampling* and *Gibbs sampling*. Both of these methods have potential application to conventional multivariate analysis as well as in Bayesian computation, so we briefly outline their mechanics. For a much fuller account see Gelfand and Smith (1990) and Smith and Roberts (1993), from which papers this summary is extracted.

We will describe the methods in relation to a collection of random variables $U_1, U_2, \ldots, U_k$, but it should be understood that any or all of these random variables can be replaced by unknown parameters θ_i if prior or posterior distributions are to be evaluated. Both sampling methods assume that functional forms are specified for various joint distributions of the U_i and, more pertinently, various conditional distributions of some U_i given the values of other U_j, and also that samples of U_i can be straightforwardly and efficiently generated from these distributions given specified values of the appropriate conditioning variables.

6.12 First consider substitution sampling. If there exists a set of values $\boldsymbol{U}^{(j)} = (U_1^{(j)}, U_2^{(j)}, \ldots, U_k^{(j)})$, we generate an 'updated' set $\boldsymbol{U}^{(j+1)}$ by means of the following steps.

(1) Draw $U_2^{(j1)}, U_3^{(j1)}, \ldots, U_k^{(j1)}$ from $f(U_2, U_3, \ldots, U_k \mid U_1^{(j)})$.
(2) Draw $U_1^{(j1)}, U_3^{(j2)}, \ldots, U_k^{(j2)}$ from $f(U_1, U_3, \ldots, U_k \mid U_2^{(j1)})$.
(3) Draw $U_1^{(j2)}, U_2^{(j2)}, U_4^{(j3)}, \ldots, U_k^{(j3)}$ from $f(U_1, U_2, U_4, \ldots, U_k \mid U_3^{(j2)})$, and so on.

Conduct k such draws, the last being $U_1^{(j,k-1)}, \ldots, U_{k-1}^{(j,k-1)}$ from $f(U_1, U_2, \ldots, U_{k-1} \mid U_k^{(j,k-1)})$. Then set $\boldsymbol{U}^{(j+1)} = (U_1^{(j,k-1)}, U_2^{(j,k-1)}, \ldots, U_k^{(j,k-1)})$. Thus one such cycle requires $k(k-1)$ generated variates. The whole process can be started by generating U_1^0 from some arbitrary distribution $f(U_1)$, one cycle of the above steps yielding $\boldsymbol{U}^{(1)}$, and letting the process run for i cycles to end up at $\boldsymbol{U}^{(i)}$. If we repeat the entire procedure m times we obtain m i.i.d. k-tuples $(U_{1j}^{(i)}, U_{2j}^{(i)}, \ldots, U_{kj}^{(i)})$, $(j = 1, \ldots, m)$ and independence between but not within the js. The density estimator for $f(U_s)$ $(s = 1, \ldots, k)$ is then given by

$$\hat{f}(U_s) = \frac{1}{m} \sum_{j=1}^{m} f(U_s \mid U_t = U_{tj}^{(i)}; t \neq s). \tag{6.12}$$

The estimated densities converge to the true ones, and the differences can be made arbitrarily small for sufficiently large i and m (see Tanner and Wong, 1987).

Note that implementation of the substitution-sampling algorithm does not require specification of the full joint distribution, but rather the conditional distributions of $k-1$ of the elements given the value of the kth. Of course, to obtain an observation from, say, $f(U_1, U_2, \ldots, U_{k-1} \mid U_k)$ we will in general need to sample a succession of values from reduced conditional distributions such as $f(U_{k-1} \mid U_k), f(U_{k-2} \mid U_{k-1}, U_k)$, and so on. Thus implementation of each step of the algorithm requires the specification, in general, of a full conditional and many additional reduced conditional distributions. The Gibbs sampler, introduced by Geman and Geman (1984), is a much simpler process which requires drawing only a single value from a full conditional distribution at each stage. Given an arbitrary set of starting values $U_1^{(0)}, U_2^{(0)}, \ldots, U_k^{(0)}$, we draw $U_1^{(1)}$ from $f(U_1 \mid U_2^{(0)}, \ldots, U_k^{(0)})$, then $U_2^{(1)}$ from $f(U_2 \mid U_1^{(1)}, U_3^{(0)}, \ldots, U_k^{(0)})$, $U_3^{(1)}$ from $f(U_3 \mid U_1^{(1)}, U_2^{(1)}, U_4^{(0)}, \ldots, U_k^{(0)})$ and so on, up to $U_k^{(1)}$ from $f(U_k \mid U_1^{(1)}, U_2^{(1)}, \ldots, U_{k-1}^{(1)})$. Thus each variable is visited in the natural order and the cycle requires just k random variate generations. After i such iterations we arrive at $(U_1^{(i)}, \ldots, U_k^{(i)})$, and repeating the whole procedure m times we obtain m i.i.d. k-tuples $(U_{1j}^{(i)}, U_{2j}^{(i)}, \ldots, U_{kj}^{(i)})$, $(j = 1, \ldots, m)$ as for the substitution sampling. The density estimator for $f(U_s)$ $(s = 1, \ldots, k)$ is thus again given by equation (6.12).

6.13 Gelfand and Smith (1990) discuss a range of examples, giving details of the implementation of these sampling techniques in a variety of practical cases. Most of them involve multivariate quantities, but of particular interest in the present context are the sections on multinomial models, hierarchical models, and multivariate normal sampling. Casella and George (1992) also list a number of diverse applications of these methods. Smith (1991) provides an overview of, and comparison between, all the computational methods reviewed above. He concludes that the choice between using analytical approximation and numerical integration rests largely on the dimensionality and complexity of the problem; that quadrature can be effective for up to about nine dimensions if the functions are relatively well-behaved but beyond that (or if the functions are badly behaved) Monte Carlo methods are generally necessary; and that use of importance sampling for high-dimensional problems is something of an art form, but that if a good procedure can be found then it is likely to be more efficient computationally than a Markov chain based iterative sampling procedure. However, in very complex problems it may be too difficult to identify a suitable importance sampling strategy, while the Markov chain based methods, in particular the Gibbs sampler, are typically very easy to implement (although convergence can be very slow and convergence criteria can be misleading – see the contribution by Diaconis and Rosenthal to the paper by Smith and Roberts, 1993).

Interval and region estimation

6.14 Point estimation, as discussed above, is in essence merely a rational and systematic procedure for making a guess at the value of an unknown parameter. Although this guess is therefore an 'informed' one, the vagaries of sampling will ensure that it is almost always 'wrong' in absolute terms. Many statisticians therefore prefer to identify an *interval* for a univariate parameter, or a *region* for a multivariate parameter, within which the true value of the parameter is almost certain to lie. We will restrict attention exclusively here to the multivariate case. In the frequentist approach to inference, $R(\boldsymbol{x})$ is said to be a $100(1-\alpha)\%$ *confidence region* for the unknown parameter $\boldsymbol{\theta}$ if, before the sample is selected, $\Pr[\boldsymbol{\theta} \in R(\boldsymbol{x})] = 1-\alpha$ where this probability is calculated under the true, but unknown, value of $\boldsymbol{\theta}$. Interpretation of this confidence region is made in relation to long-run relative frequency: if samples of given size were to be selected repeatedly from the same population under identical conditions, and the region $R(\boldsymbol{x})$ calculated each time, then a proportion $1-\alpha$ of all these regions would include the true value of $\boldsymbol{\theta}$. In the Bayesian approach to inference, $R(\boldsymbol{\theta})$ is said to be a $100(1-\alpha)\%$ *credible region* for $\boldsymbol{\theta}$ if $\Pr[\boldsymbol{\theta} \in R(\boldsymbol{\theta})] = 1-\alpha$ where this probability is calculated under the posterior distribution for $\boldsymbol{\theta}$, $\pi(\boldsymbol{\theta}|\boldsymbol{x}_1, \boldsymbol{x}_2, \ldots, \boldsymbol{x}_n)$. Here we refer directly to the probability of $\boldsymbol{\theta}$ being in a preassigned interval conditional on the data observed in the current experiment, so the interpretation of such intervals is just the naturally intuitive one. We now consider each of these forms of region estimates in practice.

6.15 Assume first that the data vectors $\boldsymbol{x}_1, \boldsymbol{x}_2, \ldots, \boldsymbol{x}_n$ form a random sample from a multivariate normal distribution with mean vector $\boldsymbol{\mu}$ and dispersion matrix $\boldsymbol{\Sigma}$. We have established in **6.3** that the maximum likelihood estimates of $\boldsymbol{\mu}$ and $\boldsymbol{\Sigma}$ are $\bar{\boldsymbol{x}}$ and $\frac{1}{n}\boldsymbol{A}$ respectively. Also, the sampling distributions of $\bar{\boldsymbol{x}}$ and $\boldsymbol{A}$ are $N(\boldsymbol{\mu}, \frac{1}{n}\boldsymbol{\Sigma})$ and $W(n-1, \boldsymbol{\Sigma})$ respectively. Moreover, these two statistics are independent (mirroring the familiar result from univariate theory that $\bar{x}$ and $\sum(x_i - \bar{x})^2$ are independent if $x_1, \ldots, x_n$ is a random sample from a normal distribution). A general result in multivariate distribution theory states that the quadratic form $\boldsymbol{x}'\boldsymbol{C}^{-1}\boldsymbol{x}$ has $p/(k-p+1)$ times an F distribution on p and $(k-p+1)$ degrees of freedom whenever the p-element vector $\boldsymbol{x}$ has a $N(\boldsymbol{0}, \boldsymbol{\Sigma})$ distribution independently of the $p \times p$ nonsingular matrix $\boldsymbol{C}$ which has a $W(k, \boldsymbol{\Sigma})$ distribution. For proof of this result see Theorems 3.5.1 and 3.5.2 of

Mardia *et al* (1979); defining the quantity

$$T^2 = n(n-1)(\bar{\boldsymbol{x}}-\boldsymbol{\mu})'\boldsymbol{A}^{-1}(\bar{\boldsymbol{x}}-\boldsymbol{\mu}), \tag{6.13}$$

it thus follows that $(n-p)T^2/[p(n-1)]$ has an F distribution on p and $(n-p)$ degrees of freedom.

The quantity T^2 is known as the *one-sample Hotelling's* T^2 (see also **6.23**), and it can be used directly to construct a confidence region for $\boldsymbol{\mu}$. Using the distributional result just given, it is evident that if we write $F^{\alpha}_{p,n-p}$ for the point exceeded by $100\alpha\%$ of the F distribution on p and $n-p$ degrees of freedom then, before the sample is selected,

$$\Pr\left[n(n-1)(\bar{\boldsymbol{x}}-\boldsymbol{\mu})'\boldsymbol{A}^{-1}(\bar{\boldsymbol{x}}-\boldsymbol{\mu}) \leqslant \frac{(n-1)p}{(n-p)}F^{\alpha}_{p,n-p}\right] = 1-\alpha, \tag{6.14}$$

whatever the values of the unknown $\boldsymbol{\mu}$ and $\boldsymbol{\Sigma}$. For a particular sample, $\bar{\boldsymbol{x}}$ and $\boldsymbol{S}=\frac{1}{n-1}\boldsymbol{A}$ can be calculated and the inequality

$$n(\bar{\boldsymbol{x}}-\boldsymbol{\mu})'\boldsymbol{S}^{-1}(\bar{\boldsymbol{x}}-\boldsymbol{\mu}) \leqslant \frac{(n-1)p}{(n-p)}F^{\alpha}_{p,n-p} \tag{6.15}$$

will define an ellipsoidal region within the space of all possible values of $\boldsymbol{\mu}$. This space is p-dimensional, with a particular value $\boldsymbol{\mu}_0$ represented by a point whose coordinates are given by the individual elements of $\boldsymbol{\mu}_0$. This ellipsoidal region is the $100(1-\alpha)\%$ confidence region for $\boldsymbol{\mu}$.

Corresponding confidence region theory does not exist for the dispersion matrix $\boldsymbol{\Sigma}$, mainly because the space of all $(p \times p)$ symmetric positive definite matrices does not admit particularly useful regions from the point of view either of relating to applications or of interpretation. Confidence statements in multivariate analysis are thus generally restricted to ones about location parameters only.

6.16 The above confidence ellipsoid for $\boldsymbol{\mu}$ is difficult to visualise if $p \geqslant 4$. Two possible courses of action are then to investigate elements of $\boldsymbol{\mu}$ singly by means of *simultaneous confidence intervals*, or in pairs by means of *simultaneous bivariate confidence regions*. The idea here is to make a set of separate confidence statements, each of which provides a readily visualised interval or region, such that all of the separate statements hold *simultaneously* with a specified probability. The general technique was introduced by Scheffé (1953). The following specific results are available, and are proved for example by Johnson and Wichern (1982); we assume throughout that $\boldsymbol{x}_1, \boldsymbol{x}_2, \ldots, \boldsymbol{x}_n$ is a random sample from a $N_p(\boldsymbol{\mu},\boldsymbol{\Sigma})$ population with $\boldsymbol{\Sigma}$ positive definite.

(1) Simultaneously for all $\boldsymbol{l}$, the intervals

$$\left(\boldsymbol{l}'\bar{\boldsymbol{x}} - \sqrt{\left[\frac{p(n-1)}{n(n-p)}F^{\alpha}_{p,n-p}\boldsymbol{l}'\boldsymbol{S}\boldsymbol{l}\right]}, \boldsymbol{l}'\bar{\boldsymbol{x}} + \sqrt{\left[\frac{p(n-1)}{n(n-p)}F^{\alpha}_{p,n-p}\boldsymbol{l}'\boldsymbol{S}\boldsymbol{l}\right]}\right)$$

will contain $\boldsymbol{l}'\boldsymbol{\mu}$ with probability $1-\alpha$.

(2) Using the successive choices $\boldsymbol{l}' = (1, 0, \ldots, 0)$, $\boldsymbol{l}' = (0, 1, \ldots, 0)$, and so on up to $\boldsymbol{l}' = (0, 0, \ldots, 1)$ in 1, the intervals

$$\bar{x}_i - \sqrt{\left[\frac{p(n-1)}{(n-p)} F^{\alpha}_{p,n-p}\right]} \sqrt{\frac{s_{ii}}{n}} < \mu_i < \bar{x}_i + \sqrt{\left[\frac{p(n-1)}{(n-p)} F^{\alpha}_{p,n-p}\right]} \sqrt{\frac{s_{ii}}{n}}$$

hold simultaneously for $i = 1, \ldots, p$ with probability $1 - \alpha$, where $\boldsymbol{S} = (s_{ij})$.

(3) Simultaneously for all $p \times 2$ matrices $\boldsymbol{L}$ of rank two, the ellipses defined by

$$n(\boldsymbol{L}'\bar{\boldsymbol{x}} - \boldsymbol{L}'\boldsymbol{\mu})'(\boldsymbol{L}'\boldsymbol{S}\boldsymbol{L})^{-1}(\boldsymbol{L}'\bar{\boldsymbol{x}} - \boldsymbol{L}'\boldsymbol{\mu}) < \frac{p(n-1)}{n(n-p)} F^{\alpha}_{p,n-p}$$

will contain $\boldsymbol{L}'\boldsymbol{\mu}$ with probability $1 - \alpha$.

(4) Taking all elements of $\boldsymbol{L}$ above to be zero, except those in positions $(i, 1)$ and $(j, 2)$ which have value 1,

$$s_{jj}(\bar{x}_i - \mu_i)^2 - 2s_{ij}(\bar{x}_i - \mu_i)(\bar{x}_j - \mu_j) + s_{ii}(\bar{x}_j - \mu_j)^2 \leqslant \frac{Dp(n-1)}{n(n-p)} F^{\alpha}_{p,n-p}$$

contains (μ_i, μ_j) for all $i \neq j$ with probability $1 - \alpha$, where $D = s_{ii}s_{jj} - s_{ij}^2$.

Example 6.3

Johnson and Wichern (1982, p194) give the scores obtained by each of $n = 87$ college students for the subtest x_1 = social science and history of the College Level Examination Program and the subtests x_2 = verbal, x_3 = science of the College Qualification Test. Summary statistics for these data were

$$\bar{\boldsymbol{x}}' = (527.74, 54.69, 25.13)$$

and

$$\boldsymbol{S} = \begin{pmatrix} 5691.34 & 600.51 & 217.25 \\ 600.51 & 126.05 & 23.37 \\ 217.25 & 23.37 & 23.11 \end{pmatrix}.$$

Here $\frac{p(n-1)}{n-p} F^{\alpha}_{p,n-p} = \frac{3(87-1)}{(87-3)} F^{\alpha}_{3,84} = \frac{3(86)}{84}(2.7) = 8.29$ for $\alpha = 0.05$, so from (6.15) a 95% confidence region for $\boldsymbol{\mu}$ is given by the ellipsoid

$$87(\bar{\boldsymbol{x}} - \boldsymbol{\mu})'\boldsymbol{S}^{-1}(\bar{\boldsymbol{x}} - \boldsymbol{\mu}) \leqslant 8.29.$$

This is difficult to visualise directly, so we might wish to obtain some simultaneous confidence statements about the individual μ_i or about (μ_i, μ_j) pairs. Using item 2 above we have

$$527.74 - \sqrt{(8.29)}\sqrt{\left(\frac{5691.34}{87}\right)} \leqslant \mu_1 \leqslant 527.74 + \sqrt{(8.29)}\sqrt{\left(\frac{5691.34}{87}\right)},$$

or

$$504.45 \leqslant \mu_1 \leqslant 551.03$$

Similarly,

$$51.22 \leqslant \mu_2 \leqslant 58.16$$

and

$$23.65 \leqslant \mu_3 \leqslant 26.61$$

The above three statements hold simultaneously with probability 0.95. They produce wider confidence intervals than those we would have obtained on applying the usual univariate theory to the individual μ_i; this is the price paid for ensuring that the three statements hold *simultaneously* with the given confidence level.

Alternatively, from item 4 we obtain

$$126.05(527.74-\mu_1)^2-1201.02(527.74-\mu_1)(54.69-\mu_2)+5691.4(54.69-\mu_2)^2$$

$$\leqslant 35211.65,$$

$$23.11(527.74-\mu_1)-434.50(527.74-\mu_1)(25.13-\mu_3)+5691.4(25.13-\mu_3)^2$$

$$\leqslant 8322.64,$$

and

$$23.11(54.69-\mu_2)^2-46.74(54.69-\mu_2)(25.13-\mu_3)+126.05(25.13-\mu_3)^2$$

$$\leqslant 233.59.$$

These three statements also hold simultaneously with probability 0.95. They can be used to plot simultaneous confidence ellipses for (μ_i, μ_j) pairs; see Johnson and Wichern (1982, p201) for some further details.

6.17 The above theory is appropriate when the data vectors $\boldsymbol{x}_1, \boldsymbol{x}_2, \ldots, \boldsymbol{x}_n$ are a random sample from a multivariate normal distribution, but this assumption may not be warranted in some applications. Providing that the sample size is large, we can still use the same confidence intervals and regions by invoking the multivariate central limit theorem (see **2.7**). However, in small and medium-sized samples such asymptotic approximations may be very inaccurate so we need to consider other approaches. One general way to obtain confidence regions, without making specific assumptions about the parent distribution of the data, is through the computer-intensive data resampling technique known as *bootstrapping*. This was introduced by Efron (1979); good reviews of the general ideas, along with specific details of the associated methodology, are provided by Efron (1982), Efron and Gong (1983), Efron and Tibshirani (1986) and Hinkley (1988). A review of the application of bootstrap methodology to confidence interval calculation is given by DiCiccio and Romano (1988), and some more recent developments together with further references may be found in Efron (1987, 1990 and 1992).

Although very much has been written on this technique since its introduction in 1979, nearly all the development has been concerned with univariate problems involving scalar parameters only. Where vector parameters have been considered, the interest has essentially remained in the univariate case and the focus has almost exclusively been on scalar functions of these parameters. We now outline briefly the basic ideas as they pertain to the multivariate situation.

6.18 Suppose that a random sample of data vectors $\boldsymbol{x}_1, \boldsymbol{x}_2, \ldots, \boldsymbol{x}_n$ has been used to obtain an estimate $\hat{\boldsymbol{\theta}}$ of a vector parameter $\boldsymbol{\theta}$. A *bootstrap sample* of size n is formed by sampling with replacement from these data vectors, i.e. by successively choosing, with equal probability $1/n$, one of the vectors. (A typical bootstrap sample will thus contain repeats of some $\boldsymbol{x}_i$, while other $\boldsymbol{x}_i$ will appear just once or not at all.) This process is repeated a number of times, yielding k such bootstrap samples; current recommendations are for k to lie between 100 and 1000, a sample of size 200 usually being sufficient. Let $\hat{\boldsymbol{\theta}}_{(i)}$ be the estimate of $\boldsymbol{\theta}$ computed from the ith bootstrap sample, and let $\bar{\boldsymbol{\theta}}$ be the mean of these k values. Then the bootstrap samples are samples from the empirical distribution function $\hat{F}$ of the data, and represent potential future samples from the underlying true distribution function F. Thus the $\hat{\boldsymbol{\theta}}_{(i)}$ represent potential future observations from the sampling distribution of $\hat{\boldsymbol{\theta}}$. An estimate of bias of $\hat{\boldsymbol{\theta}}$ is therefore given by $\hat{\boldsymbol{\theta}} - \bar{\boldsymbol{\theta}}$, while a $100(1-\alpha)\%$ confidence region can be taken to be any region that encloses $100(1-\alpha)\%$ of the $\hat{\boldsymbol{\theta}}_{(i)}$ values.

In the univariate case the obvious choice is given by ranking the $\hat{\theta}_{(i)}$ values and taking the interval marked off by the appropriate lower and upper percentiles. In the multivariate case, the $\hat{\boldsymbol{\theta}}_{(i)}$ values can be 'ordered' by peeling them in shells using a sequence of convex hulls (Barnett, 1976), thus yielding a percentile confidence region for $\boldsymbol{\theta}$. Trimming by convex hulls has satisfying distribution-free characteristics, but their construction in the multidimensional case can be heavy computationally. Titterington (1979) considers trimming by ellipsoids, in particular minimum content ones, and describes the computation of these ellipsoids. This provides a viable alternative method. An even simpler approach is to assume approximate normality of the $\hat{\boldsymbol{\theta}}_{(i)}$ (see Davison *et al*, 1986), and use ellipsoids of the form

$$(\boldsymbol{\theta} - \bar{\boldsymbol{\theta}})' \boldsymbol{S}_{(B)}^{-1} (\boldsymbol{\theta} - \bar{\boldsymbol{\theta}}) \leqslant C$$

where

$$\boldsymbol{S}_{(B)} = \sum_{i=1}^{B} (\hat{\boldsymbol{\theta}}_{(i)} - \bar{\boldsymbol{\theta}})(\hat{\boldsymbol{\theta}}_{(i)} - \bar{\boldsymbol{\theta}})'$$

and C is evaluated from percentage points of the $F_{p,B-p}$ distribution.

The above description is of the simple *percentile* method for confidence region construction, but in the past decade an almost bewildering array of modifications to this method, as well as alternative methods, have been proposed. This literature is confined mainly to the construction of confidence intervals for univariate parameters, but most methods can be extended to the multivariate case in the way outlined above. A thorough survey and comprehensive reference list is provided by Hall (1988) in his theoretical comparison of bootstrap confidence intervals. The chief methods that he focuses on are the percentile method, the percentile-t method, a hybrid of these two, a bias-corrected method, and an accelerated bias-corrected method. He also discusses the distinction between parametric and non-parametric bootstrap intervals, and develops an alternative approach based on 'shortest' bootstrap intervals. He points out that some of the methods can lead to serious errors in coverage rates, and confirms a previous conjecture of Efron that accelerated bias-correction is second-order correct in a variety of multivariate circumstances. Percentile-t and accelerated bias-correction emerge as the most promising of the methods studied. The main warning to be drawn from this study is that non-critical use of bootstrapping for confidence region construction should be avoided.

Hall (1992) links the concepts of bootstrap intervals and Edgeworth expansions, discussing also the question of coverage rates and providing further material relevant to multivariate regions. Some applications of bootstrapping in the calculation of multivariate confidence regions have been given by Weinberg *et al* (1984), Krzanowski and Radley (1989), and Weihs (1992).

6.19 In the Bayesian approach, there is very little to add to what has already been given in **6.7** to **6.13**. The $100(1-\alpha)\%$ credible region for $\boldsymbol{\theta}$ is given by the region R of $\boldsymbol{\theta}$ values such that I of (6.8), with $u(\boldsymbol{\theta}) = 1$ and with the integral in the numerator evaluated over R, is equal to $1-\alpha$. All the preceding numerical techniques can be employed if required. For exact analytical expressions in a number of standard situations, including that of sampling from a multivariate normal distribution, see Box and Tiao (1965 and 1973) or Press (1972a and 1982).

Hypothesis testing

6.20 Estimation, whether point or interval, is concerned with finding plausible values for the unknown parameter $\boldsymbol{\theta}$. By contrast, in *hypothesis testing* we wish to establish whether or not the sample data are consonant with a previously held theory about $\boldsymbol{\theta}$, or to choose between several possible theories. Each such theory can usually be expressed in the form $\boldsymbol{\theta} \in \boldsymbol{\Theta}_i$, where $\boldsymbol{\Theta}_i$ is some region of the parameter space. The Bayesian approach provides a direct attack on the problem, as in this approach we can derive a posterior probability that $\boldsymbol{\theta} \in \boldsymbol{\Theta}_i$ given sample data. If this probability is sufficiently high then the data support the theory, but if this probability is low then the data do not support it; choice among a set of theories can thus be made by picking the one whose corresponding probability is highest.

However, there are two distinct ways of obtaining such posterior probabilities. The easiest is to specify a prior distribution for the parameter $\boldsymbol{\theta}$, obtain the posterior distribution in the usual way, and then derive the posterior probability that $\boldsymbol{\theta} \in \boldsymbol{\Theta}_i$ by integrating this posterior distribution over $\boldsymbol{\Theta}_i$. Integration of the posterior distribution can be achieved with the help of the various techniques discussed earlier, so this approach does not involve any new ideas. The second possibility, dating back to Jeffreys (1939), is to specify a prior *probability* for each theory $\boldsymbol{\theta} \in \boldsymbol{\Theta}_i$ and then deduce the corresponding posterior probabilities through multiplication by the likelihood. This approach can involve more complications, and further discussion can be found in most Bayesian texts (e.g. Lee, 1989). In addition to its use in standard hypothesis testing problems, it forms the basis of Duncan's k-ratio t-test for multiple comparisons in experimental design and analysis. For a good suvey of this latter area, and discussion of the specific Bayesian approach, see Duncan (1975). For the remainder of this chapter, however, we will concentrate exclusively on the frequentist approach to general hypothesis testing.

6.21 In the frequentist approach we are required to specify *two* hypotheses concerning $\boldsymbol{\theta}$. The hypothesis $\boldsymbol{\theta} \in \boldsymbol{\Theta}$ is referred to as the *null* hypothesis, denoted H_0. The plausibility of this hypothesis must be assessed in relation to some alternative possibility, which is called the *alternative* hypothesis and is denoted H_a. A common device in practice is to use the general alternative which allows $\boldsymbol{\theta}$ to take any value not specified by the null hypothesis, in which case we wish to test $H_0: \boldsymbol{\theta} \in \boldsymbol{\Theta}$ against $H_a: \boldsymbol{\theta} \notin \boldsymbol{\Theta}$. The test is conducted by finding a *test statistic* T and an associated *rejection region* of the sample space. If the value of the test statistic for the data at hand falls in the rejection region then the null hypothesis is *rejected* in favour of the alternative hypothesis. Non-rejection is equivalent to compatibility of the null hypothesis with the data, so the complement of the rejection region is often called the *acceptance* region. Such a procedure gives rise to two possible errors: the *type one* error is when the null hypothesis is falsely rejected, while the *type two* error is when an incorrect null hypothesis is not rejected. The probability of the first error is the *size* of the test, while one minus the probability of the second error is the *power* of the test.

Optimal theory of hypothesis testing concerns identification of *uniformly most powerful* tests. A full account of this theory and its application to scalar parameters in the univariate case may be found in Stuart and Ord (1991) or Lehman (1986). In multivariate analysis, however, uniformly most powerful tests exist only in rather artificial situations so recourse must usually be made to other methods. These include the formulation of a general criterion which enables reasonable (but possibly sub-optimal) tests to be derived in a wide variety of circumstances, and the restriction of tests to a subclass within which optimal ones exist. Two popular general principles which enable multivariate tests to be obtained are the *likelihood ratio* and the *union-intersection* principles (see Appendix, **A.6** and **A.7**), while the class of available tests is most usefully restricted by countenancing only *unbiased* or *invariant* tests. The former are tests in which the power under all alternatives is never less than the size, while the latter are tests based on statistics that are invariant under a natural group of transformations. Although invariance is a big restriction, and uniformly most powerful invariant tests form a narrower class than uniformly most powerful unbiased ones, it is perhaps a more intuitively natural criterion in the multivariate case. For example, if (x, y) has a bivariate normal distribution with correlation coefficient ρ, then it is reasonable to base tests of hypothesis about ρ on a statistic (such as the sample correlation coefficient) which is invariant under the transformations $\tilde{x} = a_1x + b_1, \tilde{y} = a_2y + b_2$ for arbitrary constants a_1, a_2, b_1, b_2. It turns out that it is sometimes possible to find uniformly most powerful tests within this restricted class of tests. If such a test exists, then it is often the same as the likelihood ratio test. For general theory and some applications see Muirhead (1982, Chapter 6) and Anderson (1984).

We now survey the main tests that are of practical interest. First we consider a single sample from a multivariate normal distribution and develop tests about the parameters of this distribution, then we extend these results to several-sample problems, and finally we discuss possible methods of obtaining tests in general non-normal situations. The central approach is the likelihood ratio, not only because of the invariance argument outlined above but also because likelihood ratio tests can be derived for many situations in which union-intersection tests do not exist or are not unique.

Single-sample normal data: tests of the mean

6.22 Suppose that $\boldsymbol{x}_1, \boldsymbol{x}_2, \ldots, \boldsymbol{x}_n$ is a random sample from a p-variate normal distribution with mean vector $\boldsymbol{\mu}$ and dispersion matrix $\boldsymbol{\Sigma}$, and that H_0 and H_a are hypotheses under which maximum likelihood estimates of $\boldsymbol{\mu}$ are $\hat{\boldsymbol{\mu}}$ and $\bar{\boldsymbol{x}}$ respectively. The maximum likelihood estimate of $\boldsymbol{\Sigma}$ under H_a is $\frac{1}{n}\boldsymbol{A}$ (**3.20** and **6.3**), while under H_0 it is $\frac{1}{n}\boldsymbol{A} + \boldsymbol{dd}'$, where $\boldsymbol{d} = \hat{\boldsymbol{\mu}} - \bar{\boldsymbol{x}}$ (Exercise 6.5). The log-likelihood of the sample is

$$l(\boldsymbol{\mu}, \boldsymbol{\Sigma}) = -\frac{n}{2}\log|2\pi\boldsymbol{\Sigma}| - \frac{1}{2}\sum_{i=1}^{n}(\boldsymbol{x}_i - \boldsymbol{\mu})'\boldsymbol{\Sigma}^{-1}(\boldsymbol{x}_i - \boldsymbol{\mu}), \tag{6.16}$$

which can be simplified (Mardia *et al*, 1979, p97) to

$$l(\boldsymbol{\mu}, \boldsymbol{\Sigma}) = -\frac{n}{2}\log|2\pi\boldsymbol{\Sigma}| - \frac{1}{2}\mathrm{tr}\boldsymbol{\Sigma}^{-1}\boldsymbol{A} - \frac{n}{2}(\bar{\boldsymbol{x}} - \boldsymbol{\mu})'\boldsymbol{\Sigma}^{-1}(\bar{\boldsymbol{x}} - \boldsymbol{\mu}). \tag{6.17}$$

Substituting the appropriate expressions for $\boldsymbol{\mu}$ and $\boldsymbol{\Sigma}$ under each hypothesis, and subtracting the derived log-likelihoods, it readily follows that the likelihood ratio test statistic λ for H_0 versus H_a is given by

$$\omega = 2\log\lambda = n\boldsymbol{d}'\boldsymbol{\Sigma}^{-1}\boldsymbol{d} \tag{6.18}$$

if $\boldsymbol{\Sigma}$ is known, and

$$\omega = 2\log\lambda = n\log(1 + n\boldsymbol{d}'\boldsymbol{A}^{-1}\boldsymbol{d}) \tag{6.19}$$

if $\boldsymbol{\Sigma}$ is unknown. In particular cases it may be possible to obtain the exact null distribution of λ, ω, or some other monotonic transformation that is used as the test statistic, and hence to derive the exact critical region for a size α test. If exact results are difficult to obtain, then the asymptotic null distribution given by (A.25) of the Appendix may be invoked.

6.23 The above general result may be used to obtain a test statistic in a variety of situations; the following are the most commonly occurring ones. In each case the alternative hypothesis is the general H_a: not H_0.

(1) $H_0 : \boldsymbol{\mu} = \boldsymbol{\mu}_0$, $\boldsymbol{\Sigma}$ known.
Here $\hat{\boldsymbol{\mu}} = \boldsymbol{\mu}_0$, so using (6.18) we obtain $\omega = n(\bar{\boldsymbol{x}} - \boldsymbol{\mu}_0)'\boldsymbol{\Sigma}^{-1}(\bar{\boldsymbol{x}} - \boldsymbol{\mu}_0)$. Furthermore, from the sampling distribution of $\bar{\boldsymbol{x}}$ (**2.7**) and equation (2.30), this statistic has an exact χ_p^2 distribution under H_0 so that the critical region for a size α test can be readily obtained. (Note that in this case, the asymptotic distribution coincides with the exact distribution).

(2) $H_0 : \boldsymbol{\mu} = \boldsymbol{\mu}_0$, $\boldsymbol{\Sigma}$ unknown.
Once again $\hat{\boldsymbol{\mu}} = \boldsymbol{\mu}_0$, but now we use (6.19) to obtain $\omega = n\log[1 + n(\bar{\boldsymbol{x}} - \boldsymbol{\mu}_0)'\boldsymbol{A}^{-1}(\bar{\boldsymbol{x}} - \boldsymbol{\mu}_0)]$. This statistic is equivalent to $n(\bar{\boldsymbol{x}} - \boldsymbol{\mu}_0)'\boldsymbol{S}^{-1}(\bar{\boldsymbol{x}} - \boldsymbol{\mu}_0)$ (where

$S = \frac{1}{n-1}A$), which is known as *Hotelling's one-sample T^2 statistic* and which has $p(n-1)/(n-p)$ times an F distribution on p and $n-p$ degrees of freedom under H_0. Thus the critical region for an exact size α test can again be obtained.

(3) $H_0 : \boldsymbol{H\mu} = \boldsymbol{h}$ for prespecified $\boldsymbol{H}, \boldsymbol{h}$; $\boldsymbol{\Sigma}$ known.
This hypothesis specifies linear constraints on the elements of $\boldsymbol{\mu}$, so maximising the likelihood under H_0 requires the use of Lagrange multipliers. We find (Mardia *et al*, 1979, p106) that $\hat{\boldsymbol{\mu}} = \bar{\boldsymbol{x}} - \boldsymbol{\Sigma H}'(\boldsymbol{H\Sigma H}')^{-1}(\boldsymbol{H}\bar{\boldsymbol{x}} - \boldsymbol{h})$, whence $\boldsymbol{d} = \boldsymbol{\Sigma H}'(\boldsymbol{H\Sigma H}')^{-1}(\boldsymbol{H}\bar{\boldsymbol{x}} - \boldsymbol{h})$ and

$$\omega = (\boldsymbol{H}\bar{\boldsymbol{x}} - \boldsymbol{h})'(\boldsymbol{H\Sigma H}')^{-1}(\boldsymbol{H}\bar{\boldsymbol{x}} - \boldsymbol{h}).$$

Under H_0 the observations $\boldsymbol{y}_i = \boldsymbol{Hx}_i$ are i.i.d. $N_q(\boldsymbol{h},\boldsymbol{H\Sigma H}')$ random vectors, where $q < p$ is the number of elements of $\boldsymbol{h}$, so that by the same argument as in 1 above ω has an exact χ^2_q distribution under H_0.

(4) $H_0 : \boldsymbol{H\mu} = \boldsymbol{h}$ for prespecified $\boldsymbol{H}, \boldsymbol{h}$; $\boldsymbol{\Sigma}$ unknown.
Use of (6.19), with obvious changes to 3 in which $\frac{1}{n}\boldsymbol{A}$ replaces $\boldsymbol{\Sigma}$, yields the test statistic

$$\omega = n\log(1 + n\boldsymbol{d}'\boldsymbol{A}^{-1}\boldsymbol{d})$$

where $\boldsymbol{d} = \boldsymbol{AH}'(\boldsymbol{HAH}')^{-1}(\boldsymbol{H}\bar{\boldsymbol{x}} - \boldsymbol{h})$. In similar fashion to 2 above we can show that this test is equivalent to one based on the statistic $n\boldsymbol{d}'\boldsymbol{S}^{-1}\boldsymbol{d}$ $= n(\boldsymbol{H}\bar{\boldsymbol{x}} - \boldsymbol{h})'(\boldsymbol{HSH}')^{-1}(\boldsymbol{H}\bar{\boldsymbol{x}} - \boldsymbol{h})$, which has $q(n-1)/(n-q)$ times an F distribution on q and $n-q$ degrees of freedom under H_0.

No general result, such as the one given at the start of **6.22** for likelihood ratio tests, exists for the union-intersection principle, so a union-intersection test statistic has to be derived *ab initio* for each distinct situation. However, as regards mean vectors, the same tests are obtained using the union-intersection principle as have been obtained by the likelihood ratio approach in each of the situations above. The power function of Hotelling's one-sample T^2 has been extensively tabulated by Tiku (1967,1972); see also Das Gupta and Perlman (1974).

Example 6.4
The blackbody CIE (Commission International d'Éclairage) chromaticity specification for a colour temperature of 4000 deg K is $x = 0.3804$ and $y = 0.3768$. In ten colour-matching trials (Jackson, 1959, 1962) one subject had mean chromaticity values $\bar{x} = 0.3745$ and $\bar{y} = 0.3719$, and covariance matrix $\boldsymbol{S} = 10^{-5}\begin{pmatrix} 1.843 & 1.799 \\ 1.799 & 1.836 \end{pmatrix}$. If we wish to test whether the observations can be treated as coming from a bivariate normal population with mean given by the 4000 deg K standards, then we use case 2 above. Here $\bar{\boldsymbol{x}}' = (0.3745, 0.3719), \boldsymbol{\mu}_0' = (0.3804, 0.3768)$, and $n = 10$. Thus $(\bar{\boldsymbol{x}} - \boldsymbol{\mu}_0)' = (-0.0059, -0.0049)$ and $\boldsymbol{S}^{-1} = (10^5 \div 0.14735) \times \begin{pmatrix} 1.836 & -1.799 \\ -1.799 & 1.843 \end{pmatrix}$, from which we obtain $T^2 = 28.1214$. Since $p = 2$ and $n = 10$ then $(n-p)T^2/p(n-1) = 12.5$, and under the null hypothesis this should be compatible with observations from an $F_{2,8}$

Table 6.1 Weights of cork borings in directions N, E, S, and W for 28 trees, reproduced with permission from Rao (1948).

N	E	S	W	N	E	S	W
72	66	76	77	91	79	100	75
60	53	66	63	56	68	47	50
56	57	64	58	79	65	70	61
41	29	36	38	81	80	68	58
32	32	35	36	78	55	67	60
30	35	34	26	46	38	37	38
39	39	31	27	39	35	34	37
42	43	31	25	32	30	30	32
37	40	31	25	60	50	67	54
33	29	27	36	35	37	48	39
32	30	34	28	39	36	39	31
63	45	74	63	50	34	37	40
54	46	60	52	43	37	39	50
47	51	52	43	48	54	57	43

distribution. Critical values of this distribution from tables are 4.46 (95% point), 8.65 (99% point) and 18.5 (99.9% point), so we can conclude that the observations differ significantly from the 4000 deg K standards at the 1 per cent level.

Example 6.5

The data in Table 6.1, taken from Rao (1948), give weights (in centigrams) of cork borings from the north (N), east (E), south (S) and west (W) of the trunks of 28 trees in a block of plantations. The sample mean vector and covariance matrix are given by

$$\bar{\boldsymbol{x}}' = (50.535, 46.179, 49.679, 45.179),$$

and

$$\boldsymbol{S} = \begin{pmatrix} 290.41 & 223.75 & 288.49 & 226.27 \\ 223.75 & 219.93 & 229.06 & 171.37 \\ 288.49 & 229.06 & 350.00 & 259.54 \\ 226.27 & 171.37 & 259.54 & 226.00 \end{pmatrix}.$$

It is of interest to test whether the population mean weights are the same in the N–S and E–W directions. Writing $\boldsymbol{\mu}' = (\mu_1, \mu_2, \mu_3, \mu_4)$ for the population mean vector, we need to test the hypothesis $H_0 : \mu_1 = \mu_3, \mu_2 = \mu_4$. Now H_0 can be expressed as $\boldsymbol{H\mu} = \boldsymbol{h}$ for $\boldsymbol{H} = \begin{pmatrix} 1 & 0 & -1 & 0 \\ 0 & 1 & 0 & -1 \end{pmatrix}$ and $\boldsymbol{h} = \boldsymbol{0}$, so that $\boldsymbol{H}\bar{\boldsymbol{x}} - \boldsymbol{h} = (0.857, 1.000)'$ and $\boldsymbol{HSH}' = \begin{pmatrix} 61.27 & 26.96 \\ 26.96 & 99.50 \end{pmatrix}$.

Hence we use case 4 above with $q = 2$. We find $[n(n-q)/q(n-1)](\boldsymbol{H}\bar{\boldsymbol{x}} - \boldsymbol{h})'(\boldsymbol{HSH}')^{-1}(\boldsymbol{H}\bar{\boldsymbol{x}} - \boldsymbol{h}) = 0.2212$. Under H_0 this should be compatible with observations from an $F_{2,6}$ distribution. Critical values of this distribution are 3.39 (5% significance) and 5.57 (1% significance), so we conclude that H_0 is perfectly tenable.

Single-sample normal data: tests of dispersion

6.24 Suppose that $\boldsymbol{x}_1, \boldsymbol{x}_2, \ldots, \boldsymbol{x}_n$ is a random sample from a p-variate normal distribution with mean vector $\boldsymbol{\mu}$ and dispersion matrix $\boldsymbol{\Sigma}$, and that H_0 and H_a are hypotheses under which maximum likelihood estimates of $\boldsymbol{\Sigma}$ are $\hat{\boldsymbol{\Sigma}}$ and $\boldsymbol{C} = \frac{1}{n}\boldsymbol{A}$ respectively. The maximum likelihood estimate of $\boldsymbol{\mu}$ is always $\bar{\boldsymbol{x}}$, and must therefore be so under both hypotheses. The log-likelihood of the sample is given by (6.17). Substituting $\bar{\boldsymbol{x}}$ for $\boldsymbol{\mu}$ and $\hat{\boldsymbol{\Sigma}}$, $\boldsymbol{C}$ in turn for $\boldsymbol{\Sigma}$ under each hypothesis, then subtracting the resulting log-likelihoods, it readily follows that the likelihood ratio test statistic λ for H_0 versus H_a is given by

$$\omega = 2\log\lambda = n\mathrm{tr}\hat{\boldsymbol{\Sigma}}^{-1}\boldsymbol{C} - n\log|\hat{\boldsymbol{\Sigma}}^{-1}\boldsymbol{C}| - np. \tag{6.20}$$

If a is the arithmetic and g is the geometric mean of the eigenvalues of $\hat{\boldsymbol{\Sigma}}^{-1}\boldsymbol{C}$, then $\mathrm{tr}(\hat{\boldsymbol{\Sigma}}^{-1}\boldsymbol{C}) = pa$ and $|\hat{\boldsymbol{\Sigma}}^{-1}\boldsymbol{C}| = g^p$ so that

$$\omega = np(a - \log g - 1). \tag{6.21}$$

This general result can be used in the same way as the previous one for the mean, to obtain likelihood ratio test statistics for various hypotheses about $\boldsymbol{\Sigma}$. However, exact null distributions of these statistics are now much harder to obtain and recourse has to be made more frequently to the asymptotic distribution given by (A.25). Also, it is rarely the case that $\boldsymbol{\mu}$ is known in practice, so it is usually assumed that $\boldsymbol{\mu}$ is unknown when deriving the tests.

6.25 The following tests can be obtained readily from the above result. Again, the alternative hypothesis in each case is the general H_a: not H_0.

(1) $H_0 : \boldsymbol{\Sigma} = \boldsymbol{\Sigma}_0$, $\boldsymbol{\mu}$ unknown.
Here $\hat{\boldsymbol{\Sigma}} = \boldsymbol{\Sigma}_0$, so that $\omega = 2\log\lambda = n\mathrm{tr}(\boldsymbol{\Sigma}_0^{-1}\boldsymbol{C}) - n\log|\boldsymbol{\Sigma}_0^{-1}\boldsymbol{C}| - np = np(a - \log g - 1)$ where a and g are the arithmetic and geometric means of the eigenvalues of $\boldsymbol{\Sigma}_0^{-1}\boldsymbol{C}$. While some progress has been made in finding the exact null distribution of this statistic (see Anderson, 1984, and Korin, 1968), the results are not easy to use. Asymptotically, ω has a $\chi^2_{\frac{1}{2}p(p+1)}$ distribution under H_0 from (A.25).

(2) $H_0 : \boldsymbol{\Sigma} = k\boldsymbol{\Sigma}_0$, k and $\boldsymbol{\mu}$ unknown.
The maximum likelihood estimate of k is given by $\hat{k} = \mathrm{tr}(\boldsymbol{\Sigma}_0^{-1}\boldsymbol{C})/p$ (Exercise 6.7). Then $\omega = np(a - \log g - 1)$, where a and g are the arithmetic and geometric means of the eigenvalues of $\boldsymbol{\Sigma}_0^{-1}\boldsymbol{C}/\hat{k}$. Let a_0 and g_0 be the arithmetic and geometric means of the eigenvalues of $\boldsymbol{\Sigma}_0^{-1}\boldsymbol{C}$. Then $a = a_0/\hat{k}$ and $g = g_0/\hat{k}$. But $\hat{k} = a_0$, so that $a = 1$ and $g = g_0/a_0$. Hence $\omega = np\log(a_0/g_0)$, and this has an asymptotic $\chi^2_{\frac{1}{2}(p-1)(p+2)}$ distribution under H_0. The special case of $\boldsymbol{\Sigma}_0 = \boldsymbol{I}$ is known as the 'test of sphericity'. In this case we have $a_0 = \frac{1}{p}\,\mathrm{tr}\,\boldsymbol{S}$ and $g_0 = |\boldsymbol{S}|^{\frac{1}{p}}$.

(3) H_0: $\boldsymbol{\Sigma}$ is diagonal, $\boldsymbol{\mu}$ is unknown.
This is the hypothesis that all the variables are uncorrelated with each other. Under H_0, the mean and variance of each variable are estimated separately, so that $\hat{\boldsymbol{\mu}} = \bar{\boldsymbol{x}}$ and $\hat{\boldsymbol{\Sigma}} = \mathrm{diag}(c_{11}, c_{22}, \ldots, c_{pp})$ where $\boldsymbol{C} = (c_{ij})$.

Thus $\hat{\boldsymbol{\Sigma}}^{-1}\boldsymbol{C} = \boldsymbol{R}$, the sample correlation matrix. This has trace p, so from (6.20) we find $\omega = -n \log |\boldsymbol{R}|$. Under H_0, ω has an asymptotic $\chi^2_{\frac{1}{2}p(p-1)}$ distribution; Box (1949) showed that the χ^2 approximation is improved if n is replaced by $n' = n - \frac{1}{6}(2p + 11)$.

(4) Independence of a subset of the variables from the rest.
Suppose that the vector $\boldsymbol{x}$ of variables is partitioned into two subvectors $\boldsymbol{x}_1$, $\boldsymbol{x}_2$ having p_1 and p_2 elements respectively. Then $\boldsymbol{\Sigma}$ is partitioned conformally as $\begin{pmatrix} \boldsymbol{\Sigma}_{11} & \boldsymbol{\Sigma}_{12} \\ \boldsymbol{\Sigma}_{21} & \boldsymbol{\Sigma}_{12} \end{pmatrix}$, and this hypothesis is $H_0 : \boldsymbol{\Sigma}_{12} = \boldsymbol{0}$. Under H_0 the likelihood splits into two factors, each of which can be maximised separately. Thus if $\boldsymbol{C}$ is partitioned conformally as $\begin{pmatrix} \boldsymbol{C}_{11} & \boldsymbol{C}_{12} \\ \boldsymbol{C}_{21} & \boldsymbol{C}_{12} \end{pmatrix}$, then $\hat{\boldsymbol{\Sigma}}_{ij} = \boldsymbol{C}_{ij}$ and $\hat{\boldsymbol{\Sigma}} = \begin{pmatrix} \boldsymbol{C}_{11} & \boldsymbol{0} \\ \boldsymbol{0} & \boldsymbol{C}_{22} \end{pmatrix}$. Thus $\hat{\boldsymbol{\Sigma}}^{-1}\boldsymbol{C} = \begin{pmatrix} \boldsymbol{I} & \boldsymbol{C}_{11}^{-1}\boldsymbol{C}_{12} \\ \boldsymbol{C}_{22}^{-1}\boldsymbol{C}_{21} & \boldsymbol{I} \end{pmatrix}$, from which it follows that $\mathrm{tr}(\hat{\boldsymbol{\Sigma}}^{-1}\boldsymbol{C}) = p$ and, using standard results for determinants of partitioned matrices as given for example by Mardia *et al* (1979 p457), that $|\hat{\boldsymbol{\Sigma}}^{-1}\boldsymbol{C}| = |\boldsymbol{C}_{22} - \boldsymbol{C}_{21}\boldsymbol{C}_{11}^{-1}\boldsymbol{C}_{12}|/|\boldsymbol{C}_{22}|$. Hence, from (6.20), the test statistic becomes $\omega = -n \log(|\boldsymbol{C}_{22} - \boldsymbol{C}_{21}\boldsymbol{C}_{11}^{-1}\boldsymbol{C}_{12}|/|\boldsymbol{C}_{22}|) = -n \log(|\boldsymbol{I} - \boldsymbol{C}_{22}^{-1}\boldsymbol{C}_{21}\boldsymbol{C}_{11}^{-1}\boldsymbol{C}_{12}|) = -n \log \prod_{i=1}^{k}(1 - \lambda_i)$, where the λ_i are the non-zero eigenvalues of $|\boldsymbol{I} - \boldsymbol{C}_{22}^{-1}\boldsymbol{C}_{21}\boldsymbol{C}_{11}^{-1}\boldsymbol{C}_{12}|$ and $k = \min(p_1, p_2)$. The likelihood ratio statistic ($\exp^{2\omega}$) here is Wilks' criterion (Appendix, **A8**). Providing that $n - 1 \geqslant p_1 + p_2$, its exact distribution is given by Mardia *et al* (1979, p135). For general p_1, p_2, the asymptotic null distribution of $-(n - \frac{1}{2}[p_1 + p_2 + 3]) \log(|\boldsymbol{I} - \boldsymbol{C}_{22}^{-1}\boldsymbol{C}_{21}\boldsymbol{C}_{11}^{-1}\boldsymbol{C}_{12}|)$ is chi-squared on p_1p_2 degrees of freedom (cf Appendix, A32).

No straightforward union-intersection tests appear to exist for cases 2 or 3, but see Olkin and Tomsky (1975) for some modified versions. Following the general pattern of relationships between the likelihood ratio and the union-intersection principles (cf Appendix, **A.7**), in the other cases the union-intersection statistic is a function of the extreme roots of $\hat{\boldsymbol{\Sigma}}^{-1}\boldsymbol{C}$ whereas the likelihood ratio test statistic was a function of *all* the roots of this quantity. Thus for case 1 the union-intersection test rejects H_0 if either $\lambda_p < c_1$ or $\lambda_1 > c_2$, where λ_i is the ith largest root of $\boldsymbol{\Sigma}_0^{-1}\boldsymbol{C}$ and c_1, c_2 are chosen to make the size of test α, while in case 4 the union-intersection test rejects H_0 if the largest root of $\boldsymbol{C}_{22}^{-1}\boldsymbol{C}_{21}\boldsymbol{C}_{11}^{-1}\boldsymbol{C}_{12}$ exceeds a suitable constant. The null distribution of the test statistic in the latter case follows from the properties of the Wishart distribution and its eigenvalues (Mardia *et al*, 1979 p136), but no exact results are yet available for the former case.

Properties of the above statistics, such as unbiasedness and invariance, are discussed by Giri (1977, Chapter 8) and Muirhead (1982, Chapters 8 and 11). Muirhead also details modifications to the statistics in order to ensure unbiased tests, and establishes asymptotic null and non-null distributional results. A general review of all the tests, along with some significance levels, is provided by Krishnaiah and Lee (1980). Further exact, asymptotic and approximate distributional results are given by Korin and Stevens (1973), Nagarsenker and Pillai (1973a,b), Olkin and Siotani (1976), Lee *et al* (1977), Mathai and Katiyar (1979) and Mudholkar *et al* (1982). In general, all these tests depend critically on normality of the data while corresponding inference for the mean (**6.23**) is much more robust.

Another test in this general group is that for conditional independence between two variables given the values of the rest. This is effectively the test of zero partial correlation between those two variables given the values of the rest, and from **2.6** it can be seen that this is the same as the test that an appropriate element of the inverse (population) covariance matrix is zero. Models in which selected elements of inverse covariance matrices are set to zero were first studied by Dempster (1972), who called them covariance selection models. More recently, such models have formed the subset of graphical Gaussian models within the general area of graphical modelling (Whittaker, 1990). Graphical modelling enables nested series of such models to be set up, and a likelihood ratio test between two models in such a series can be obtained by calculating appropriate deviances (**2.22**). For full technical details see Chapter 6 of Whittaker (1990).

6.26 In some situations neither a likelihood ratio nor a union-intersection test can be obtained easily, and recourse must be made to heuristic arguments. One such case of practical interest is the test of population equicorrelation among all the variables, for which Lawley (1963) derived the following test (asymptotically equivalent to the likelihood ratio statistic). Let r_{ij} be the sample correlation between $\boldsymbol{x}_i$ and $\boldsymbol{x}_j$, and write $\bar{r} = \frac{2}{p(p-1)}\sum_{i=1}^{p}\sum_{j=i}^{p} r_{ij}$, $\bar{r}_k = \frac{1}{p-1}\sum_{i \neq k} r_{ik}, s = 1 - \bar{r}$, and $t = \frac{(p-1)^2(1-s^2)}{p-(p-2)s^2}$. Then the test statistic is given by $Q = \frac{n-1}{s^2}[\sum_{i=1}^{p}\sum_{j=i}^{p}(r_{ij} - \bar{r})^2 - t\sum_{k=1}^{p}(\bar{r}_k - \bar{r})^2]$, and under the null hypothesis of population equicorrelation Q has an approximate χ^2 distribution on $\frac{1}{2}(p+1)(p-2)$ degrees of freedom.

Note that the test of equicorrelation allows arbitrary variances for each of the variables. If we additionally constrain all the variances to be equal under H_0 then the hypothesis becomes that of the *intraclass correlation model*, $H_0 : \boldsymbol{\Sigma} = \sigma^2[(1-\rho)\boldsymbol{I} + \rho\boldsymbol{e}\boldsymbol{e}']$, where σ, ρ are unknown and $\boldsymbol{e} = (1, 1, \ldots, 1)'$. A likelihood ratio test *does* exist for this hypothesis, having been derived by Wilks (1946). It is based on the statistic

$$\lambda = |\boldsymbol{S}|/(s^p[1-r]^{p-1}[1+(p-1)r]),$$

where $\boldsymbol{S} = (s_{ij}), s = \frac{1}{p}\sum_{i=1}^{p} s_{ii}$, and $r = \frac{2}{sp(p-1)}\sum_{i=1}^{j-1}\sum_{j=2}^{p} s_{ij}$. Box (1949, 1950) has shown that under H_0, $\omega = -[n - 1 - p(p+1)^2(2p-3)/6(p-1)(p^2+p-4)]\log\lambda$ has an asymptotic chi-square distribution on $\frac{1}{2}p(p+1) - 2$ degrees of freedom. Assumption of an intraclass correlation structure is necessary for certain procedures in the analysis of repeated measures or growth curves (see Volume 2).

Example 6.6

Returning to the blackbody chromaticity data of Example 6.4, we might ask whether the subject's x and y observations could be treated as independent and having equal variance. This requires a test of sphericity (case 2). Eigenvalues of $\boldsymbol{S}$ turn out to be 3.6385 and 0.0405, with arithmetic mean $a_0 = 1.8395$ and geometric mean $g_0 = 0.3839$. Here $n = 10$ and $p = 2$, so that $\omega = 31.34$ and $\frac{1}{2}(p-1)(p+2) = 2$. Critical values of the χ_2^2 distribution are 5.99 (5% significance) and 9.21 (1% significance), so we can safely reject the null hypothesis of sphericity (even though the sample size is far from asymptotic!)

Example 6.7
Returning next to the cork boring data of Example 6.5, we consider a test of intraclass correlation (i.e. equal variances and equal pairwise correlations). From the (4×4) covariance matrix $\boldsymbol{S}$ given in Example 6.5, and using the definitions above, we find $s = 270.085, r = 0.863$ and $|\boldsymbol{S}| = 207,222,725$. Hence $\lambda = 0.422$ and $\omega = 22.20$, with $\frac{1}{2}p(p+1)-2 = 8$. Critical values of the χ_8^2 distribution are 15.5 (5% significance) and 20.09 (1% significance), so we conclude that an intraclass correlation structure is not an appropriate assumption for these data.

Multi-sample normal data

6.27 We now suppose that we have independent samples from each of k separate normal populations, and consider various tests about the parameters of these populations. To be specific, let $\boldsymbol{x}_{i1}, \boldsymbol{x}_{i2}, \ldots, \boldsymbol{x}_{in_i}$ be a random sample from a p-variate normal distribution with mean vector $\boldsymbol{\mu}_i$ and dispersion matrix $\boldsymbol{\Sigma}_i$ for $i = 1, \ldots, k$. It is readily seen that the log likelihood function in this case can be written

$$l(\boldsymbol{\mu}_1, \ldots, \boldsymbol{\mu}_k, \boldsymbol{\Sigma}_1, \ldots, \boldsymbol{\Sigma}_k) = -\frac{1}{2}\sum_{i=1}^{k}\{n_i \log|2\pi\boldsymbol{\Sigma}_i| + n_i \mathrm{tr}\boldsymbol{\Sigma}_i^{-1}(\boldsymbol{C}_i + [\bar{\boldsymbol{x}}_i - \boldsymbol{\mu}_i][\bar{\boldsymbol{x}}_i - \boldsymbol{\mu}_i]')\},$$

where $\boldsymbol{C}_i = \frac{1}{n_i}\boldsymbol{A}_i = \frac{1}{n_i}\sum_{j=1}^{n_i}(\boldsymbol{x}_{ij} - \bar{\boldsymbol{x}}_i)(\boldsymbol{x}_{ij} - \bar{\boldsymbol{x}}_i)'$ is the maximum likelihood estimate of $\boldsymbol{\Sigma}_i$ and $\bar{\boldsymbol{x}}_i = \frac{1}{n_i}\sum_{j=1}^{n_i}\boldsymbol{x}_{ij}$ is the maximum likelihood estimate of $\boldsymbol{\mu}_i$.

Consider first the null hypothesis that the means $\boldsymbol{\mu}_i$ are all equal (to $\boldsymbol{\mu}$), assuming that the dispersion matrices $\boldsymbol{\Sigma}_i$ are all equal (to $\boldsymbol{\Sigma}$). This hypothesis is equivalent to saying that the k populations are identical, so that the maximum likelihood estimates of $\boldsymbol{\mu}$ and $\boldsymbol{\Sigma}$ are given by $\bar{\boldsymbol{x}} = \frac{1}{n}\sum_{i=1}^{k}\sum_{j=1}^{n_i}\boldsymbol{x}_{ij}$ and $\frac{1}{n}\boldsymbol{T} = \frac{1}{n}\sum_{i=1}^{k}\sum_{j=1}^{n_i}(\boldsymbol{x}_{ij} - \bar{\boldsymbol{x}})(\boldsymbol{x}_{ij} - \bar{\boldsymbol{x}})'$, where $n = \sum_{i=1}^{k} n_i$. If the null hypothesis is not true, then using the unconstrained likelihood above we find that the maximum likelihood estimates of $\boldsymbol{\mu}_i$ and $\boldsymbol{\Sigma}$ are given by $\bar{\boldsymbol{x}}_i = \frac{1}{n_i}\sum_{j=1}^{n_i}\boldsymbol{x}_{ij}$ and $\frac{1}{n}\boldsymbol{W} = \frac{1}{n}\sum_{i=1}^{k}\sum_{j=1}^{n_i}(\boldsymbol{x}_{ij} - \bar{\boldsymbol{x}}_i)(\boldsymbol{x}_{ij} - \bar{\boldsymbol{x}}_i)'$. Writing $\boldsymbol{B} = \boldsymbol{T} - \boldsymbol{W} = \sum_{i=1}^{k} n_i(\bar{\boldsymbol{x}}_i - \bar{\boldsymbol{x}})(\bar{\boldsymbol{x}}_i - \bar{\boldsymbol{x}})'$, then the matrix $\boldsymbol{B}$ is the 'hypothesis' matrix $\boldsymbol{H}$ while the matrix $\boldsymbol{W}$ is the 'error' matrix $\boldsymbol{E}$ in the terminology of Appendix **A8**. Test statistics for the hypothesis, and their null distributions, are thus given by equations (A.31)–(A.37). In particular, the likelihood ratio criterion is Wilks' statistic

$$\Lambda = |\boldsymbol{W}|/|\boldsymbol{B}+\boldsymbol{W}| = |\boldsymbol{I}+\boldsymbol{B}\boldsymbol{W}^{-1}|^{-1} = \prod_{i=1}^{p}(1-l_i) \tag{6.22}$$

where $l_1 \geqslant l_2 \geqslant \ldots \geqslant l_p$ are the eigenvalues of $\boldsymbol{W}\boldsymbol{T}^{-1}$, while the union-intersection principle yields l_1 as the test statistic.

Simplification occurs in the case of two samples, i.e. $k = 2$. Here

$$\begin{aligned} \boldsymbol{B} &= n_1(\bar{\boldsymbol{x}}_1-\bar{\boldsymbol{x}})(\bar{\boldsymbol{x}}_1-\bar{\boldsymbol{x}})' + n_2(\bar{\boldsymbol{x}}_2-\bar{\boldsymbol{x}})(\bar{\boldsymbol{x}}_2-\bar{\boldsymbol{x}})' \\ &= (n_1n_2/n)(\bar{\boldsymbol{x}}_1-\bar{\boldsymbol{x}}_2)(\bar{\boldsymbol{x}}_1-\bar{\boldsymbol{x}}_2)', \end{aligned}$$

so that

$$|\boldsymbol{I}+\boldsymbol{B}\boldsymbol{W}^{-1}| = 1 + (n_1n_2/n)(\bar{\boldsymbol{x}}_1-\bar{\boldsymbol{x}}_2)'\boldsymbol{W}^{-1}(\bar{\boldsymbol{x}}_1-\bar{\boldsymbol{x}}_2).$$

The second term here is Hotelling's two-sample T^2 statistic (Appendix equation (A.5)), and so the likelihood ratio test is based on this statistic. Moreover, $\boldsymbol{B}\boldsymbol{W}^{-1}$ has rank one so there is only one non-zero eigenvalue c_1, which is easily shown to be equal to $(n_1n_2/n)(\bar{\boldsymbol{x}}_1-\bar{\boldsymbol{x}}_2)'\boldsymbol{W}^{-1}(\bar{\boldsymbol{x}}_1-\bar{\boldsymbol{x}}_2)$ (Exercise 6.8). Thus the union-intersection test is also based on Hotelling's T^2; the null distribution of this statistic is given in the Appendix (**A1**).

Ito and Schull (1964) have studied the effect of unequal dispersion matrices on this test. They have found that if n_1 and n_2 are both large and approximately equal then the effect on size and power is minimal providing that the eigenvalues of $\boldsymbol{\Sigma}_1\boldsymbol{\Sigma}_2^{-1}$ lie in the range (0.5, 2), but there can be a seriously deleterious effect when n_1 and n_2 are markedly different. In this case the test described in **6.29** is more appropriate.

Example 6.8

Measurements of cranial length and cranial breadth for samples of male and female frogs (Seal 1964, p106) gave the following summary statistics. For the male sample the number of observations was $n_1 = 14$, the mean vector was $\bar{\boldsymbol{x}}_1' = (21.821, 22.843)$, and the sum of squares and products matrix was

$$\boldsymbol{A}_1 = \begin{pmatrix} 240.226 & 248.234 \\ 248.234 & 269.822 \end{pmatrix}.$$

For the female sample, the corresponding values were $n_2 = 35$, $\bar{\boldsymbol{x}}_2' = (22.860, 24.397)$, and

$$\boldsymbol{A}_2 = \begin{pmatrix} 601.230 & 689.850 \\ 689.850 & 829.850 \end{pmatrix}.$$

Thus

$$\boldsymbol{C}_1 = \frac{1}{14}\boldsymbol{A}_1 = \begin{pmatrix} 17.159 & 17.731 \\ 17.731 & 19.273 \end{pmatrix}$$

and

$$\boldsymbol{C}_2 = \frac{1}{35}\boldsymbol{A}_2 = \begin{pmatrix} 17.178 & 19.710 \\ 19.710 & 23.710 \end{pmatrix},$$

so it seems reasonable to assume equal dispersion matrices in male and female populations. To test for equality of means in the two populations we calculate $(\bar{\boldsymbol{x}}_1 - \bar{\boldsymbol{x}}_2)' = (-1.039, -1.554)$ and, from equation (A.1)

$$\boldsymbol{W} = \frac{1}{47}(\boldsymbol{A}_1 + \boldsymbol{A}_2) = \begin{pmatrix} 17.903 & 19.959 \\ 19.959 & 23.397 \end{pmatrix},$$

so that $\boldsymbol{W}^{-1} = \begin{pmatrix} 1.1405 & -0.9729 \\ -0.9729 & 0.8727 \end{pmatrix}$, $T^2 = 1.969$, and $\frac{(n_1+n_2-p-1)}{(n_1+n_2-2)p}T^2 =$ 0.964. This value is clearly not significant when referred to the F distribution on 2 and 46 degrees of freedom, so the mean vectors of male and female frog populations can be taken to be equal.

6.28 To use the above theory we must assume homogeneity of dispersion matrices. In Example 6.8 this seemed to be a reasonable assumption to make, but in general we might first wish to verify its reasonableness by testing the null hypothesis $H_0 : \boldsymbol{\Sigma}_i = \boldsymbol{\Sigma}$ for all i against the general alternative H_a: at least one $\boldsymbol{\Sigma}_i \neq \boldsymbol{\Sigma}$. Test statistics and their null distributions are given for this case in the Appendix (**A8**, equations A.28 to A.30). Percentage points, and power of tests, may be calculated with the help of formulae given by Nagarsenker (1978); see also Muirhead (1982, Section 8.2).

Now suppose that the null hypothesis is rejected by this test. In view of the alternative hypothesis, there may nevertheless be *some* similarity among the $\boldsymbol{\Sigma}_i$, and any similarity that exists should be exploited in subsequent parametric analyses. Several nested series of hypotheses, and associated tests of them, have therefore been suggested in recent years for establishing the relationships between a set of dispersion matrices. Flury (1988) proposed the following sequence:

$$H_0 : \boldsymbol{\Sigma}_1 = \boldsymbol{\Sigma}_2 = \ldots = \boldsymbol{\Sigma}_k;$$

$$H_p : \boldsymbol{\Sigma}_i = \rho_i \boldsymbol{\Sigma}_1, \ i = 2, \ldots, k;$$

$$H_c : \boldsymbol{\Sigma}_i = \boldsymbol{\Psi}\boldsymbol{\Delta}_i\boldsymbol{\Psi}', \ i = 1, \ldots, k$$

for orthogonal $\boldsymbol{\Psi}$ and diagonal $\boldsymbol{\Delta}_i$;

$$H_a : \text{arbitrary } \boldsymbol{\Sigma}_i.$$

Thus H_0 is the hypothesis of equality of dispersion matrices, H_p is the hypothesis of proportionality of dispersion matrices, and H_c is the hypothesis of common (population) principal components (**4.5**). Note also that H_p can be obtained from H_c on setting $\boldsymbol{\Delta}_i = \rho_i \boldsymbol{\Delta}_1$ for $i = 2, \ldots, k$. Furthermore, only *some* of the principal components might be common to all $\boldsymbol{\Sigma}_i$ while the others might differ from population to population, so we can add the hypothesis of *partial* common principal components between H_c and H_a. Formally, this is stated as

$$H_{pc} : \boldsymbol{\Sigma}_i = \boldsymbol{\Psi}_{(i)}\boldsymbol{\Delta}_i\boldsymbol{\Psi}'_{(i)}, \ i = 1, \ldots, k$$

for orthogonal $\boldsymbol{\Psi}_{(i)} = (\boldsymbol{\Psi}_1, \boldsymbol{\Psi}_{(i),2})$ and diagonal $\boldsymbol{\Delta}_i$. Flury (1988) provides maximum likelihood estimates of the parameters under each of these hypotheses, and likelihood ratio tests of each hypothesis against the next one in the sequence. An alternative possibility is to replace H_c plus H_{pc} by the hypothesis

$$H_{ec} : \boldsymbol{\Sigma}_i = \boldsymbol{\Phi}_i\boldsymbol{\Sigma}\boldsymbol{\Phi}'_i$$

for diagonal $\boldsymbol{\Phi}_i$. This is the hypothesis of common correlation matrices in the k populations; Manly and Rayner (1987) and Rayner *et al* (1990) adopt this approach, and provide maximum likelihood estimates and likelihood ratio tests for this modified sequence of hypotheses. For other tests of equality of correlation matrices, see Modarres and Jernigan (1992).

6.29 Finally we return to the two-sample test of location, but now relax the requirement for the dispersion matrices to be equal. Thus we suppose that $\boldsymbol{x}_{11}, \boldsymbol{x}_{12}, \ldots, \boldsymbol{x}_{1n_1}$ is a sample from $N(\boldsymbol{\mu}_1, \boldsymbol{\Sigma}_1)$ while $\boldsymbol{x}_{21}, \boldsymbol{x}_{22}, \ldots, \boldsymbol{x}_{2n_2}$ is a sample from $N(\boldsymbol{\mu}_2, \boldsymbol{\Sigma}_2)$, and we wish to test the hypothesis $H_0 : \boldsymbol{\mu}_1 = \boldsymbol{\mu}_2$ against the general alternative $H_a : \boldsymbol{\mu}_1 \neq \boldsymbol{\mu}_2$. This is the multivariate version of the *Behrens–Fisher problem.* Solutions of various degrees of approximation exist in the univariate case, see Welch (1937,1947) and Scheffé (1943) for example. Extensions of these solutions to the multivariate case have been provided by Bennett (1951) and James (1954), while the following relatively straightforward approximate multivariate test has been suggested by Yao (1965). Let $\bar{\boldsymbol{x}}_i$ and $\boldsymbol{S}_i$ $(i = 1, 2)$ be the two sample means and (unbiased) covariance matrices, and write $\boldsymbol{d} = \bar{\boldsymbol{x}}_1 - \bar{\boldsymbol{x}}_2$, $\boldsymbol{S} = \boldsymbol{S}_1/n_1 + \boldsymbol{S}_2/n_2$. Then the test statistic is given by $U = \boldsymbol{d}'\boldsymbol{S}^{-1}\boldsymbol{d}$, and $[(f - p + 1)/fp]U$ has an approximate $F_{p,f-p+1}$ distribution under H_0 where $f = \sum_{i=1}^{2}(\boldsymbol{d}'\boldsymbol{S}^{-1}\ \boldsymbol{S}_i\boldsymbol{S}^{-1}\boldsymbol{d})^2/(U^2[n_i^3 - n_i^2])$. Some comparisons among the different tests have been provided by Subrahmaniam and Subrahmaniam (1973, 1975).

Example 6.9

Srivastava and Carter (1983, p54) give measurements for the thorax length and the elytra length of two species of flea beetle, the data being extracted from those provided by Lubischew (1962). For these measurements we have $n_1 = 10, \bar{\boldsymbol{x}}_1' = (194.9, 263.4)$, $\boldsymbol{S}_1 = \begin{pmatrix} 330.32 & 325.27 \\ 325.27 & 354.71 \end{pmatrix}$, $n_2 = 13, \bar{\boldsymbol{x}}_2' = (178.5, 292.9)$, and $\boldsymbol{S}_2 = \begin{pmatrix} 109.27 & 189.79 \\ 189.79 & 505.41 \end{pmatrix}$. It seems evident that the population dispersion matrices should not be taken as equal, so to test for equality of mean vectors we will use Yao's procedure. We find $U = 118.5$ for f calculated as 16. Hence $[(f - p + 1)/(fp)]U = 55.5$, which exceeds considerably the critical values at either the 5% or the 1% significance levels from the F distribution on 2 and 16 degrees of freedom so that the means of the two species can be taken to be different. Note that the multivariate test is far more powerful than separate univariate tests, because $\bar{x}_{11} > \bar{x}_{21}$ and $\bar{x}_{12} < \bar{x}_{22}$ while x_1, x_2 have high positive correlation.

Non-normality

6.30 All the above tests have assumed normality of data. Three distinct lines of research can be identified as providing help for the practitioner faced with non-normal data: studies of robustness of the above tests to non-normality, production of tests for specific forms of non-normal data, and development of computer-based procedures which overcome dependence on distributional assumptions. We now consider briefly each of these topics.

6.31 Robustness of the single-sample Hotelling statistic to non-normality has been considered by Arnold (1964), Mardia (1970), Everitt (1979) and Srivastava and Awan (1982). The consensus view is that the test is reasonably robust with regard to the nominal significance level when the underlying distribution is symmetrical, but true significance levels tend to increase progressively with increasing skewness and dimensionality. Everitt (1979) also considers Hotelling's two-sample statistic (assuming equal dispersion matrices). Here, while skewness is again a dominant factor, the test is conservative in that non-normality tends to decrease rather than increase true significance levels. Moreover, the test statistic has the correct asymptotic distribution when $\Sigma_1 = \Sigma_2$ irrespective of the underlying distribution of the difference in sample means, and this asymptotic robustness holds approximately for moderately sized samples. Thus non-normality is less of a problem than inequality of dispersion matrices.

By contrast, it is the kurtosis of the underlying distributions that governs robustness to non-normality of tests on dispersion matrices, with positive kurtosis tending to make significance levels greater than the nominal values and negative kurtosis having the opposite effect. Some of the main results here have been established by Ito (1969), Layard (1972,1974) and Muirhead and Waternaux (1980).

Good summaries of all these robustness studies, along with some detailed results, may be found in Muirhead (1982) and Seber (1984). Layard (1972) also develops robust large-sample tests for dispersion matrices by transforming the problem from tests of matrices to tests of means.

6.32 As regards the production of tests for specific forms of non-normal data, very few results appear to exist as yet in the literature. One recent focus of interest has been on establishing test statistics when the samples come more generally from a distribution within the elliptic family (equation 6.2) rather than just from the normal distribution. Available results in this case have been summarised in Chapter 5 of Fang and Zhang (1990), who list likelihood ratio tests and their null distributions for all the above situations as well as deriving some invariance properties of these distributions.

6.33 Once we move outside the elliptic family there appear to be very few analytical results available and recourse must be made to a computer-based method of inference. One possibility is to try and set up a permutation test. Such tests are appropriate when all permutations of the data are equally likely under the null hypothesis, but a certain type of pattern is more likely under the alternative hypothesis. For example, if H_0 is the hypothesis of equality of means in two univariate populations that have equal variances while H_a is the alternative that the second mean is greater than the first, and random samples are available from both populations, then under H_0 all permutations of the observed sample values between the two groups would be equally likely but under H_a the values in the second sample will be 'bigger' than those in the first sample. If such a pattern is present when H_0 is true, then this is purely a chance event. A permutation test requires us first to choose a statistic which measures the extent to which the data show the pattern in question. Thus in the above example we might choose $S = \bar{x}_2 - \bar{x}_1$; the larger the observed value s_0 of S, the more evidence there is in favour of H_a. The value of S is then calculated for all possible permutations of the data between the two samples, yielding the *permutation distribution* of S. If H_0 is true then all possible orderings of the data were equally likely to have occurred, so the value s_0 obtained for the actual samples should appear as a 'typical' value from this permutational distribution. If, on the other hand, s_0 appears to be 'extreme' (in the direction of H_a) with regard to this distribution then H_0 is discredited and H_a is considered to be the more reasonable situation. A formal significance level is provided by the proportion of values in the permutational distribution that are more 'extreme' than s_0. Thus, continuing the example, H_0 would be rejected at the 5% level if s_0 appeared in the *top* 5% of the permutational distribution.

Obtaining all possible permutations of the data may be computationally prohibitive, in which case a (large) sample of random permutations will be adequate. Also, bootstrapping (**6.18**) is a viable alternative to permuting the data. For a full discussion of such tests, including permutational versions of the common multivariate situations, see Manly (1991). One example of a permutational test, in the context of multivariate analysis of variance, is Mardia's (1971) test of generalised T^2 (see **7.5**). More recently, Krzanowski (1993b) has given a permutational test of equality of correlation matrices.

Exercises

6.1 Let $\boldsymbol{x}_1, \boldsymbol{x}_2, \ldots, \boldsymbol{x}_n$ be a random sample from the elliptic distribution with density given by (6.2) where $\psi(z) = c(1+z)^{-(np+1)/2}$ (i.e. a matrix distribution of t-type with power np, see equation 2.37). Show that the maximum likelihood estimators of $\boldsymbol{\mu}$ and $\boldsymbol{\Sigma}$ are given by $\bar{\boldsymbol{x}}$ and $\frac{1}{np}\boldsymbol{S}$ respectively.

(Fang and Zhang, 1990 p130)

6.2 Let $\boldsymbol{x}_1, \boldsymbol{x}_2, \ldots, \boldsymbol{x}_n$ be a random sample from a p-variate normal distribution with mean $\boldsymbol{\mu}$ and dispersion matrix $\boldsymbol{\Sigma}$. Assuming a joint prior distribution for $(\boldsymbol{\mu}, \boldsymbol{\Sigma})$ of the form (6.4), verify that the joint posterior distribution of the sample mean $\bar{\boldsymbol{x}}$ and sample sum of squares and products matrix $\boldsymbol{A}$ is given by (6.5). Hence show that the marginal posterior distribution of $\boldsymbol{\mu}$ is the multivariate t-distribution (6.6) with mean $\bar{\boldsymbol{x}}$, while the marginal posterior distribution of $\boldsymbol{\Sigma}$ is an inverted Wishart distribution with parameter $\boldsymbol{A}$, degrees of freedom $n+p$, and mean $\frac{1}{n-p-2}\boldsymbol{A}$.

(Press, 1972a p130)

6.3 Let $\boldsymbol{x}_1, \boldsymbol{x}_2, \ldots, \boldsymbol{x}_n$ be a random sample from a $(q+1)$-category multinomial distribution in which the kth element, x_{kj}, of $\boldsymbol{x}_j$ is 1 if the jth individual is from category k and 0 otherwise. Suppose also that $\Pr(x_{kj} = 1) = p_k$ for $k = 1, 2, \ldots, q+1$ and $j = 1, 2, \ldots, n$. Then for large n, use of the central limit theorem establishes that $\sqrt{n}(\hat{\boldsymbol{p}} - \boldsymbol{p})$ is approximately normally distributed with mean $\mathbf{0}$ and dispersion matrix $\boldsymbol{\Sigma} = (\sigma_{ij})$, where $\sigma_{ij} = p_i(1-p_i)$ for $i = j$ and $-p_ip_j$ for $i \neq j$, $\boldsymbol{p}' = (p_1, p_2, \ldots, p_{q+1})$, and $\hat{\boldsymbol{p}} = \frac{1}{n}\sum_{j=1}^{n} \boldsymbol{x}_j$. Obtain approximate simultaneous $100(1-\alpha)\%$ confidence regions for all linear combinations $\boldsymbol{l}'\boldsymbol{p} = l_1p_1 + l_2p_2 + \ldots + l_{q+1}$ for large n.

(Johnson and Wichern, 1982 p208)

6.4 Let $\boldsymbol{x}_{11}, \boldsymbol{x}_{12}, \ldots, \boldsymbol{x}_{1n_1}; \boldsymbol{x}_{21}, \boldsymbol{x}_{22}, \ldots, \boldsymbol{x}_{2n_2}$ be independent random samples from p-variate normal distributions with means $\boldsymbol{\mu}_1$ and $\boldsymbol{\mu}_2$ and common dispersion matrix $\boldsymbol{\Sigma}$. Show that a $100(1-\alpha)\%$ confidence region for the difference $\boldsymbol{\mu}_1 - \boldsymbol{\mu}_2$ in means is given by

$$([\bar{\boldsymbol{x}}_1 - \bar{\boldsymbol{x}}_2] - [\boldsymbol{\mu}_1 - \boldsymbol{\mu}_2])'\boldsymbol{S}^{-1}([\bar{\boldsymbol{x}}_1 - \bar{\boldsymbol{x}}_2] - [\boldsymbol{\mu}_1 - \boldsymbol{\mu}_2]) \leqslant c$$

where

$$c = \frac{(n_1 + n_2)(n_1 + n_2 - 2)p}{n_1n_2(n_1 + n_2 - p - 1)} F^{\alpha}_{p, n_1+n_2-p-1}$$

and

$$\boldsymbol{S} = \frac{1}{n_1 + n_2 - 2}\left[\sum_{j=1}^{n_1}(\boldsymbol{x}_{1j} - \bar{\boldsymbol{x}}_1)'(\boldsymbol{x}_{1j} - \bar{\boldsymbol{x}}_1) + \sum_{j=1}^{n_2}(\boldsymbol{x}_{2j} - \bar{\boldsymbol{x}}_2)'(\boldsymbol{x}_{2j} - \bar{\boldsymbol{x}}_2)\right].$$

(Johnson and Wichern, 1982 p239)

6.5 Suppose that $\boldsymbol{x}_1, \boldsymbol{x}_2, \ldots, \boldsymbol{x}_n$ is a random sample from a p-variate normal distribution with mean vector $\boldsymbol{\mu}$ and dispersion matrix $\boldsymbol{\Sigma}$, and that H_0 and H_a are hypotheses under which maximum likelihood estimates of $\boldsymbol{\mu}$ are $\hat{\boldsymbol{\mu}}$ and $\bar{\boldsymbol{x}}$ respectively. Show that the maximum likelihood estimate of $\boldsymbol{\Sigma}$ under H_0 is $\frac{1}{n}\boldsymbol{A} + \boldsymbol{d}\boldsymbol{d}'$, where $\boldsymbol{A} = \sum_{i=1}^{n}(\boldsymbol{x}_i - \bar{\boldsymbol{x}})(\boldsymbol{x}_i - \bar{\boldsymbol{x}})'$ and $\boldsymbol{d} = \hat{\boldsymbol{\mu}} - \bar{\boldsymbol{x}}$.

(Mardia *et al*, 1979 p131)

6.6 Let $\boldsymbol{x}_1, \boldsymbol{x}_2, \ldots, \boldsymbol{x}_n$ be a random sample from a p-variate normal distribution with mean $\boldsymbol{\mu}$ and dispersion matrix $\boldsymbol{\Sigma}$, and write $y_i = \boldsymbol{a}'\boldsymbol{x}_i$ for $i = 1, 2, \ldots, n$ and $\boldsymbol{a}' = (a_1, a_2, \ldots, a_p)$. Deduce the distribution of the y_i and write down the usual test statistic $t(\boldsymbol{a})$ for the null hypothesis $H_0 : \boldsymbol{a}'\boldsymbol{\mu} = \boldsymbol{a}'\boldsymbol{\mu}_0$ against the general alternative $H_a : \boldsymbol{a}'\boldsymbol{\mu} \neq \boldsymbol{a}'\boldsymbol{\mu}_0$. By finding the maximum of t^2 over $\boldsymbol{a}$, show that the union-intersection test of the multivariate hypothesis $H_0 : \boldsymbol{\mu} = \boldsymbol{\mu}_0$ against the general alternative $H_a : \boldsymbol{\mu} \neq \boldsymbol{\mu}_0$ is given by Hotelling's T^2 (as defined in **6.23**).

(Krzanowski, 1988a p243)

Verify that T^2 is invariant under all affine transformations $\boldsymbol{y} = \boldsymbol{B}\boldsymbol{x} + \boldsymbol{c}$ where $\boldsymbol{B}$ is $(p \times p)$ and non-singular.

6.7 Suppose that $\boldsymbol{x}_1, \boldsymbol{x}_2, \ldots, \boldsymbol{x}_n$ is a random sample from a p-variate normal distribution with mean vector $\boldsymbol{\mu}$ and dispersion matrix $k\boldsymbol{\Sigma}_0$, where $\boldsymbol{\mu}$ and k

are unknown. Show that the maximum likelihood estimate of k is given by $\hat{k} = \mathrm{tr}(\boldsymbol{\Sigma}_0^{-1}\boldsymbol{C})/p$ where $\boldsymbol{C} = \frac{1}{n}\sum_{i=1}^{n}(\boldsymbol{x}_i - \bar{\boldsymbol{x}})(\boldsymbol{x}_i - \bar{\boldsymbol{x}})'$.

(Mardia *et al*, 1979 p107)

6.8 Verify that, in the special case of two samples in **6.27**, the non-zero eigenvalue c_1 of $\boldsymbol{B}\boldsymbol{W}^{-1}$ is equal to $(n_1 n_2/n)(\bar{\boldsymbol{x}}_1 - \bar{\boldsymbol{x}}_2)'\boldsymbol{W}^{-1}(\bar{\boldsymbol{x}}_1 - \bar{\boldsymbol{x}}_2)$ and hence that the union-intersection test of equality of mean vectors is based on Hotelling's two-sample T^2 statistic.

7

Multivariate Linear Models

The univariate linear model

7.1 This section summarises the properties and applications of the univariate linear model. For a much fuller treatment, see Stuart and Ord (1991), Chapters 26–29.

The model may be written

$$\underset{n\times 1}{\boldsymbol{y}} = \underset{n\times(q+1)}{\boldsymbol{X}} \quad \underset{(q+1)\times 1}{\boldsymbol{\beta}} + \underset{n\times 1}{\boldsymbol{\epsilon}}$$

Here, $\boldsymbol{y}$ is a vector of dependent variables, and the aim is prediction of a random variable y as a linear function of $(x_1, \ldots, x_q)$, The matrix $\boldsymbol{X}$ contains the values of these variables, and of $x_0 = 1$, giving the constant term in the regression equation (it is sometimes appropriate to omit this when $q = 1$, but not otherwise). $\boldsymbol{\beta}$ is a vector of unknown parameters, to be estimated. $\boldsymbol{\epsilon}$ is a vector of residuals, and the assumption underlying ordinary least squares estimation is that

$$E(\boldsymbol{\epsilon}) = \underset{n\times 1}{\boldsymbol{0}}$$

$$\text{cov}(\boldsymbol{\epsilon}) = \underset{n\times n}{\sigma^2\boldsymbol{I}}$$

where σ^2 is an unknown parameter.

The assumptions concern only the residuals, and the scope of the model is very wide.

(1) The x variables may be continuous variables fixed by the experimenter.
(2) The x variables may be continuous random variables. Since we are concerned with inference conditional upon their values, this does not affect the model. (It may, however, affect such problems as the treatment of missing values).

(3) The x variables may be functionally dependent. For example, if they are powers of a single variable x, the model is a polynomial regression. The 'linear' model is linear in the parameters $\boldsymbol{\beta}$, not necessarily in the predictor variables that are actually observed. The only restriction is that the x variables may not be *linearly* dependent, otherwise the estimates of the elements of $\boldsymbol{\beta}$ are not unique.

(4) The x variables may be dummies, separating the data into groups. The linear model then gives an analysis of variance between and within groups.

(5) The x variables may be divided into two groups, and the question is the way in which one group affects y when the effect of the other group has been eliminated. A particular case is when one group are dummies, and the other are 'covariates', leading to the analysis of covariance.

(6) The x variables may follow a multivariate distribution, and the y variable may be binary. If the binary variable affects the means, but not the covariance matrix, of the x variables, the assumptions of the model hold. This calculation gives Fisher's linear discriminant function (see Volume 2).

Least squares estimation minimises

$$S_\beta = (\boldsymbol{y} - \boldsymbol{X\beta})'(\boldsymbol{y} - \boldsymbol{X\beta})$$

giving

$$\hat{\boldsymbol{\beta}} = (\boldsymbol{X}'\boldsymbol{X})^{-1}\boldsymbol{X}'\boldsymbol{y}$$

and if $\hat{\boldsymbol{y}} = \boldsymbol{X}\hat{\boldsymbol{\beta}}$, $\boldsymbol{y} - \hat{\boldsymbol{y}} = \boldsymbol{e}$,

$$\hat{\sigma}^2 = \frac{\boldsymbol{e}'\boldsymbol{e}}{n - q - 1}.$$

The fundamental theorem of least squares, due to Gauss, but often referred to as the Gauss–Markov theorem (see Stuart and Ord, 1991, 19.6) states that the estimates $\hat{\boldsymbol{\beta}}$ are minimum variance unbiased linear estimates, and the same is true of any linear combination of them—that is, of any prediction $\hat{y}$. Then the mean and covariance matrix of the estimated parameters are $E(\hat{\boldsymbol{\beta}}) = \boldsymbol{\beta}$ and $\text{cov}(\hat{\boldsymbol{\beta}}) = \sigma^2(\boldsymbol{X}'\boldsymbol{X})^{-1}$, and unbiased estimates of the elements of this matrix are given by replacing σ^2 by $\hat{\sigma}^2$.

If it is further assumed that $\boldsymbol{\epsilon} \sim N(\boldsymbol{0}, \sigma^2\boldsymbol{I})$, the usual exact inferential procedures are justified. The least squares estimates are also maximum likelihood. Confidence intervals for the elements of $\boldsymbol{\beta}$ and prediction intervals for y are based on the t distribution, tests of null hypotheses and confidence intervals for $\boldsymbol{\beta}$ or subsets of its elements are based on the F distribution. Further, the central limit theorem ensures that these results are asymptotically valid even if the residuals are not normally distributed. Provided the least-squares assumptions hold, inference may be based on the normal distribution and the χ^2 distribution in large samples without risk of serious error.

All the properties, and all the applications, of the general univariate linear model have their counterpart in multivariate analysis.

The multivariate linear model

7.2 The multivariate linear model has the form

$$\underset{n \times p}{\boldsymbol{Y}} = \underset{n \times (q+1)}{\boldsymbol{X}} \quad \underset{(q+1) \times p}{\boldsymbol{\beta}} + \underset{n \times p}{\boldsymbol{\epsilon}}$$

where

$$E(\boldsymbol{\epsilon}) = \underset{n \times p}{\mathbf{0}}$$

$$\operatorname{cov}(\operatorname{vec} \boldsymbol{\epsilon}) = \underset{p \times p}{\boldsymbol{\Sigma}} \otimes \underset{n \times n}{\boldsymbol{I}}$$

in the notation of **2.27**.

This equation is the natural extension of the univariate linear model to the multivariate case where there are p dependent variates. The residuals of each p-variate observation—the rows of $\boldsymbol{\epsilon}$—are independent, but the residuals of the individual $\boldsymbol{y}$ values have an unknown covariance matrix $\boldsymbol{\Sigma}$. Different responses in the same individual item may be correlated.

Given any estimate $\hat{\boldsymbol{\beta}}$ of $\boldsymbol{\beta}$, the matrix of residual sums of squares and products is

$$(\boldsymbol{Y} - \boldsymbol{X}\hat{\boldsymbol{\beta}})'(\boldsymbol{Y} - \boldsymbol{X}\hat{\boldsymbol{\beta}}).$$

Differentiating with respect to $\hat{\boldsymbol{\beta}}$ gives

$$-2\boldsymbol{X}'(\boldsymbol{Y} - \boldsymbol{X}\hat{\boldsymbol{\beta}}),$$

and setting this equal to zero gives

$$\hat{\boldsymbol{\beta}} = (\boldsymbol{X}'\boldsymbol{X})^{-1}\boldsymbol{X}'\boldsymbol{Y}. \tag{7.1}$$

This equation minimises both the determinant $|(\boldsymbol{Y} - \boldsymbol{X}\hat{\boldsymbol{\beta}})'(\boldsymbol{Y} - \boldsymbol{X}\hat{\boldsymbol{\beta}})|$ and the trace $\operatorname{tr}[(\boldsymbol{Y} - \boldsymbol{X}\hat{\boldsymbol{\beta}})'(\boldsymbol{Y} - \boldsymbol{X}\hat{\boldsymbol{\beta}})]$. This means that the estimates $\hat{\boldsymbol{\beta}}$ are exactly those that would be obtained by separate regression of each y variable on the set of x values. In fact, most of the theory of univariate multiple regression, including the standard errors of the estimated coefficients, is unchanged. Gauss's theorem on least squares shows that the estimates $\hat{\boldsymbol{\beta}}$ and the predictions $\hat{\boldsymbol{Y}}$ are unbiased and have minimum variance in the class of unbiased linear estimates. Differences arise in significances tests and in confidence intervals because of the multiplicity of the tests and the non-independence of the error structure.

The predicted values are now given by

$$\hat{\boldsymbol{Y}} = \boldsymbol{X}\hat{\boldsymbol{\beta}} = \boldsymbol{X}(\boldsymbol{X}'\boldsymbol{X})^{-1}\boldsymbol{X}'\boldsymbol{Y}, \tag{7.2}$$

and the residuals by

$$\hat{\boldsymbol{\epsilon}} = \boldsymbol{Y} - \hat{\boldsymbol{Y}}. \tag{7.3}$$

The usual analysis of variance for univariate regression is replaced by a multivariate analysis of variance as in Table 7.1.

Here, $\hat{\boldsymbol{Y}}_c$ and $\boldsymbol{Y}_c$ are the matrices of deviations from the means of the p variables ($\boldsymbol{Y}_c = \boldsymbol{Y} - \frac{1}{n}\mathbf{1}\mathbf{1}'\boldsymbol{Y}$), and each sum of squares in the univariate analysis

Table 7.1 Analysis of variance for multivariate regression

	d.f.	S.O.P.
Regression	q	$\hat{\boldsymbol{Y}}_c'\hat{\boldsymbol{Y}}_c$
Residual	n-q-1	$\hat{\boldsymbol{\epsilon}}'\hat{\boldsymbol{\epsilon}}$
Total	n-1	$\boldsymbol{Y}_c'\boldsymbol{Y}_c$

of variance becomes a $p \times p$ matrix in the multivariate form. The elements of

$$\hat{\Sigma} = \frac{\hat{\epsilon}'\hat{\epsilon}}{n-q-1}$$

are unbiased estimates of the Σ, the covariance matrix of the residuals, and

$$\widehat{\text{cov}}\,(\text{vec } \boldsymbol{\beta}) = \hat{\Sigma} \otimes (\boldsymbol{X}'\boldsymbol{X})^{-1}.$$

The total and residual matrices are of rank p in practical cases when n is reasonably large and the variables are not linearly related. The regression matrix is of rank p or q, whichever is smaller.

The further assumption that the errors have a multivariate normal distribution,

$$\epsilon \sim N(\mathbf{0}, \Sigma), \tag{7.4}$$

implies that $\hat{\boldsymbol{\beta}}$ and $\hat{Y}$ also have multivariate normal distributions, and justifies significance tests and confidence intervals based on that assumption. Least squares estimation is also maximum likelihood estimation under multivariate normality, and likelihood ratio tests are available. The distribution of other test statistics is also known when the distribution is multivariate normal (see Appendix). These tests are exact, or based on tabulated values that can be regarded as exact, but even if multivariate normality does not hold exactly, the multivariate central limit theorem means that they are asymptotically valid.

Multivariate calibration

7.3 The calibration model, in its simplest form, involves using the relationship between variables X and Y to predict values of x, when the experimental data available consist of observations of y, with random error, corresponding to known values of x. This problem arises in the calibration of an instrument. Observations of the response y correspond to fixed x values, perhaps controlled by an accurate, but cumbersome device, and the y values later observed are used to estimate new x values.

Of course, if each observation can be regarded as a random observation from the bivariate distribution of a random variable (x, y), no problem arises; it is simply required to estimate the regression of x on y. This situation is sometimes referred to as the *unconditional model* (Stuart and Ord, 1991, **28.77**), or *random calibration* (Brown, 1982). The difficulty is that it is the controlled variable in the original data that is to be predicted in the subsequent use of the instrument. In these circumstances, it is appropriate to use the estimated regression of y on x as a relationship for prediction of x. This is the *conditional model* (Stuart and Ord, 1991), or *controlled calibration* (Brown, 1982).

The extension to multivariate observations $\boldsymbol{x}$ and $\boldsymbol{y}$ was apparently first discussed by Williams (1959), and the methodology of the multivariate case was developed by Brown (1982). Typically, $\boldsymbol{x}$ may represent an exact chemical analysis of certain substances, and $\boldsymbol{y}$ physical observations on them, related to the chemical composition and much easier to obtain than the full analysis. The distinction between the two models still applies. Perhaps the most important applications are in spectroscopic analysis; modern methods of automatic data recording make the collection of spectroscopic data a routine process, and these data can then be related to traditional chemical analyses.

Another problem arises here, however. The vector $\boldsymbol{x}$ may well consist of 1000 or more 'variables' (spectral energies in different frequency bands), and often there will be more variables than independent observations. In these circumstances, the problem becomes indeterminate, and the distinction between models becomes blurred (Sundberg and Brown, 1989). Denham and Brown (1993) discuss ways of resolving this indeterminacy, and give two practical examples of calibration with many x-variables. The possible approaches will be examined in Part 2.

Inference in the multivariate linear model

7.4 Overall significance tests are based on the multivariate analysis of variance. Writing

$$\begin{aligned} \boldsymbol{W} &= \hat{\boldsymbol{\epsilon}}'\hat{\boldsymbol{\epsilon}} \\ \boldsymbol{T} &= (\boldsymbol{Y} - \frac{1}{n}\mathbf{1}\mathbf{1}'\boldsymbol{Y})'(\boldsymbol{Y} - \frac{1}{n}\mathbf{1}\mathbf{1}'\boldsymbol{Y}) \end{aligned}$$

the tests of the null hypothesis that there is no relationship ($\boldsymbol{\beta} = \mathbf{0}$) depend on the eigenvalues of $\boldsymbol{T}^{-1}\boldsymbol{W}$. On the null hypothesis, these are both Wishart matrices derived from multivariate normal variates with the same covariance matrix $\boldsymbol{\Sigma}$, and the various possible tests, given by Wilks' criterion, the Lawley–Hotelling trace, Pillai's trace, and the minimum eigenvalue (or the maximum eigenvalue of $\boldsymbol{H}\boldsymbol{T}^{-1}$), are discussed in the Appendix, **A.8**.

The most usual, and most flexible, test is based on Wilks' criterion, $L = |\boldsymbol{T}^{-1}\boldsymbol{W}|$. This is the likelihood ratio test, against the general alternative $\boldsymbol{\beta} \neq \mathbf{0}$. The distribution has been much studied, and the usual χ^2 approximation with adjustments to the degrees of freedom, or the Box (1949) F approximation, is usually satisfactory.

Roy's (1957) union-intersection test suggests as a test criterion the maximum eigenvalue of $\boldsymbol{H}\boldsymbol{T}^{-1}$, where $\boldsymbol{H} = \boldsymbol{T} - \boldsymbol{W}$. This test is usually more powerful than the likelihood ratio test when there is a single non-zero eigenvalue, that is, when the two sets of observed variables are related to a single underlying variable.

The Lawley–Hotelling trace tr $(\boldsymbol{H}\boldsymbol{W}^{-1})$ usually give P-values intermediate between the likelihood ratio test and the maximum root test. Pillai's trace, tr $(\boldsymbol{HT}^{-1})$, is most powerful when the eigenvalues are nearly equal (for details, see the Appendix).

Tables of significance points for these tests are available in various textbooks; Anderson (1984) gives them in a particularly convenient form. The statistical packages SPSS and SAS give all four statistics with the corresponding P-values.

Canonical variables have been discussed in Chapter 4. They are useful in multivariate regression only if the smaller eigenvalues are non-significant, so that the corresponding canonical variables can be ignored, and if those that are retained can be reasonably interpreted.

The problems of outliers, points of high leverage, and influential points that are encountered in multiple regression arise also in the multivariate case. The usual techniques for regression diagnostics can be used for their detection in the individual regression equations for each of the dependent variables; see, for example, Atkinson (1985).

The specific problems of multivariate regression diagnostics have not received much attention; Gnanadesikan and Kettenring (1972), Gnanadesikan (1977) and Atkinson and Mulira (1993) discuss multivariate outlier detection, and Critchley (1985) discusses the problem of influence in principal component analysis. For robust estimation, see Chapter 5.

Multivariate analysis of variance

7.5 Apart from its use in multivariate regression, the multivariate analysis of variance has three principal applications.

(1) It is the structure underlying Fisher's linear discriminant analysis (see Part 2), and provides the basis for inferential arguments about the significance of differences between groups and the importance of particular variables. The assumptions involved are those of multivariate normality and equality of covariance matrices within groups. These assumptions are seldom strictly true in practice, but the method is reasonably robust and usually works well with small data sets. With large data sets, the problem of estimating large numbers of parameters for more realistic models can be overcome, and it is usually possible to find better methods.

(2) Planned experiments to test the effects of different treatments may involve multivariate data. The multivariate analysis of variance has then exactly the form of the univariate analysis of variance, with the sums of squares replaced by matrices of sums of squares and products; the form is identical with that of an analysis of covariance, but the aim is to compare multivariate means, rather than means of one variable adjusted for the effects of the others.

(3) A special case of the last application occurs when one or more variables are observed at different set times. This is the problem of 'repeated measures' or 'growth curve analysis'; for a detailed treatment, see Part 2. One way of comparing time series with observations at fixed times is to regard the sequence of observations as a single multivariate observation. This approach is implemented in SPSS and BMDP. The analysis is optimal when there is adequate replication and the number of time points—the

Table 7.2 Multivariate analysis of variance

	d.f.	S.O.P.
Treatments	q	$\boldsymbol{H}$
Error	$m-q$	$\boldsymbol{W}$
Total	m	$\boldsymbol{T}$

number of variates—is small. Otherwise, estimation of the covariance matrix without taking account of the time structure may be inefficient. It is often better to fit a time-series model, which amounts to imposing constraints on the structure of the covariance matrix.

The multivariate analysis of variance has the structure given in Table 7.2. The 'Total' matrix is the sum of the treatments and error matrices; $\boldsymbol{T} = \boldsymbol{H} + \boldsymbol{W}$. If this is the complete analysis of variance table, $m = n - 1$, but if the effects of blocks have been removed, or if all the matrices have been adjusted for covariates, m must be adjusted accordingly.

The analysis assumes that the components of $\boldsymbol{W}$ within each treatment are homogeneous, and in particular that the variances and covariances are independent of the means. If this is not so, there is a multivariate Behrens–Fisher problem, and interpretation becomes difficult. If there are obvious differences that cannot be removed by transformations (see Chapter 3) this is unavoidable. Again, formal testing of the homogeneity of the variance-covariance matrices within treatments may be possible, but is not appropriate; the test for homogeneity is much more sensitive to non-normality than the multivariate analysis of variance itself, and will often show heterogeneity when the analysis is perfectly appropriate.

Example 7.1
Snedecor (1946) gives an example of a Latin square experiment on the effects of spacing on the yield and the average number of culms produced by millet (Li *et al*, 1936). He used it as an illustration of analysis of covariance, with yields adjusted for differences in the number of culms, but expressed doubts about the the appropriateness of the adjustment. The example does not appear in later editions of the book, by Snedecor and Cochran.
The analysis of variance and covariance has the form of Table 7.3.
Here, x_1 and x_2 stand for culms and yield respectively. Snedecor shows that the effect of spacing on yield is not significant at the 5% level, whether or not adjusted for culms. The multivariate analysis of variance tests the null hypothesis that spacing has no effect on culms or spacing. Notice that the analysis of variance on x_1 does give a significant variance ratio, but the multivariate test makes allowance for the number of variates being tested.
The means are shown in Table 7.4.
The analysis depends on the Error matrix of sums of squares and products

Table 7.3 Multivariate analysis of Latin square

	d.f.	x_1^2	x_1x_2	x_2^2
Total	24	12.5428	51.99	36571.36
Rows	4	2.0445	139.07	13601.36
Columns	4	0.3434	1.54	6146.16
Spacing	4	6.1378	−132.62	4156.56
Error	12	4.0171	44.00	12667.28
Spacing + Error	16	10.1549	−88.62	16823.84

Table 7.4 Table of means

	Spacing (ins)				
Means	2.	4.	6.	8.	10.
x_1 (Culms)	2.89	3.62	3.75	3.74	4.45
x_2 (Yield)	269.8	262.8	252.4	238.2	237.6
$x_2 - 99.4x_1$	-17.5	-97.1	-120.4	-133.6	-204.8

and on the corresponding 'Spacing + Error' matrix—just as in the analysis of covariance, the Row and Column matrices are simply removed. Writing:

$$\boldsymbol{W} = \begin{pmatrix} 4.0171 & 44.00 \\ 44.00 & 12667.28 \end{pmatrix} \quad \boldsymbol{T} = \begin{pmatrix} 10.1549 & -88.62 \\ -88.62 & 16823.84 \end{pmatrix}$$

Wilks' criterion is given by $L = |\boldsymbol{W}|/|\boldsymbol{T}|$.

$$|\boldsymbol{W}| = 48949.7305 \tag{7.5}$$
$$|\boldsymbol{T}| = 162990.9084 \tag{7.6}$$

Then $L = 0.3003$, with $p = 2$, $q = 4$, $m = 16$. The approximate likelihood ratio test gives

$$\left(-16 + \frac{7}{2}\right) \log L = 15.04 \sim \chi_8^2.$$

Since $p = 2$, an exact test is possible (Mardia *et al*, 1979 p83); see also **A.1**:

$$\frac{11}{4}\frac{1-\sqrt{L}}{\sqrt{L}} = 2.27 \sim F_{(8,22)}.$$

Both tests agree in giving a P-value just greater than 0.05. Solving the quadratic equation $|\boldsymbol{H} - t\boldsymbol{T}| = 0$ gives the eigenvalues $t_1 = 0.6764$, $t_2 = 0.0719$. Interpolation in the tables of the maximum eigenvalue (see Anderson, 1984, or Pearson and Hartley, 1972, tables 48 and 49) gives the 5% point as about 0.64, so the result is just significant. The Lawley–Hotelling trace (2.168) is just significant; the Pillai trace (0.748) is not.

Table 7.5 Test criteria

Roy's maximum root test	t_1
The Lawley–Hotelling trace	$\frac{t_1}{1-t_1} + \frac{t_2}{1-t_2}$
Wilks' criterion	$(1 - t_1)(1 - t_2)$
The Pillai trace	$t_1 + t_2$

Table 7.6 Comparison of four tests; critical values

Roy	t_1	=	0.3344
Lawley–Hotelling	$\frac{t_1}{1-t_1} + \frac{t_2}{1-t_2}$	=	0.6086
leading to	$t_1 + t_2 - \frac{2.6086}{1.6086} t_1 t_2$	=	0.3783
Wilks	$(1 - t_1)(1 - t_2)$	=	0.6007
leading to	$t_1 + t_2 - t_1 t_2$	=	0.3993
Pillai	$t_1 + t_2$	=	0.4331

In this case the maximum root test is more powerful than the other tests, and the reason is clear from the table of means; the two variates show the same pattern of variation—with opposite sign—across the treatments. The first canonical variable is proportional to $x_2 - 99.4x_1$, and the corresponding contrast among the means is almost the linear component associated with the spacings.

Of course, in this case the conclusions suggested by the different tests are practically the same, but this may not be so when the number of variates is high. In general, when the groups are ordered, as in the regression situation when a single dominant source of variation is suspected, it is worth examining the largest eigenvalue as well as the likelihood ratio.

Finally, the Bartlett decomposition of the likelihood ratio χ^2 gives the test of the smaller eigenvalue as $\chi_3^2 = 0.93$. This result confirms that the second canonical variable gives no useful information. Notice that the contribution of the first eigenvalue is $\chi^2 = 14.10$. If this were tested as χ^2 with 5 degrees of freedom it would give a misleadingly low P-value, close to 1%. This effect, too, can be much more serious when there is a higher number of variates.

Example 7.2

The four tests discussed depend on the values of the eigenvalues t_i of $\boldsymbol{HE}^{-1}$. When $p = 2$, they are shown in Table 7.5.

For a specific example, suppose $q = 5$, and the residual degrees of freedom are 35. Now the critical values can be read from the tables, giving the results in Table 7.6.

It is clear that when $t_2 = 0$, Roy's test rejects the null hypothesis for the lowest value of t_1, followed by Lawley–Hotelling, Wilks and Pillai in that order. It is easily verified that at the opposite extreme, when $t_1 = t_2$, the order is reversed. This reflects, in general, what may be expected of the power of the tests. When there is a single non-zero eigenvalue, so that the means are collinear, Roy's test is most powerful; when the eigenvalues are nearly equal, so that the means are at the vertices of a regular simplex, Pillai's test is best, and the other tests are intermediate. This result is true for reasonably large samples when the eigenvalues are large enough for the sample values to correspond approximately to the population values.

It is clear that

(1) Roy's maximum root depends only on t_1, and will give the lowest P-value of the four criteria when t_2 is zero or very small.
(2) Wilks' maximum likelihood criterion is sensitive to general deviations from the null hypothesis; it will seldom give the lowest P-value, but will detect any pattern of non-zero population eigenvalues.
(3) The Lawley–Hotelling trace is intermediate between the maximum root test and the likelihood ratio test, in the sense that it gives more weight than the latter to the largest t values.
(4) The Pillai trace gives the lowest P-value of the four criteria when the sample eigenvalues are nearly equal.

These conclusions relate to the *sample* eigenvalues. They are directly relevant to the power only when the sample eigenvalues and eigenvectors are reasonable approximations to the population values—and in this case all the tests are likely to detect departures from the null hypothesis. When the power is low, the first sample eigenvector may be quite unrelated to the corresponding population vector, and Roy's criterion may not be powerful even against a single non-zero population eigenvalue (Pillai and Jayachandran, 1967).

Most of the published work on the power of these tests is based on simulation studies. These are inevitably of limited applicability, because the number of possible variables—the dimensionality, sample size and eigenvalue structure—is so large. The same is true of studies of robustness. Mardia (1970) examined the effect of skewness and kurtosis on Hotelling's T^2, the Lawley–Hotelling trace when $p = 2$. Mardia (1971) also studied the robustness of the Pillai trace, and derived an approximate randomisation test for it, based on the ideas of Pitman (1937a, 1937b, 1938) and Box and Watson (1962). Normal theory (Pillai, 1955) gives an approximate test of the form

$$\frac{V}{p} \sim B\left(\frac{pq}{2}, \frac{1}{2}p(n-1-q)\right).$$

The permutation test has the same form, with the parameters of the Beta distribution modified using Mardia's (1970) coefficient of multiple kurtosis.

The general conclusions of these studies are that

(1) The effect of skewness is more serious than that of kurtosis.
(2) Long tailed distributions tend to give conservative tests (P-values that are too large).
(3) Effects of non-normality become progressively more serious as dimensionality increases.

Multivariate analysis of covariance

7.6 The extension of the analysis of covariance to the multivariate case is straightforward. The matrices $\boldsymbol{W}$ and $\boldsymbol{T}$ in Table 7.2 are replaced by matrices adjusted for the covariates, and $\boldsymbol{H}$ is $\boldsymbol{T} - \boldsymbol{W}$, as before. The degrees of freedom for $\boldsymbol{W}$ and $\boldsymbol{T}$ are each reduced by the number of covariates fitted, and the analysis on the adjusted table is the same as an ordinary multivariate analysis of variance.

Applications are not as common as might be expected. In discriminant analysis, say in a problem of medical diagnosis, it is easy to imagine that some of the observed variables affect the symptoms but are unconnected with the diseases involved. This assumption would suggest an analysis of covariance, but in practice it is seldom possible to classify variables in this way.

The most important application of multivariate analysis of covariance is in the analysis of repeated measures, or growth curves, discussed at length in Volume 2. Wishart (1938) first discussed the possibility of fitting simple models with $k < p$ parameters to the responses, with a different set of parameters for each case. Then, a multivariate analysis of variance can be carried out on the $n \times k$ matrix of fitted parameters. In the simplest case, low order polynomials are fitted; Wishart fitted straight lines, and did an analysis on the slopes, disregarding the intercepts.

The analysis of parameters of fitted curves is a natural approach to many problems of this type, but it appears that data are being wasted. The k parameters fitted correspond to polynomials of order $k - 1$, while the p observations could be used to fit polynomials of order $p - 1$. If orthogonal polynomials are fitted, the original $n \times p$ data matrix $\boldsymbol{X}$ could be replaced by another $n \times p$ matrix of coefficients of orthogonal polynomials. The first k columns are used in the analysis of variance. Leech and Healy (1959) first pointed out that the remaining $p-k$ columns could be regarded as covariates, by hypothesis unaffected by treatments, but providing information that could be used to make more accurate comparisons among the sets of k coefficients. The idea was developed by Rao (1965, 1966).

The procedure, then, is to fit orthogonal polynomials of order p to each individual growth curve, and then carry out a multivariate analysis of covariance on the k coefficients defining the response to treatments, using one or more of the remaining $p - k$ coefficients as covariates. This method of analysis is efficient and straightforward, but one caution is necessary. In practice, both the value of k and the coefficients to be used as covariates are selected in the light of the data. This means that inference is at best approximate; significance levels are affected by choosing variables to fit the model.

Simultaneous inference

7.7 When several groups are compared, or when a regression depends on a number of explanatory variables, a single overall test of significance is often supplemented by further tests involving subsets of the groups or variables. If each of these tests has error rate α, the error rate for the whole analysis will be larger than α. This multiple comparison problem is well known in univariate statistics, and many statisticians believe that the appropriate procedure is to ensure that the probability of making a type I error should be controlled at a fixed level α *for the whole experiment.*

This view was proposed by Tukey (1949) and Scheffé (1953). Earlier, Fisher advocated, for example, testing individual comparisons using t-tests *provided that* the overall F-test gave a significant result.

The subject is still controversial. Critics of the 'error rate per experiment' concept point out:

(1) In structured experiments, such as factorial designs, nobody has seriously questioned the appropriateness of examining individual degrees of freedom, representing main effects, linear components, interactions and so on without considering the simultaneous inference problem.
(2) An 'experiment' is not a well-defined entity. A group of experiments planned to investigate certain treatments could be regarded as a single experiment.
(3) The trend in experimental design over the last 50 years has been towards complex experiments designed to involve many different factors or comparisons. Should this trend be reversed, since individual experiments to answer single questions give greater power?

Duncan (1965) developed the argument against the error rate per experiment. If an experiment is designed to answer a number of questions, decision theory regards a significance test as associated with losses from the type I and II errors, and α is chosen in the light of these losses. Further, the losses associated with different questions should be regarded as additive, so that simultaneous inference becomes a problem in empirical Bayesian decision theory. The mathematical treatment is complex, but the outcome is very like a smoothed version of Fisher's procedure; conclusions in analysis of variance depend on the value of F, and on individual t tests. There is not a sharp break according to whether or not F is significant, but the critical t values increase as the value of F gets smaller. This approach is dismissed with some scorn by Tukey (1991).

Control of the error rate per experiment in univariate statistics is achieved in various ways; for a full treatment, see Chew (1977). Not all of these are available in the multivariate situation. In particular, the most popular simultaneous test procedures in comparisons among univariate treatment means are based on the Studentised range, and this has no simple analogy for multivariate means.

A very general method of controlling the error rate depends on the Bonferroni inequalities. The well-known identity

$$\Pr(\cup A_i) = \sum \Pr(A_i) - \sum \Pr(A_i \cap A_j) + \sum \Pr(A_i \cap A_j \cap A_k) - \ldots$$

can be regarded as a sequence of approximations—the first sum, the difference between the first two sums, and so on. The Bonferroni inequalities state that the error in each successive approximation has the opposite sign to that of the next term, and decreases in absolute value when that term is included.

The practical conclusion is that if k significance tests are carried out with type I error rate α/k, the overall error rate is less than alpha. This inequality gives a very simple way of controlling the error rate; unfortunately, if k is not very small, the test is extremely conservative. If something is known about the structure of the tests—if, for example, they are independent—the test can be 'sharpened', but this is not generally possible. In multivariate analysis of variance, if formal significance tests between pairs of means are required and if the significance level is to be controlled for the whole experiment, the Bonferroni method is often recommended. In practice, the number of groups is usually not very large, and the procedure is not unreasonably conservative. Most computer programs give P-values for comparing individual means, and multiplying these values by the number of comparisons gives an appropriate significance level.

Scheffé (1953, 1959) suggested quite a different approach. In an analysis of variance, the group means can be regarded as an observation from a multivariate normal distribution, and a multivariate confidence region can be constructed. This formulation leads to a confidence interval for any linear combination of the means, and in particular a significance test for any contrast among them.

In practice, this is not what is required. Simple comparisons between pairs, or groups, of means are the main interest, and for such comparisons Scheffé's test is so conservative as to be practically useless. A similar approach, however, can be taken to a set of regression coefficients, and the resulting tests are much more reasonable.

The direct application of multivariate normal theory to multiple tests was studied by Gabriel (1968, 1969). The basic procedure is simply to test each comparison as if it were based on p variables, with q degrees of freedom associated with the hypothesis, and n degrees of freedom for error. Thus, a comparison between two means still involves q degrees of freedom if there are $q + 1$ treatments in the original experiment. This is a natural extension of Scheffé's test. The F statistic in that test is replaced by a multivariate test statistic; Gabriel examines the use of Roy's test, the Lawley–Hotelling trace, Pillai's trace and the likelihood-ratio (Wilks') test, and concludes that Roy's test has clear advantages. Later work by Mudholkar *et al* (1974b) suggests that this may not always be the case.

For variable selection in multivariate regression or in multivariate analysis of variance, stepwise programs are widely available (stepwise discriminant analysis in the statistical packages SPSS and BMDP). These select variables in the same way as in stepwise regression analysis, with the default 'F to enter' set to an approximate 5% level for that single test. This default value can be changed. The aim is to find a best subset of variables, in the sense that no variable is included unnecessarily, no further variable would give significant improvement, and no subset of the same size is as good. There is no guarantee that this is achieved, and it is not clear that it is a sensible aim.

Aitkin (1974) examined the problem of variable selection in multiple (univariate) regression. His approach was to find all 'adequate' subsets, in the sense that they were not significantly improved by including the complete set of variables. Significance was judged by a test with error rate controlled for the whole experiment; this means that the critical multiple correlation for a subset does not depend on its size. A minimum adequate subset is then an adequate subset that does not contain another adequate subset.

The conclusion is then not that a particular subset is best, but that one or more subsets are as informative as the complete set of regressor variables. This idea was extended to multivariate regression by McKay (1977, 1979). The methods have the minor drawback that they involve the examination of all subsets—not a serious difficulty for modern computers unless there are very many variables—and that the simultaneous test procedures are conservative. The last point implies that variables with some explanatory power may be omitted, but of course the overall significance level can be controlled. The advantage is that a choice of subsets is available, and the decision about which to use can depend on factors such as ease of collection.

Presentation of means

7.8 The estimated Mahalanobis distance between two groups has the form

$$D_{ij}^2 = (\bar{\boldsymbol{x}}_i - \bar{\boldsymbol{x}}_j)' \boldsymbol{V}^{-1} (\bar{\boldsymbol{x}}_i - \bar{\boldsymbol{x}}_j) \tag{7.7}$$

where $V_{ij} = \dfrac{1}{m-q} \boldsymbol{W}_{ij}$.

The null hypothesis that $\Delta = 0$ can be tested using the F distribution,

$$\left(\frac{1}{n_i} + \frac{1}{n_j} \right)^{-1} D_{ij}^2 \sim F_{p,n}. \tag{7.8}$$

The resulting P-value may be adjusted to give a simultaneous test using the Bonferroni inequality as described in the last section.

The result is easily generalised to give a test of any contrast among the means. Suppose $\boldsymbol{a} = (a_1, \ldots, a_{q+1})'$ with $\sum_{i=1}^{q+1} a_i = 0$, and $\bar{\boldsymbol{x}}$ is a vector containing the $q+1$ means. Then

$$\left[\sum \left(\frac{a_i^2}{n_i} \right) \right]^{-1} \boldsymbol{a}' \bar{\boldsymbol{x}} \boldsymbol{V}^{-1} \bar{\boldsymbol{x}}' \boldsymbol{a} \sim F_{p,n}. \tag{7.9}$$

The usual graphical display to show the groups is a canonical variable plot, showing the first two canonical variables, as described in Chapter 4. The data points should appear as approximately circular clusters around their respective means, if the assumption of multivariate normality within groups, with equal dispersion matrices is justified.

This plot gives the two-dimensional projection that maximises $\sum n_i n_j d_{ij}^2$, where d_{ij} is the projection of the Mahalanobis distance on to the plane. It thus spreads the means as widely as possible, when the groups are of equal size. When the numbers vary, the representation of the distances between small groups may be underrepresented; see Example 4.4.

The canonical plot is given by many computer programs, such as SPSS and BMDP discriminant analysis.

Selection of variables

7.9 In a linear model relating $\boldsymbol{y} = (y_1, \dots, y_p)'$ and $\boldsymbol{x} = (x_1, \dots, x_q)'$, some of the x-variables may be redundant in the sense that they contribute nothing to the prediction of the ys. The variable x_i is irrelevant to the relationship if the multiple correlation of x_i conditional on $(x_1, \dots, x_{i-1}, x_{i+1}, \dots, x_q)$ with $\boldsymbol{y}$ is zero. This is the obvious multivariate generalisation of the corresponding problem in univariate multiple regression. It is equivalent to the condition $\beta_{ki} = 0, \ \forall k$. If the residuals have a multivariate normal distribution, it implies the conditional *independence* of x_i and $\boldsymbol{y}$.

This conditional independence can be tested by a standard F-test, of the regression of $x_{i.1,\dots,i-1,i+1,\dots,q}$ on $\boldsymbol{y}$. If the result is not significant, x_i may be dropped from the relationship. This test is perfectly valid for a specified x_i, but of course questions of multiple testing arise when it is applied to all the x-variables, and when it is applied to x-variables after some have already been eliminated.

Stepwise methods ignore this problem. They proceed either upwards or downwards. The upwards stepwise method selects first the x-variable with the highest multiple correlation with $\boldsymbol{y}$, and adjusts $\boldsymbol{y}$ and the remaining x-variables for its effect. It then repeats the process until none of the remaining adjusted x-variables is significantly related to $\boldsymbol{y}$. There is usually provision for eliminating variables that have been included at an early stage, but have been made redundant by the inclusion of later variables. Downwards stepwise methods proceed by eliminating variables one at a time from the relationship in the same way. Most standard computer packages include programs for stepwise linear discrimination.

A recently developed approach to the investigation of conditional independence is that of independence graphs. These are concerned with the independence structure of the data set as a whole, rather than specifically with the redundancy of variables in a multivariate linear model. Perhaps the most important application is in log-linear models for contingency tables, in deciding which interaction terms can be omitted from the model. They apply also to conditional independence models for multivariate normal distributions, and to the conditional Gaussian distribution. Whittaker (1990) gives a general account of the methods. The computer program MIM (Edwards, 1987, 1992) makes it possible to construct such graphs, and they may be used for subset selection. Krusińska (1991, 1992) has discussed the relationship between graph-theoretic methods for the conditional Gaussian model and the location model for discriminant analysis.

This approach is much more flexible than the stepwise method, and makes it possible to select one of several 'adequate' subsets. It does not, however, take account of the multiple testing problem, though the significance level for the individual tests may be chosen to make some allowance for it.

The multivariate generalisation of Aitkin's (1974) simultaneous test procedure concentrates on finding adequate subsets of $\boldsymbol{x}$ for the prediction of $\boldsymbol{y}$ (or of subsets of $\boldsymbol{y}$). Suppose the matrix of sums of squares and products of $\boldsymbol{x}$ and $\boldsymbol{y}$, about the mean values, is $\boldsymbol{S}$ and it is partitioned into $\begin{matrix} \boldsymbol{S}_{xx} & \boldsymbol{S}_{xy} & \boldsymbol{S}_{yy} \\ q \times q & p \times q & p \times p \end{matrix}$.

Now write

$$H = S'_{xy}S_{xx}^{-1}S_{xy} \tag{7.10}$$
$$T = S_{yy} \tag{7.11}$$
$$W = S_{yy} - S'_{xy}S_{xx}^{-1}S_{xy} \tag{7.12}$$

The eigenvalues of HW^{-1} or HT^{-1} give tests for the multivariate regression. Suppose now H^* is defined in the same way as H for a subset of the variables x. Then the eigenvalues of $(H - H^*)W^{-1}$ give tests of whether x contains information about y not included in the subset represented in H^*.

The extension to multivariate regression of Aitkin's procedure is described by McKay (1977). Tests are based on the eigenvalues of $(H - H^*)W^{-1}$. Any subset for which the test is *not* significant is 'adequate', and adequate subsets that contain no smaller adequate subsets are minimal adequate; a suitable subset can be chosen from these. The simultaneous test procedure is described in detail for Roy's maximum root test and for the likelihood ratio criterion. The tests are based on p, q and $n - q - 1$ degrees of freedom, so that the critical value for the chosen test is independent of the size of the subset being considered. This ensures that the overall significance level is controlled at a chosen level α or lower.

As with all simultaneous test procedures, the tests are 'conservative' in the sense that the probability of wrong rejection of the null hypothesis is less than α. In the present context, this means that subsets may be accepted as adequate even when a single test of conditional independence of one or more x-variables not in the subset would give a significant result. It may therefore be advisable not to choose too small a value of α. For other reasons, concerned with demonstrating the difference between the two criteria discussed, McKay (1977) uses a 10% significance level; this may be a good practical choice.

Redundancy indices and redundancy analysis

7.10 In a canonical variable analysis, the first canonical variable of the xs, say $a'x$, is the linear combination that has maximum correlation with a linear combination of the y variables. When y is adjusted for this variable, the resulting variables $y^* = y|a'x$ have minimum *generalised variance*; that is, $a'x$ is chosen to minimise $|S_{y^*y^*}|$. The effect on the total variance of the y variables, in the sense of $\text{tr}S_{yy}$, is less obvious. This change may be of some interest, and has been studied particularly in the psychometric literature. It depends, of course, on the scale of the y variables, just as principal components are scale dependent, and is usually only of interest when they are standardised, so that S_{yy} is a correlation matrix.

Stewart and Love (1968) defined the *redundancy*, or redundancy index, of a set of variables conditional on another variable as the proportion of the total variance—the trace of the covariance matrix—accounted for by adjusting for that variable. In particular, suppose x and y are standardised to unit variance, and the first pair of canonical variables are a'_1x and b'_1y, both standardised to have unit variance. The redundancy index of y conditional on the first canonical variable is the product of two parts:

(i) The proportion of the variance of $\boldsymbol{b}_1'\boldsymbol{y}$ accounted for by $\boldsymbol{a}_1'\boldsymbol{x}$, that is, λ_1, the squared canonical correlation.
(ii) The proportion of $\mathrm{tr}(\boldsymbol{R}_{yy})$ removed by regression on $\boldsymbol{b}_1'\boldsymbol{y}$ (writing $\boldsymbol{R}_{yy}$ for the correlation matrix, the matrix $\boldsymbol{S}_{yy}$ in standardised form). Now the vector of correlations of $\boldsymbol{b}_1'\boldsymbol{y}$ with the individual terms of $\boldsymbol{y}$ is $\boldsymbol{b}'\boldsymbol{R}_{yy}$, and the reduction in the trace is the sum of squares of these correlations.

Then the redundancy of $\boldsymbol{y}$ conditional on the first canonical variable is given by

$$R(\boldsymbol{y}|\boldsymbol{x})_1 = \frac{\boldsymbol{b}_1'\boldsymbol{R}_{yy}\boldsymbol{R}_{yy}\boldsymbol{b}_1}{p}\lambda_1 \tag{7.13}$$

where λ_1 is the largest eigenvalue, the square of the first canonical correlation. In the same way, the corresponding redundancy of $\boldsymbol{x}$ is

$$R(\boldsymbol{x}|\boldsymbol{y})_1 = \frac{\boldsymbol{a}_1'\boldsymbol{R}_{xx}\boldsymbol{R}_{xx}\boldsymbol{a}_1}{q}\lambda_1. \tag{7.14}$$

These two redundancies are, of course, unequal. They depend on the correlation structure of $\boldsymbol{y}$ and $\boldsymbol{x}$ respectively, as well as on the canonical correlations. Redundancies can be defined for the other canonical variables in the same way, and the sum of the redundancies of either set of variables is the proportion of the trace of the covariance matrix accounted for by the other set.

$$\sum_i R(\boldsymbol{y}|\boldsymbol{x})_i = \frac{\mathrm{tr}\boldsymbol{S}_{yx}\boldsymbol{S}_{xx}^{-1}\boldsymbol{S}_{xy}}{\mathrm{tr}\boldsymbol{S}_{yy}} \tag{7.15}$$

$$= \frac{\mathrm{tr}\boldsymbol{R}_{yx}\boldsymbol{R}_{xx}^{-1}\boldsymbol{R}_{xy}}{\mathrm{tr}\boldsymbol{R}_{yy}} \tag{7.16}$$

Van den Wollenberg (1977) first suggested the idea of choosing linear functions of $\boldsymbol{x}$ to maximise the redundancy of $\boldsymbol{y}$ conditional upon them. The problem may be written in terms of the $n \times p$ and $n \times q$ centred data matrices $\boldsymbol{Y}$ and $\boldsymbol{X}$ as:

$$\text{Maximise} \quad \frac{1}{n^2}\boldsymbol{a}'\boldsymbol{X}'\boldsymbol{Y}\boldsymbol{Y}'\boldsymbol{X}\boldsymbol{a} \quad \text{subject to} \quad \boldsymbol{a}'\boldsymbol{X}'\boldsymbol{X}\boldsymbol{a} = n.$$

The maximisation leads to the characteristic equation

$$(\boldsymbol{X}'\boldsymbol{Y}\boldsymbol{Y}'\boldsymbol{X} - n\lambda\boldsymbol{X}'\boldsymbol{X})\boldsymbol{a} = 0 \tag{7.17}$$

or

$$|(\boldsymbol{X}'\boldsymbol{X})^{-1}(\boldsymbol{X}'\boldsymbol{Y}\boldsymbol{Y}'\boldsymbol{X}) - \lambda\boldsymbol{I}| = 0. \tag{7.18}$$

To each eigenvalue λ there corresponds an eigenvector and the set of linear functions $\boldsymbol{a}'\boldsymbol{x}$ so derived constitute an alternative to the canonical variables associated with $\boldsymbol{x}$. There are $\min(p, q)$ of these *redundancy variables*, spanning the same space as the canonical variables, but not being, in general, the same.

In the same way, a set of redundancy variables can be derived from the y variables, spanning the same space as the canonical variables of the ys. There is, however, no particular relationship between the ith redundancy variables of $\boldsymbol{x}$ and $\boldsymbol{y}$, and in general the corresponding eigenvalues are different. The redundancy variables of $\boldsymbol{x}$ are the same as the canonical variables only if the y

variables are uncorrelated. If the x and y variables are exactly linearly related, so that the canonical variables are undefined, the redundancy variables are the principal components.

This is known as a redundancy analysis, or a redundancy factoring analysis. It has some features in common with canonical analysis, with principal components, and with principal component regression. From the statistical point of view it has the disadvantages of being scale dependent, and of being affected by the inclusion of highly correlated variables. It can be regarded as an alternative to canonical analysis when it is felt that the total variance $\mathrm{tr}\boldsymbol{S}_{yy}$ is a more realistic measure of variability than the generalised variance $|\boldsymbol{S}_{yy}|$.

Exercise

7.1 If $\boldsymbol{y}$ consists of a set of binary variables classifying the observations into groups, show that the first two canonical variables give the projection that maximises $\sum n_i n_j d_{ij}^2$, where d_{ij} is the projection of the Mahalanobis distance on to the plane (see 7.7). Show that the same result is true for the redundancy variables, if d_{ij} is the projection of the Euclidean distance.

8

Nonlinear Methods

8.1 Most of the techniques discussed so far in this volume can be described as *linear*, because they conform to one or more of the following descriptions: they utilise *linear* transformations of the measured variables; they seek *linear* structure in the data; or they replace one high-dimensional set of coordinates by another which has a one-to-one *linear* relation with it. While these techniques do enable a great variety of multivariate problems to be solved a number of gaps nevertheless remain, so that attention has increasingly been turned towards nonlinear generalisation. The last ten years have seen some vigorous research in this area, but much of this work has been dispersed among a number of substantive areas (notably psychology) so that it still remains relatively unfamiliar to many statisticians. Also, there is no unique definition of a nonlinear multivariate system, so that different interpretations can be found under the single umbrella. Our purpose here therefore is to collect together as many of these methods as seem to afford useful potential for statisticians, and to provide a brief survey of the current state of development. We first describe nonlinear generalisations of two specific multivariate techniques, and then outline two approaches that lead to general systems of nonlinear multivariate analysis.

Nonlinear principal components

8.2 Principal component analysis being probably the most common descriptive multivariate technique for seeking linear structure in data, it is unsurprising to find a number of attempts at generalising it in order to handle nonlinear structures. An early attempt was made by Gnanadesikan and Wilk (1969 — see also Gnanadesikan, 1977), who called the technique *generalised principal components*. The idea was a very simple one, namely to augment the list of variables by adding quadratic and perhaps higher order terms and then to perform ordinary principal component analysis on the expanded set of variables. For instance, if two variables x_1 and x_2 are present, then one might do a principal component analysis on the five variables x_1, x_2, x_1^2, x_2^2 and x_1x_2. Gnanadesikan (1977) illustrated this procedure on an artificial set of data which lay exactly on a circle. The equation of the circle being $(x_1 - \mu_1)^2 + (x_2 - \mu_2)^2 = r^2$, the covariance matrix of the expanded list of five variables had a zero latent root and the coefficients of the associated latent vector recovered exactly the equation of the circle. However, Flury (1994) points out some difficulties with this idea; the linear and quadratic terms are not in the same units of measurement, and the results will depend heavily on shifts of origin and scale. Moreover, he has conducted a number of experiments in which he added small random errors to Gnanadesikan's data and found that it then became essentially impossible to recover the nonlinear structure from the eigenvectors of the expanded covariance matrix. These drawbacks perhaps account for the fact that little use appears to have been made of this technique in practical applications.

8.3 Gnanadesikan and Wilk's technique cannot really be termed a generalisation of principal component analysis, but rather an application of the existing technique to transformed and augmented data. A true generalisation should consider some particular properties of the method and then define more general models for which the same properties are still valid. This is the approach adopted by Hastie and Stuetzle (1989). Their aim is to provide a nonlinear summary of a set of multivariate data by finding a smooth one-dimensional *curve* passing through the 'middle' of the data, in the sense that orthogonal projections of all points on to this curve have minimum total displacement. This then provides a generalisation of the first principal component which is known to be the best-fitting *line* for such data in the orthogonal least-squares sense. To provide the theoretical framework for the analysis, they first define a general property of multivariate distributions which is satisfied by principal components in certain special cases. This property suggests a computational algorithm for theoretical distributions, which in turn leads to a method for fitting such a *principal curve* to a set of data. The following description gives an outline of the main technical details.

8.4 A one-dimensional curve in p-dimensional space is a vector $\boldsymbol{f}(\lambda)$ of p functions of a single variable λ. These functions are the *coordinate* functions, and λ provides an ordering along the curve. The vector $\boldsymbol{f}'(\lambda)$ is tangent to the curve at λ and is known as the velocity vector at λ. Any smooth curve with Euclidean norm $\| \boldsymbol{f}' \| > 0$ can be reparameterised so that $\| \boldsymbol{f}' \| \equiv 1$, in which case it is called a *unit speed* curve. The vector $\boldsymbol{f}''(\lambda)$ is called the acceleration of the curve at λ, and for a unit-speed curve is orthogonal to the velocity vector. In this case $\boldsymbol{f}''/\|\boldsymbol{f}''\|$ is called the principal normal to the curve at λ. If $\boldsymbol{v}$ is a unit vector, then $\boldsymbol{f}(\lambda) = \boldsymbol{v}_0 + \lambda \boldsymbol{v}$ is a unit-speed straight line where $\boldsymbol{v}_0$ can be assumed orthogonal to $\boldsymbol{v}$.

Given these preliminaries, Hastie and Stuetzle (1989) first consider a p-dimensional random variable $\boldsymbol{x}$ having density h and finite second moments, and a smooth unit-speed curve $\boldsymbol{f}(\lambda)$. They then say that the curve $\boldsymbol{f}$ is *self-consistent*, or a *principal curve* of h, if

$$E[\boldsymbol{x} \mid \boldsymbol{f}^{-1}(\boldsymbol{x}) = \lambda] = \boldsymbol{f}(\lambda), \tag{8.1}$$

where

$$\boldsymbol{f}^{-1}(\boldsymbol{x}) = \sup_{\lambda}\{\lambda : \| \boldsymbol{x} - \boldsymbol{f}(\lambda) \| = \inf_{\mu} \| \boldsymbol{x} - \boldsymbol{f}(\mu) \|\}. \tag{8.2}$$

The quantity $\boldsymbol{f}^{-1}(\boldsymbol{x})$ defined in this way is the value of λ for which $\boldsymbol{f}(\lambda)$ is closest to $\boldsymbol{x}$. Thus $\boldsymbol{f}$ is a principal curve if, for all λ, $\boldsymbol{f}(\lambda)$ is the average of all those observations that have $\boldsymbol{f}(\lambda)$ as their closest point on the curve. For ellipsoidal distributions, the principal components are all principal curves; for a spherically symmetric distribution, any line through the mean vector is a principal curve; and for any two-dimensional spherically symmetric distribution, a circle with centre at the origin and radius $E \parallel \boldsymbol{x} \parallel$ is also a principal curve. Furthermore, if a straight line is self-consistent then it must be a principal component (Exercise 8.1).

The above discussion suggests an iterative projection-expectation algorithm for finding $\boldsymbol{f}$ given the distribution h of $\boldsymbol{x}$. Start with a smooth curve, and consider a hyperplane orthogonal to this curve at each point. Find the conditional expectation of $\boldsymbol{x}$ over those points of each hyperplane that are no nearer to any other part of the curve as determined by orthogonal projection. If these conditional expectations coincide everywhere with the curve then it is a principal curve so the process should terminate, otherwise the conditional expectations define a new curve and the process can be repeated. Formally we can write

$$\boldsymbol{f}_{i+1}(\lambda) = E[\boldsymbol{x} \mid \boldsymbol{f}_i^{-1}(\boldsymbol{x}) = \lambda], \tag{8.3}$$

where $\boldsymbol{f}_i$ is the curve on the ith iteration. The process can be started by setting $\boldsymbol{f}_0(\lambda) = \bar{\boldsymbol{x}} + \boldsymbol{a}\lambda$, where $\boldsymbol{a}$ is the first linear principal component of h, and stopped when the conditional expectations are 'sufficiently close' to the current curve. Hastie and Stuetzle define an expected distance criterion for judging when to stop the process.

8.5 The above discussion is in terms of principal curves for theoretical probability distributions, but in practice we will be faced with finite multivariate data sets. Thus we will need to *estimate* $\boldsymbol{f}$ from the data set $\boldsymbol{x}_1, \ldots, \boldsymbol{x}_n$, by estimating $E[\boldsymbol{x} \mid \boldsymbol{f}^{-1}(\boldsymbol{x}) = \lambda]$. A curve $\boldsymbol{f}(\lambda)$ is now represented by the n-tuples $(\lambda_i, \boldsymbol{f}_i)$, joined up in increasing order of λ to form a polygon. As in the distribution case, the algorithm alternates between a projection step and an expectation step and is started by taking the curve to be the first principal component line. Let $\hat{\boldsymbol{f}}_i$ be the estimated $\boldsymbol{f}$ at the ith iteration, and let $\hat{\lambda}_{ij} = \hat{\boldsymbol{f}}_i^{-1}(\boldsymbol{x}_j)$ for $j = 1, \ldots, n$ be the projections of the n data points on $\hat{\boldsymbol{f}}_i$ (see Hastie and Stuetzle, 1989, for details of the calculation). This completes the projection step. The goal of the expectation step is then to estimate $\boldsymbol{f}_{i+1} = E[\boldsymbol{x} \mid \boldsymbol{f}^{-1}(\boldsymbol{x}) = \lambda]$ at the n values $\hat{\lambda}_{ij}$. A natural way would be to gather all of the observations that project on to each $\hat{\lambda}_{ij}$ and find their mean, but generally $\boldsymbol{x}_j$ is the only such observation. Hastie and Stuetzle therefore suggest using a *scatterplot smoother* at this step, and estimating the conditional expectation by averaging all observations $\boldsymbol{x}_k$ whose $\hat{\lambda}_{ik}$ is *close* to $\hat{\lambda}_{ij}$. Various different types of smoother have been described in the literature, including kernel smoothers (Watson, 1964), spline smoothers (Silverman, 1985) and locally weighted running-line smoothers (Cleveland, 1979). Hastie and Stuetzle implemented the last named, using a general *S* function given by Becker *et al* (1988), and discussed such issues as the size of the neighbourhood over which the averaging takes place (i.e. the 'span') and the relationships between principal curves and splines. Once again, a suitable distance criterion was defined and hence a stopping rule for the iterative process determined.

8.6 The above technique can thus be seen to be a method of fitting the curve $\boldsymbol{f}(\lambda)$ to a set of points by minimising the sum of squared orthogonal distances from the points to the curve, which generalises the principal component idea of fitting a straight line to the points by minimising the sum of squared orthogonal deviations. We could alternatively suppose that the data have the form

$$\boldsymbol{x} = \boldsymbol{f}(\lambda) + \boldsymbol{e}, \tag{8.4}$$

where $\boldsymbol{e}$ is a vector of random disturbances and $\boldsymbol{f}(\lambda)$ is to be estimated from the data by means of the above technique. However, Hastie and Stuetzle (1989) point out two components of bias in such an estimation procedure. The first is model bias, because if $\boldsymbol{f}(\lambda)$ has curvature then it is not a principal curve for the distribution that it generates. Thus the principal curve procedure can only find a biased version of $\boldsymbol{f}(\lambda)$, even if it is started at the generating curve. Secondly, averaging over neighbourhoods as part of the scatterplot smoothing usually has a 'flattening effect', so this introduces estimation bias. Hastie and Stuetzle discuss these two components of bias and illustrate them by a simple example. Banfield and Raftery (1992) propose a modification of the above algorithm that reduces bias and is particularly designed for estimating closed curves. Neither algorithm has been formally proved to be convergent, but both sets of authors state that no problems have been encountered in many empirical applications of the procedures.

8.7 Although the above technique has been propounded as a nonlinear generalisation of principal components, it is perhaps more correctly viewed as another method for nonlinear curve fitting to set beside such non-parametric computer-intensive variants of regression analysis as splines (De Boor, 1978), interaction splines (Barry, 1986), generalised additive models (Hastie and Tibshirani, 1990), projection pursuit regression (Friedman and Stuetzle, 1981), recursive partitioning (Breiman *et al*, 1984) and adaptive regression splines (Friedman, 1991). Hastie and Stuetzle (1989) define the concept of a two-dimensional *principal surface*, and mention briefly an extension of the curve algorithm to the fitting of two-dimensional surfaces, but no further generalisations appear to exist at present. Alternative multivariate approaches have been taken to the fitting of an equation of the form of (8.4), but these all assume parametric forms for $\boldsymbol{f}(\lambda)$ so are much more restrictive than the method of principal curves. Relevant references to this work are Shepard and Carroll (1966), Carroll (1969), and Etezadi-Amoli and McDonald (1983). Nonlinear generalisations of principal component analysis that go beyond curve fitting are described later in this chapter.

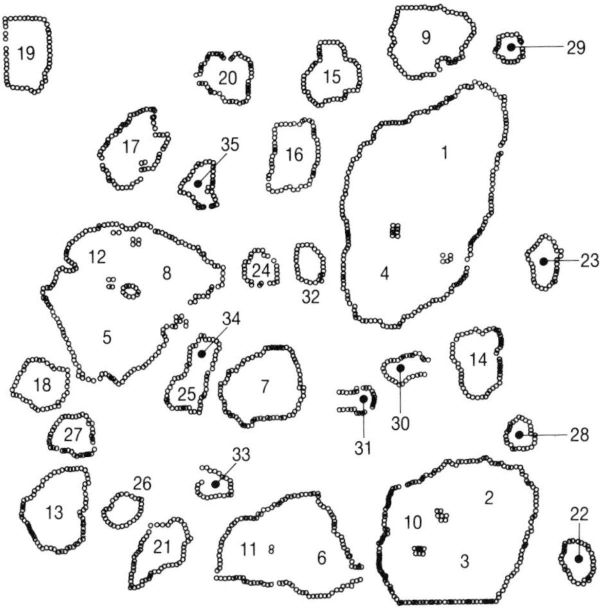

Figure 8.1 Outlines of ice floes larger than a fixed minimum size, as found by the erosion-propagation algorithm. Open circles are edge elements while solid dots or numbers are centres. Floes containing more than one centre were generally subdivided. Reproduced with permission from Banfield and Raftery (1992), *Journal of the American Statistical Association*, by the American Statistical Association. All rights reserved.

Example 8.1
Banfield and Raftery (1992) give an interesting application of principal curve analysis applied to the identification of ice floes from satellite images. They first describe a method, known as the erosion-propagation algorithm, for identifying the outlines of ice floes from a satellite image taken in the polar regions. Fig. 8.1 shows the outcome of this algorithm as applied to a typical satellite image. One problem of the algorithm is that it tends to subdivide floes, either when they are nonconvex or when they have melt points or noise in the interior. Floes in Fig. 8.1 having more than one centre were subdivided in this way. Banfield and Raftery therefore go on to describe a method for determining which of the floes identified by the algorithm should be merged. They postulate that the edge pixels for an ice floe that has not been subdivided should be (a) tightly clustered about the floe outline, as estimated by a closed principal curve, and (b) regularly spaced along the outline, so that the variance of the distances between neighbouring edge pixels should be small. Banfield and Raftery thus fit closed principal curves to the x, y coordinates of the outlines, using a robust modification of Hastie and Stuetzle's algorithm. Such a modification is needed to overcome awkward problems caused by the melt points, which can here be viewed as 'outliers'. Having fitted the curves, they decompose the within-group sum of squares V of the data

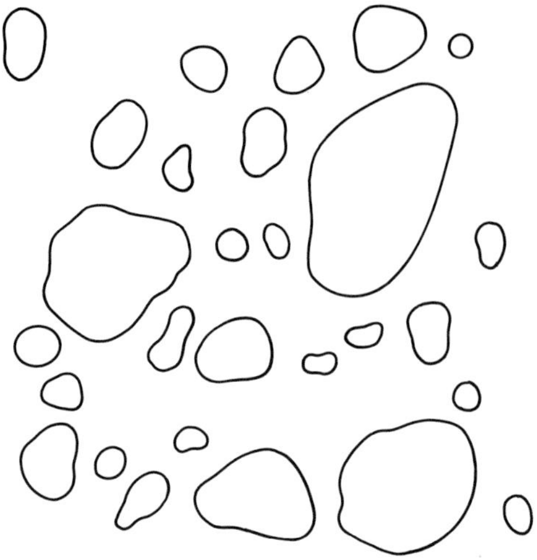

Figure 8.2 Ice floe outlines from Fig. 8.1 identified by clustering about principal curves. Reproduced with permission from Banfield and Raftery (1992), *Journal of the American Statistical Association*, by the American Statistical Association. All rights reserved.

into a term V_{about} corresponding to (a), a term V_{along} corresponding to (b), and a residual term. These terms are then combined into a single criterion, to judge whether a set of groups should be merged. Finally, the outlines of the floes are identified by refitting principal curves; the resultant ('cleaned') set of outlines from Fig. 8.1 is shown in Fig. 8.2.

Nonlinear biplots

8.8 Closely associated with principal component analysis is the idea of a *biplot*, introduced by Gabriel (1971) and described in **4.9** above. For the purposes of discussing nonlinear generalisations, we require the following summary algebra and interpretations of the linear technique. Suppose that $\boldsymbol{X}$ is a data matrix giving the values of p (quantitative) variates observed on each of n sample units. A t-dimensional biplot exhibits the units as n points and the variables as p vectors in a single t-dimensional space. This space is that of the first t principal components of the data. Moreover, if $\boldsymbol{X}$ is mean-centered, then the coordinates of the sample points are given by the rows of $\boldsymbol{Y} = \boldsymbol{U}\boldsymbol{S}_t$ and the vectors representing the variables are the directions given by the rows of $\boldsymbol{V}_t$, where $\boldsymbol{U}, \boldsymbol{S}_t$ and $\boldsymbol{V}_t$ are obtained from the singular value decomposition of $\boldsymbol{X}$:

$$\boldsymbol{X} = \boldsymbol{U}\boldsymbol{S}\boldsymbol{V}'. \tag{8.5}$$

Here $\boldsymbol{U}$ and $\boldsymbol{V}$ are orthogonal matrices of sizes $(n \times n)$ and $(p \times p)$ respectively, while $\boldsymbol{S}$ has size $(n \times p)$ and elements $s_{ii} = s_i \geqslant 0$ if $i \leqslant r = \text{rank}(\boldsymbol{X})$, $s_{ii} = 0$ if $i > r$, and $s_{ij} = 0$ if $i \neq j$; furthermore, $s_1 \geqslant s_2 \geqslant \ldots \geqslant s_r$. Then $\boldsymbol{V}_t$ is the matrix comprising the first t columns of $\boldsymbol{V}$, and $\boldsymbol{S}_t$ is obtained from $\boldsymbol{S}$ by setting s_i to zero for all $i > t$. The t-dimensional space thus obtained is the one which best approximates the Euclidean distance d_{ij} between two arbitrary units i and j, defined by

$$d_{ij}^2 = \sum_{k=1}^{p} (x_{ik} - x_{jk})^2, \tag{8.6}$$

with respect to the classical scaling discrepancy measure (5.5) [see **5.8**].

To interpret the $\boldsymbol{V}_t$ plots, one can regard the matrix $\rho \boldsymbol{I}$ as containing information on p new sample individuals. The ith row of this matrix has zero elements in all positions except the ith, which has element ρ, so the ith new individual has values equal to the variate mean for all variates except the ith. The projection of these new individuals on to the t principal dimensions of the component analysis are given by $\rho \boldsymbol{I} \boldsymbol{V}_t = \rho \boldsymbol{V}_t$. Thus each biplot vector varies *linearly* with ρ, and represents individuals all of whose weight lies in one variable. The classical biplot can therefore be interpreted as a component analysis augmented by information on the variables obtained by projecting notional sample-units that have values concentrated in a single variable.

8.9 Gower and Harding (1988) generalise the above approach, once again taking the classical scaling view of the first-stage component analysis but now allowing *any* distance function imbeddable in a Euclidean space to be used in place of the Euclidean distance (8.6). The first stage of the analysis is thus to conduct a classical scaling (**5.7**) on the $(n \times n)$ matrix of inter-unit distances d_{ij} computed by using the chosen distance function. We assume that a set of coordinates $\boldsymbol{Y}_t$ for the n points in t dimensions has been so determined. Classical scaling conventionally fixes the origin of the axes at the centroid G of the configuration, so that $\boldsymbol{Y}'\boldsymbol{1} = \boldsymbol{0}$; also $\boldsymbol{Y}$ is referred to its principal axes, so that $\boldsymbol{Y}'\boldsymbol{Y} = \boldsymbol{\Lambda}$, a diagonal matrix of ranked eigenvalues.

The second stage of the analysis now requires a generalisation of the concept of projecting the rows of $\rho \boldsymbol{I}_p$, regarded as values of notional sample-units, on to the space spanned by $\boldsymbol{Y}_t$. Let the kth row of $\rho \boldsymbol{I}_p$ be regarded as an $(n+1)$th sample individual, and let the distances $d_{i,n+1} (i = 1, \ldots, n)$ of this new individual from each of the original ones be calculated using the same metric as for the original d_{ij}. Then, using the result given by Gower (1968), the coordinates of the projection of this new individual on to the t-dimensional ordination are given by $\boldsymbol{y}_t = \frac{1}{2} \boldsymbol{\Lambda}_t^{-1} \boldsymbol{Y}_t' \boldsymbol{d}$, where $\boldsymbol{\Lambda}_t$ is the principal $(t \times t)$ submatrix of $\boldsymbol{\Lambda}$ and $\boldsymbol{d}$ is the vector whose ith element d_i is defined by

$$d_i^2 = \frac{1}{n} \sum_{j=1}^{n} d_{ij}^2 - \frac{1}{2n^2} \sum_{i=1}^{n} \sum_{j=1}^{n} d_{ij}^2 - d_{i,n+1}^2. \tag{8.7}$$

The biplot for the ith variable is then defined to be the locus of $\boldsymbol{y}_t$ as ρ varies, and for non-Euclidean choices of d_{ij} this will yield a nonlinear trajectory. Note that only the last term in (8.7) depends on ρ, and so it is only this term that changes when calculating $\boldsymbol{d}$ for different points on the trajectory. Also, setting $\rho = 0$, it is clear that the trajectories for all variables meet at the point corresponding to the mean vector of the the original variables. This unique and easily identified point can be regarded as the origin O of the nonlinear biplot; O will not normally coincide with the origin G of the ordination for non-Euclidean distances, but for the classical biplot these two points *do* coincide.

8.10 Gower and Harding (1988) discuss various issues concerning these plots. In a classical biplot only the origin and one point on each line are needed to plot the vectors representing variables, but in the nonlinear biplot a series of projections must be computed for different values of ρ and then linked. Gower and Harding suggest choosing ρ to plot from $m_k - L$ to $M_k + L$ in steps of length $l = (M_k - m_k)/100$, where $m_k = \min(x_{ik}), M_k = \max(x_{ik})$ and $L = 10l$. They also suggest graduating each trajectory, by marking on it intervals of unit deviations from the mean in the original measurement scales of the corresponding variable, and discuss the interpolation of sample points relative to these trajectories. Following these suggestions, it is possible that some trajectories may be very short, or that they may be of finite length even when ρ is allowed to increase indefinitely. Short trajectories correspond to variables that contribute little to the approximation in the given ordination, while finite trajections may arise either because the chosen distance function is bounded or because the extremes of the trajectory may move orthogonally to the space of the ordination. Both types provide useful information for interpreting the analysis.

Some further extensions of the above ideas, to permit analysis of qualitative as well as quantitative variables and to allow nonmetric scaling in place of classical scaling, have been sketched by Gower (1990b) under the name *generalised* biplots. A comprehensive treatment of the geometry underpinning these methods is given by Gower (1993). Meulman and Heiser (1993) generalise the nonlinear biplot in a different way, by embedding it within a nonlinear mapping (that uses the least-squares loss function given by equation (5.6)) rather than within a classical scaling (that uses the loss function given by equation (5.5)).

Example 8.2

Gower and Harding (1988) contrast their nonlinear biplot with the classical biplot on a set of data given by Rudeforth and Bradley (1972). At each of 15 sites (the units) the amounts of 12 trace elements (the variables) were determined and logs taken to obtain the values x_{ij}. Fig. 8.3 shows the classical biplot for these data. Projecting the range (m_k, M_k) for each variable provides more information in this figure than is given by a conventional display. In particular, the differing lengths of the trajectories highlight the relative contributions of the variables. Variables 5, 7 and 9 are best represented while the other variables have little weight, and a similar figure is obtained if the analysis is repeated using just these three variables. Also, samples g, e and k are evident outliers.

If now the L_1 distance function $d_{ij}^2 = \sum_{k=1}^{p} \mid x_{ik} - x_{jk} \mid$ is used instead of Euclidean distance (8.6), the nonlinear biplot shown in Fig. 8.4 is obtained. Points of difference to note from the previous diagram are that there is now a small displacement of the origin of the biplot (the join of all trajectories) from that (G) of the ordination; variables 5, 7 and 9 again dominate the ordination but there is now a greater contribution from the others, particularly variable 12; and the trajectories are of finite

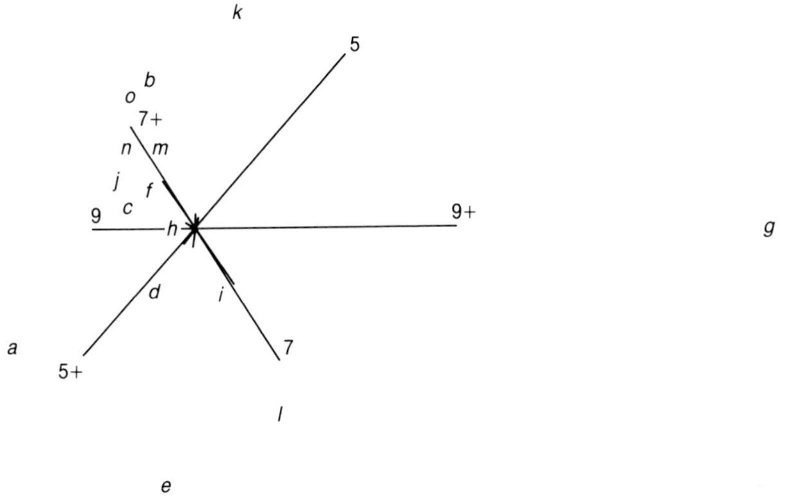

Figure 8.3 Classical biplot of soil data; the letters refer to samples and the numbers labelling the trajectories to the variables. Reproduced with permission from Gower and Harding (1988).

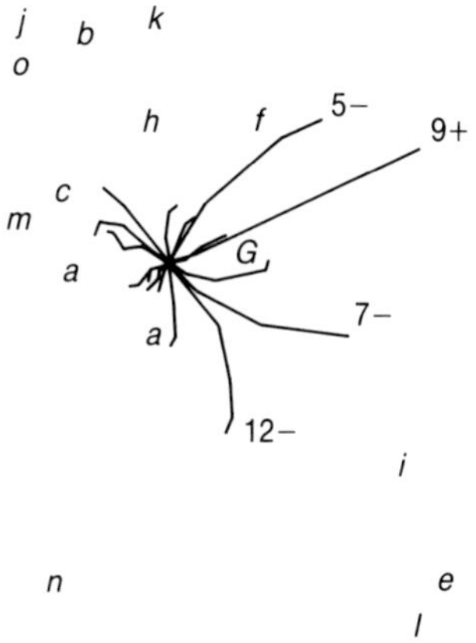

Figure 8.4 Nonlinear biplot of soil data; the letters refer to samples and the numbers labelling the trajectories to the variables. Reproduced with permission from Gower and Harding (1988).

length because of the boundedness of the L_1 distance function (since it terminates at the maximum value in the data set). However, the qualitative conclusions remain broadly as before.

General nonlinear systems

8.11 The above sections have dealt with some specific nonlinear generalisations of particular linear multivariate techniques. By contrast, Meulman (1986) and Gifi (1990) develop general nonlinear *systems* of multivariate analysis, which each encompass generalisations of a range of individual linear techniques under a unified strategy. The two systems have several features in common. They both have as objectives the approximation of a high-dimensional space by a suitable low-dimensional one; the qualification 'nonlinear' means that a nonlinear transformation of the variables is an intermediate part of the process. In addition, they both have least squares fitting of a suitable objective (loss) function as the mechanism for achieving a particular approximation. Often the function requires simultaneous optimisation over several criteria, in which case an alternating least squares algorithm (**8.13**) is used to obtain a solution.

As an incidental point, both systems adopt the same classification of multivariate techniques, based on lattice theory, into either *join*- or *meet*-techniques. Essentially, the join is the linear sum of two subspaces while the meet is their intersection. Join-techniques are those (such as principal component analysis) in which there is no *a priori* structure on the variables and each variable defines a one-dimensional subspace. The approximating space is the single subspace of the space spanned by the p variables that has minimum dimensionality. Meet-techniques, on the other hand, are those (such as canonical variate analysis) where the p variables have an *a priori* division, say into g sets. Each *set* now defines a subspace, and the approximating space is the intersecting subspace of maximum dimensionality.

However, we will not be concerned with this classification of techniques, but will rather discuss the methods of achieving the analyses. Where the two systems diverge is in their general approaches; Meulman (1986) focuses on distance properties of multivariate techniques, and looks for nonlinear generalisations of least squares *distance* fitting methods, while Gifi (1990) concentrates essentially on generalisations to qualitative variables of the familiar multivariate quantitative methods, and the nonlinearity that this entails. This difference in approaches is manifested in different loss functions to be optimised when seeking the approximating subspaces. In the Gifi system, the difference between the high-dimensional and the low-dimensional spaces is measured directly by inner products, while in Meulman's approach the difference is measured by suitable comparisons between inter-point distances in the two spaces.

We can at best only provide a fairly general overview of these two approaches, so for details of specific techniques the reader must consult the cited books and references.

The Gifi system

8.12 The lynch-pin of the Gifi system is the idea of *homogeneity analysis*, so a good starting point for a description of the system is a definition of homogeneity. Intuitively, a set of entities is thought of as *homogeneous* if they are all 'of the same type' in some sense. Suppose now that in a multivariate system we observe p variables on each of n individuals. The *individuals* would usually be described as homogeneous if the observed set of p-vectors $\boldsymbol{x}_1, \ldots, \boldsymbol{x}_n$ (giving the values of the p variables on each of the n individuals) constitutes a sample from a single population; by contrast, heterogeneity would imply that the sample could be broken down into a number of subsamples, each of which is from a different population. One of the main objectives of *cluster analysis* (see Volume 2) is to partition a heterogeneous sample into such homogeneous subsamples. For the present, however, we will be more concerned with homogeneity among the *variables*. Following Heiser and Meulman (1993), we say that a set of variables is homogeneous if the set of n-vector scores $\boldsymbol{h}_1, \ldots, \boldsymbol{h}_p$ (giving the observed scores of the n individuals on each of the p variables) are equal, up to some class of information-preserving operations and up to random deviations. By 'information-preserving operations' we mean operations such as changing the mean, rescaling, monotonic transformations and so on, that keep the information on the individuals as carried by the variables unchanged. Random deviations among the variables are measured by means of a loss function, in which the variables are compared either with each other or with a latent variable $\boldsymbol{z}$ giving the centre of the distribution.

It seems appropriate to use a least squares loss function for such a comparison. To establish a suitable base-line, first suppose that no information-preserving transformations are allowed and that we wish to measure homogeneity among the raw variables. Then we can write the loss function as

$$\sigma^2(\boldsymbol{z}) = \frac{1}{np} \sum_{j=1}^{p} \| \boldsymbol{h}_j - \boldsymbol{z} \|, \tag{8.8}$$

where $\| \boldsymbol{x} \|$ denotes the sum of squares of the elements of $\boldsymbol{x}$. The greater the mean square Euclidean distance between the vectors $\boldsymbol{h}_1, \ldots, \boldsymbol{h}_p$ and $\boldsymbol{z}$, the greater the *loss of homogeneity* $\sigma^2(\boldsymbol{z})$. It is easy to show that the minimum loss of homogeneity $\sigma^2(*)$ is achieved when $\boldsymbol{z} = \bar{\boldsymbol{h}} = \frac{1}{p}\sum_j \boldsymbol{h}_j$, the mean across variables for each individual, and that in this case

$$\sigma^2(*) = \frac{1}{n}[\frac{1}{p}\sum_j \| \boldsymbol{h}_j \| - \| \bar{\boldsymbol{h}} \|]. \tag{8.9}$$

Furthermore, if all variables are measured as deviations from their means and are standardised so that $s^2(\boldsymbol{h}_j) = n^{-1} \| \boldsymbol{h}_j \| = 1$, then $\sigma^2(*) = 1 - \bar{r}$, where $\bar{r}$ is the average of the p^2 correlations between all $\boldsymbol{h}_j$ (i.e. of all elements of the $p \times p$ correlation matrix including the self-correlations equal to 1; Gifi, 1990 p84–85). Thus loss of homogeneity attains its lowest value if all variables are perfectly correlated.

8.13 Now suppose that transformations of the variables are admitted before averaging, in order to try and improve the homogeneity over the above base-line value. First consider simple rescaling of each variable. This is equivalent to multiplying $\boldsymbol{h}_j$ by an arbitrary scalar a_j for $j = 1, \ldots, p$, and it is then natural to modify the definition of loss of homogeneity to

$$\sigma^2(\boldsymbol{a}, \boldsymbol{z}) = \frac{1}{np} \sum_{j=1}^{p} \| a_j \boldsymbol{h}_j - \boldsymbol{z} \|, \tag{8.10}$$

where $\boldsymbol{a}$ is the p-vector with elements a_j satisfying some suitable constraint (see below). To minimise loss of homogeneity we now have to estimate *two* vectors, $\boldsymbol{z}$ and $\boldsymbol{a}$, embedded in a quadratic loss function, and this can be done easily by an *alternating least squares* procedure. The idea is very straightforward: for any fixed value $\boldsymbol{a}_0$ of $\boldsymbol{a}$, the argument in **8.12** shows that $\sigma^2(\boldsymbol{a}_0, \boldsymbol{z})$ is minimised by $\boldsymbol{z}_0 = p^{-1} \sum_j a_{0j}\boldsymbol{h}_j$, where $\boldsymbol{a}_0 = (a_{01}, \ldots, a_{0p})$; on the other hand, for any fixed value $\boldsymbol{z}_0$ of $\boldsymbol{z}$, it is evident from (8.10) that the value of $\boldsymbol{a}$ minimising $\sigma^2(\boldsymbol{a}, \boldsymbol{z}_0)$ is given by the linear regression of $\boldsymbol{z}_0$ on $\boldsymbol{h}_j$. Thus for an arbitrary starting value $\boldsymbol{a}_0$ we obtain

$$\boldsymbol{z}_0 = \frac{1}{p} \sum_{j=1}^{p} a_{0j}\boldsymbol{h}_j, \tag{8.11}$$

and then an updated set of weights

$$a_j = c(\boldsymbol{h}_j, \boldsymbol{z}_0)/s^2(\boldsymbol{h}_j) \tag{8.12}$$

for $j = 1, \ldots, p$, where $c(\boldsymbol{h}_j, \boldsymbol{z}_0)$ denotes the covariance between $\boldsymbol{h}_j$ and $\boldsymbol{z}_0$.

Each step always improves loss of homogeneity, and alternating between (8.11) and (8.12) yields a convergent process. However, in order to avoid the trivial minimisation of $\sigma^2(\boldsymbol{a}, \boldsymbol{z})$ given by $a_j = 0$ for all j (and hence $\boldsymbol{z} = 0$), some convention on normalisation is required; usually, one fixes either the sum of squares of the elements of the $\boldsymbol{h}_j$, or those of $\boldsymbol{a}$, at some prechosen value. Alternatively the elements of $\boldsymbol{z}$ can be scaled to satisfy $s^2(\boldsymbol{z}) = 1$, and in this case it can be shown that $\boldsymbol{z}$ is the first principal component of the system (Bekker and De Leeuw, 1988). Successive principal components can be found by repeating the above process but restricting the weights so that previously found components are not repeated. This is done by requiring that all components are mutually uncorrelated, so that a formal statement of the procedure is as the minimisation of

$$\sigma^2(\boldsymbol{A}, \boldsymbol{Z}) = \frac{1}{npq} \sum_{j=1}^{p} \sum_{s=1}^{q} \| a_{js}\boldsymbol{h}_j - \boldsymbol{z}_s \|, \tag{8.13}$$

where q is the number of components extracted, $\boldsymbol{Z}$ is an $(n \times q)$ matrix of component scores with columns $\boldsymbol{z}_s$, $\boldsymbol{A}$ is a $(p \times q)$ matrix of weights a_{js} (for variable j on component s), and $c(\boldsymbol{z}_s, \boldsymbol{z}_t) = 0$ for all pairs s, t of components.

8.14 Extending the above idea provides another possible generalisation to nonlinearity of principal components, different from those considered previously in this chapter. If the simple rescaling $\phi_j(\boldsymbol{h}_j) = a_j\boldsymbol{h}_j$ in the loss function (8.10) is viewed as the feature that provides linearity of components, then generalisation to nonlinear principal components is obtained by permitting ϕ_j to be any nonlinear function of the variable $\boldsymbol{h}_j$. Thus the loss function to be minimised is now

$$\sigma^2(\boldsymbol{\phi}, \boldsymbol{z}) = \frac{1}{np} \sum_{j=1}^{p} \| \phi_j(\boldsymbol{h}_j) - \boldsymbol{z} \| . \tag{8.14}$$

Once again we need to impose a normalisation, and we could use $\|\boldsymbol{z}\| = 1$ or $\| \phi_j(\boldsymbol{h}_j) \| = 1$, but in this case the minimisation of $\sigma^2(\boldsymbol{\phi}, \boldsymbol{z})$ becomes trivial. By admitting all nonlinear transformations, the space of admissible transformations is enlarged to an n-dimensional space and so *any* quantification of the variables will trivially provide a perfect fit.

It is therefore evident that we must restrict the admissible transformations in some way. In particular, we have to diminish the dimensionality of the transformation space and this can be done by choosing a basis whose rank is much less than n. One possible way to do this is to restrict the transformations to be polynomials or piecewise polynomials of low order (i.e. splines). This approach has been examined by Winsberg and Ramsay (1980, 1981, 1982, 1983) and is reviewed by Winsberg (1988). However, the Gifi system uses a different approach, which provides its second distinctive feature: the transformations are restricted by choosing as basis an *indicator matrix* (see **5.21**) for each variable, having much fewer columns than n. Thus, in this system, all variables presented for analysis *must be categorical*; if some or all are continuous, then the user must first discretise them into a limited number of categories. In this case we can write $\phi_j(\boldsymbol{h}_j) = \boldsymbol{G}_j\boldsymbol{y}_j$, where $\boldsymbol{G}_j$ is the indicator matrix for $\boldsymbol{h}_j$ and $\boldsymbol{y}_j$ is a vector of coefficients, and the loss function becomes

$$\sigma^2(\boldsymbol{y},\boldsymbol{z}) = \frac{1}{p}\sum_{j=1}^{p} \parallel \boldsymbol{G}_j\boldsymbol{y}_j - \boldsymbol{z} \parallel . \tag{8.15}$$

This loss function can immediately be generalised to its multidimensional form in the same way that (8.10) was generalised to (8.13), yielding

$$\sigma^2(\boldsymbol{Y},\boldsymbol{Z}) = \frac{1}{p}\sum_{j=1}^{p} \parallel \boldsymbol{G}_j\boldsymbol{Y}_j - \boldsymbol{Z} \parallel . \tag{8.16}$$

However, it should be stressed that the nonlinear case is not as straightforward as the previous linear case, and there exist various other ways of dealing with multiplicity of solutions; Bekker and De Leeuw (1988) provide an extensive discussion.

8.15 Before considering this technique in more detail, it will prove useful later to pause briefly here over computational matters associated with the general nonlinear loss function (8.14). From the discussion in **8.12**, it is clear that the centre $\boldsymbol{z}$ of the distribution must equal the mean of the transformed variables, viz $p^{-1}\sum_j \phi_j(\boldsymbol{h}_j)$, but the optimal transformations ϕ_j are unknown. Using alternating least squares, a conditionally optimal transformation can be found separately for each variable, given the current 'best guess' $\boldsymbol{z}_0$ of $\boldsymbol{z}$ and keeping the other variables constant at their current values, because (8.14) can then be decomposed (Heiser and Meulman, 1993) into a constant and a variable term:

$$\sigma^2(\phi_j,\boldsymbol{z}_0) = constant + (np)^{-1} \parallel \boldsymbol{z}_0 - \phi_j(\boldsymbol{h}_j) \parallel . \tag{8.17}$$

The second term is minimised over choices of ϕ_j by regressing $\boldsymbol{z}_0$ on the space of transformations of the data $\boldsymbol{h}_j$. In linear PCA, $\phi_j(\boldsymbol{h}_j) = a_j\boldsymbol{h}_j$ and the regression is linear without an intercept; in nonlinear PCA we could have polynomial regression, piecewise polynomials for spline regression, isotonic regression for ordinal structure, and so on. After all variables have been processed according to their prespecified class of transformations, the alternating least squares principle tells us to continue with an updated guess $\boldsymbol{z}_0$ equal to the standardised mean of the variables unless the resulting vector of scores is close enough to the previous one to stop the process.

8.16 We now return to the technique embodied by equation (8.16) and consider its details. To do so it is instructive to return to first principles, as by doing so it will become evident how the technique is used in practice. As a by-product it will also be seen that what was derived above as a nonlinear generalisation of principal components has in fact even closer connection with correspondence analysis and multiple correspondence analysis (**5.19–5.21**).

Following the restriction outlined in **8.14**, we assume that p variables have been observed on each of n individuals, but the jth variable has only a finite number, k_j, of values or categories. The indicator matrix $\boldsymbol{G}_j$ for variable j is thus an $(n \times k_j)$ matrix, in which each row has all elements except one equal to zero, and the remaining element has value one. For the ith row, the column in which this element occurs indicates the category of variable j observed for individual i. It follows that $\boldsymbol{G}_j\boldsymbol{1}_{k_j} = \boldsymbol{1}_n$, where $\boldsymbol{1}_q$ denotes a q-vector whose elements all equal one, and that $\boldsymbol{D}_j = \boldsymbol{G}_j'\boldsymbol{G}_j$ is a diagonal matrix having on its diagonal the *marginals* of variable j. If $\boldsymbol{d}_j$ is the vector of marginals, then $\boldsymbol{d}_j = \boldsymbol{G}_j'\boldsymbol{1}_n = \boldsymbol{D}_j\boldsymbol{1}_{k_j}$. For two different variables j and l the matrix $\boldsymbol{C}_{jl} = \boldsymbol{G}_j'\boldsymbol{G}_l$ contains the *bimarginals* (the cross-table) of the two variables, and $\boldsymbol{C}_{jl}\boldsymbol{1} = \boldsymbol{d}_j$. The $(\sum k_j \times \sum k_j)$ supermatrix $\boldsymbol{C}$ which has the $\boldsymbol{C}_{jl}$ as its submatrices is the *Burt matrix* (see also **5.21**).

In line with most of the other descriptive multivariate techniques discussed in this volume, we would like to obtain a convenient q-dimensional space in which to represent both individuals and variables of the observed sample. To this end, we require *quantifications* (i.e. scales) for the individuals and variables which can be used as coordinate values in this space; the quantifications for the individuals will be termed the *object scores* and will be collected in the $(n \times q)$ matrix $\boldsymbol{Z}$, while the quantifications for the categories of variable j will be collected in the $(k_j \times q)$ matrix $\boldsymbol{Y}_j$ for $j = 1, \ldots, p$. The nonlinear multivariate analysis problem is thus to find *optimum quantifications*, and in this it can be seen to share the same objective as those methods surveyed in **5.20** that all lead to correspondence analysis. Note, however, that those methods were described for just two-way tables (i.e. bivariate samples), while the present interest is in general multivariate data sets. Tenenhaus and Young (1985) provide further synthesis of results in this area; we proceed by means of homogeneity analysis and follow the development in De Leeuw (1984) and Gifi (1990).

8.17 We thus seek optimum object scores $\boldsymbol{Z}$ and category quantifications $\boldsymbol{Y}_j$ for $j = 1, \ldots, p$. The object scores and category quantifications are said to be perfectly *consistent* if $\boldsymbol{Z} = \boldsymbol{G}_1\boldsymbol{Y}_1 = \ldots = \boldsymbol{G}_p\boldsymbol{Y}_p$. The object scores are perfectly *discriminating* if there exist p category quantifications satisfying this relationship, and conversely the category quantifications are perfectly *homogeneous* if there exist object scores for which the relationship is true.

Given a set of perfectly discriminating object scores $\boldsymbol{Z}$, the category quantifications are thus given as $\boldsymbol{Y}_j = \boldsymbol{D}_j^-\boldsymbol{G}_j'\boldsymbol{Z}$. (The Moore–Penrose generalised inverse $\boldsymbol{D}_j^-$ is needed in case some of the categories are empty.) Thus $\boldsymbol{Z}$ is perfectly discriminating if $\boldsymbol{Z} = \boldsymbol{P}_1\boldsymbol{Z} = \ldots = \boldsymbol{P}_p\boldsymbol{Z}$, where $\boldsymbol{P}_j = \boldsymbol{G}_j\boldsymbol{D}_j^-\boldsymbol{G}_j'$; object scores are perfectly discriminating if objects in the same category of a variable have the same score, and this is true for all variables.

Given a set of perfectly homogeneous category quantifications, then any

$\boldsymbol{G}_j\boldsymbol{Y}_j$ can be used to define perfectly discriminating object scores. Category quantifications are thus perfectly homogeneous if categories which contain the same object receive the same quantification.

Perfect fit will not be achieved with real data, but our aim is to get as close to it as possible. To do this we must optimise a suitable loss function, and such a function has been given already in (8.16). This is the *loss of consistency*, and can be written alternatively as

$$\sigma^2(\boldsymbol{Y},\boldsymbol{Z}) = \frac{1}{p}\sum_{j=1}^{p} \operatorname{tr}[(\boldsymbol{G}_j\boldsymbol{Y}_j - \boldsymbol{Z})'(\boldsymbol{G}_j\boldsymbol{Y}_j - \boldsymbol{Z})]. \qquad (8.18)$$

We can additionally define *loss of discrimination* as $\sigma^2(*,\boldsymbol{Z})$, the minimum of loss of consistency over category quantification, and *loss of homogeneity* as $\sigma^2(\boldsymbol{Y},*)$, the minimum of loss of consistency over object scores. Substituting the induced $\boldsymbol{Y}_j = \boldsymbol{D}_j^{-}\boldsymbol{G}_j'\boldsymbol{Z}$ into (8.18) yields

$$\sigma^2(*,\boldsymbol{Z}) = \operatorname{tr}[\boldsymbol{Z}'(\boldsymbol{I} - \boldsymbol{P}_*)\boldsymbol{Z}], \qquad (8.19)$$

where $\boldsymbol{P}_*$ is the mean of the $\boldsymbol{P}_j$, and setting $\boldsymbol{Z}= \frac{1}{p}\sum_{j=1}^{p}\boldsymbol{G}_j\boldsymbol{Y}_j$ in (8.18) yields

$$\sigma^2(\boldsymbol{Y},*) = \frac{1}{p^2}\operatorname{tr}[\boldsymbol{Y}'(\boldsymbol{C} - p\boldsymbol{D})\boldsymbol{Y}], \qquad (8.20)$$

where the $\boldsymbol{Y}_j$ are collected in the $(\sum k_j \times q)$ supermatrix $\boldsymbol{Y}$ and the $\boldsymbol{D}_j$ in the $(\sum k_j \times \sum k_j)$ supermatrix $\boldsymbol{D}$.

Homogeneity analysis is the technique that minimises these functions. The above foundations are due in essence to Guttman (1941), who also established that it does not matter which of the three loss functions is minimised, providing appropriate normalisations are chosen. Moreover, the algebra that results from any of these minimisations reduces to that already discussed for correspondence analysis in **5.19**; Tenenhaus and Young (1985) explore fully all the algebraic interrelationships among the techniques.

8.18 If the input data are purely categorical in form, then the minimisation of (8.18), (8.19) or (8.20) can be achieved analytically through the formulae of correspondence analysis, as indicated above. The major benefit and flexibility of the Gifi system, and the feature which makes numerical minimisation necessary, is the incorporation of extra information about the nature of the variables into the analysis. The information that we would want to incorporate is that a variable is *ordinal* or *numerical* instead of being merely *nominal.* Such information is handled in the Gifi system by imposing restrictions on the category quantifications and conducting constrained minimisations by alternating least squares, as outlined in **8.15** above. Moreover, any of these types of quantifications can be either *multiple* (if each dimension has a separate quantification, so that there is no connection between any of the q columns of each $\boldsymbol{Y}_j$) or *single* (if all dimensions share the same quantification, so that all the $\boldsymbol{Y}_j$ are of rank one). Thus simple homogeneity analysis as described above has *multiple nominal* quantifications.

Perfect generality is permitted in choice of restrictions. For example, between multiple nominal (all dimensions separately categorical) and multiple ordinal (all dimensions separately monotonic) we could require monotonicity only for selected dimensions, or could try different definitions of partial orders on q-space. Multiple numerical quantifications could be defined via polynomials, trigonometric polynomials, splines, etc. See Van Rijckevorsel (1982) for a discussion. These features have all been implemented in the program HOMALS, which in turn is included in the SPSS system library (SPSS, 1990), so there is ready access to the facilities.

8.19 The above system can easily be adapted to a great variety of different data structures, thereby producing a Gifi-type nonlinear generalisation of many standard linear multivariate techniques. For example, suppose that the variables are divided *a priori* into several groups. If the number of groups is two then canonical correlation analysis (Chapter 4) is a standard (linear) method of analysis which seeks the linear combinations of variables in the two groups that produce the largest correlations. If the number of groups is $g > 2$, then various generalisations of canonical analysis have been proposed (Carroll, 1968; Kettenring, 1971; Van De Geer, 1984). These all seek the linear combinations of variables in the separate groups for which the mutual correlations (i.e. the *consistencies*) are maximised in some way. This idea can be further generalised then to the nonlinear case, by allowing each variable an arbitrary nonlinear transformation before looking for the optimal weights with which to combine the transformed variables. If p_j denotes the number of variables in the jth group, $\boldsymbol{X}_j$ is the $(n \times p_j)$ data matrix for the jth group of variables, $\boldsymbol{Q}_j$ denotes this data matrix after each column has undergone an arbitrary nonlinear transformation, and $\boldsymbol{A}_j$ denotes the $(p_j \times q)$ matrix of weights for the jth group of variables, then *nonlinear generalised canonical analysis* seeks $\boldsymbol{Z}, \boldsymbol{Q}_j$ and $\boldsymbol{A}_j$ to minimise

$$\sigma^2(\boldsymbol{A}_j, \boldsymbol{Q}_j, \boldsymbol{Z}) = \sum_{j=1}^{g} \| \boldsymbol{Z} - \boldsymbol{Q}_j \boldsymbol{A}_j \|, \qquad (8.21)$$

subject to the conditions that the columns of $\boldsymbol{Z}$ are standardised and independent, and the columns of $\boldsymbol{Q}_j$ are standardised and satisfy the measurement restrictions. If furthermore we impose the Gifi restriction that the data are categorised, this objective reduces to that of finding the object scores $\boldsymbol{Z}$ and category quantifications $\boldsymbol{Y}_{ij}$ that minimise

$$\sigma^2(\boldsymbol{Y}_{ij}, \boldsymbol{Z}) = \sum_{j=1}^{g} \| \boldsymbol{Z} - \sum_{i=1}^{p_j} \boldsymbol{G}_{ij} \boldsymbol{Y}_{ij} \|, \qquad (8.22)$$

where $\boldsymbol{G}_{ij}$ and $\boldsymbol{Y}_{ij}$ are the indicator and category quantification matrices for the ith variable in the jth group, and the minimisation is conducted subject to the conditions that the columns of $\boldsymbol{Z}$ are independent and standardised. The same options as before (multiple, single; nominal, ordinal and numerical quantifications) can be allowed (Van Der Burg, De Leeuw and Verdegaal, 1988). This technique is implemented in the program OVERALS, also in the SPSS package.

Many other such nonlinear generalisations have been worked out, but are not detailed here. For a comprehensive list of possibilities, description of

Table 8.1 Fish data taken with permission from Gifi (1990) p210

	Variables																
Fish	1	2	3	4	5	6	7	8	9	10	11	12	13	14	15	16	17
1	1	1	1	1	0	0	9	0	0	9	8	9	9	9	9	9	1
2	1	0	0	0	3	0	4	0	1	8	9	9	7	7	7	6	1
3	0	0	1	1	0	1	3	0	1	9	9	9	7	8	8	9	1
4	0	1	0	0	0	2	4	0	1	9	9	9	8	9	6	9	1
5	0	0	1	1	1	2	0	2	0	1	0	0	0	3	0	3	1
6	0	0	0	1	1	0	3	0	0	1	2	2	1	2	2	3	1
7	0	0	0	0	1	0	0	1	0	1	1	1	2	2	2	3	1
8	1	1	0	1	1	0	4	0	3	0	1	3	1	0	1	0	1
9	2	2	1	3	5	1	3	1	2	2	2	3	2	4	3	6	2
10	5	5	3	2	6	1	3	1	4	3	5	6	5	4	3	3	2
11	2	2	2	2	2	5	3	1	1	3	3	3	3	5	3	9	2
12	3	4	1	2	2	2	3	7	4	2	1	2	2	4	4	6	2
13	3	5	2	2	4	4	3	1	9	3	4	4	3	4	9	6	2
14	6	2	1	2	6	4	3	1	1	0	0	0	0	2	3	3	2
15	2	2	1	2	1	2	3	1	3	4	5	5	2	4	7	6	2
16	3	3	1	1	3	0	3	2	5	4	7	4	5	5	8	6	2
18	9	9	9	8	4	0	6	5	2	2	2	3	2	2	4	3	3
19	6	6	8	8	2	8	0	6	1	1	1	2	1	2	3	3	3
20	9	8	7	9	9	0	0	9	9	0	0	1	1	1	3	0	3
21	3	4	3	4	2	0	2	0	1	6	6	7	6	8	6	9	3
22	6	6	9	7	0	0	5	8	2	4	4	5	3	7	5	3	3
23	6	6	8	8	6	9	9	6	1	4	4	4	3	4	5	6	3
24	5	1	5	5	1	0	3	3	0	5	4	4	4	6	4	9	3

methodology, and availability of software see Young *et al* (1980), Young (1981) and Gifi (1990).

Example 8.3

Gifi (1990) presents an illustration of nonlinear generalised canonical analysis using some fish data from an experiment by Amiard, with data taken in categorised form from Cailliez and Pagès (1976). Table 8.1 gives data on twenty-four fish that had been placed in one of three aquaria contaminated with radioactive strontium. Fish numbered 1–8 remained in the first aquarium for only a short period of time, fish numbered 9–17 remained in the second aquarium for a longer spell, while fish numbered 18–24 remained in the third aquarium the longest. Seventeen variables were measured on each fish: variables 1–9 were measures of radioactivity of various parts of the body of the fish after the experiment, variables 10–16 were size measurements of the fish, and variable 17 indicates the aquarium in which each fish was placed. The variables were each discretised to have ten categories (here coded 0–9 rather than 1–10 as in Gifi); fish number 17 died during the experiment so has been omitted from the table. It is of interest to determine whether the three tanks can be distinguished on the basis of the data, and if so which of the variables is primarily responsible for the distinction.

Previous analyses used the original (i.e undiscretised) data. Cailliez and Pagès (1976, pp. 280–286) showed that in a plot of the object scores from

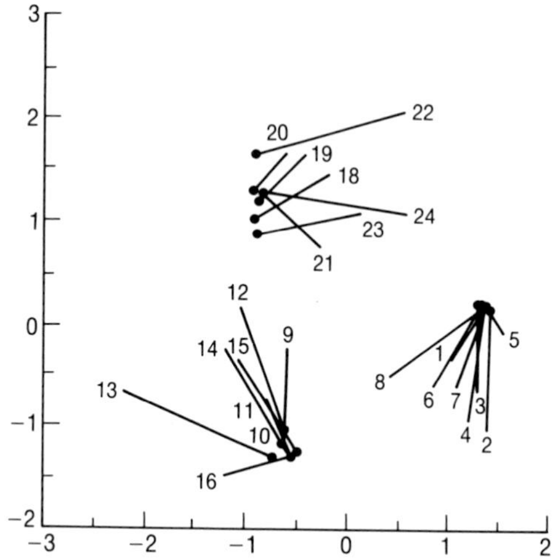

Figure 8.5 Object scores for the fish data; points labelled by numbers give fish positions for the numerical solution, and these are joined by lines to the corresponding positions in the ordinal solution. Reproduced with permission from Gifi (1990).

metric component analysis the fish from different aquaria were readily separated, although fish numbers 21 and 24 (aquarium 3) were close to the fish from aquarium 2. Plotting the component loadings produced two clusters of variables, one consisting of variables 10–14 (direct measures of fish size) and the other of variables 1, 2, 3, 4 and 8 (measurements of radioactivity of hard tissues). Bouroche and Saporta (1980 pp. 190–221) used multiple discriminant analysis but omitted variable 7. They showed that aquarium membership could be identified very well, the three group centroids being at the vertices of an equilateral triangle and individual fish lying close to their aquarium centroid. The same two groups of important variables were identified.

For nonlinear analysis the variables were grouped into three sets, the first containing variables 1–9, the second containing variables 10–16 and the third containing just variable 17. Two separate analyses were conducted: for the first analysis, variables 1–16 were treated as single numerical and variable 17 as multiple nominal, while for the second analysis the measurement level for variables 1–16 was changed to single ordinal. A two-dimensional solution was sought each time. Fig. 8.5 shows the two sets of object scores for the 23 fish: the points labelled by numbers constitute the first (numerical) solution while the unnumbered points constitute the second (ordinal) solution. (The lines joining numbers and points identify the fish in the second analysis.) We see that the clustering of aquaria is very clear in both solutions, being sharper in the ordinal than in the numerical case. This is consistent with results often encountered in multidimensional scaling, where nonmetric techniques are prone to clearer pictures in low dimensionalities than their metric counterparts. To investigate the effects of the variables, it proved to be most useful to calculate canonical loadings (i.e. the correlations of the canonical variables

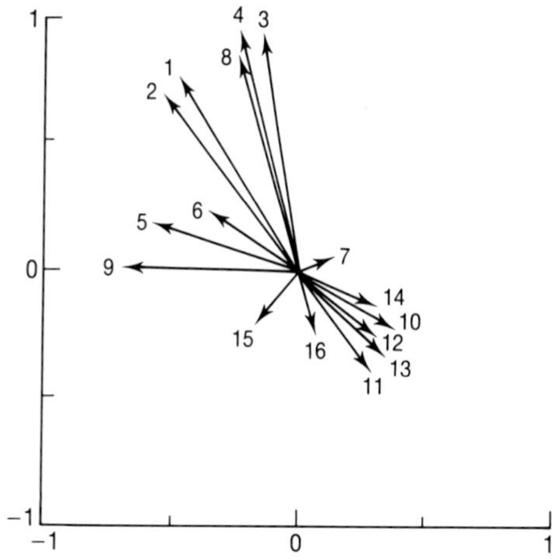

Figure 8.6 Canonical loadings for the numerical solution. Reproduced with permission from Gifi (1990).

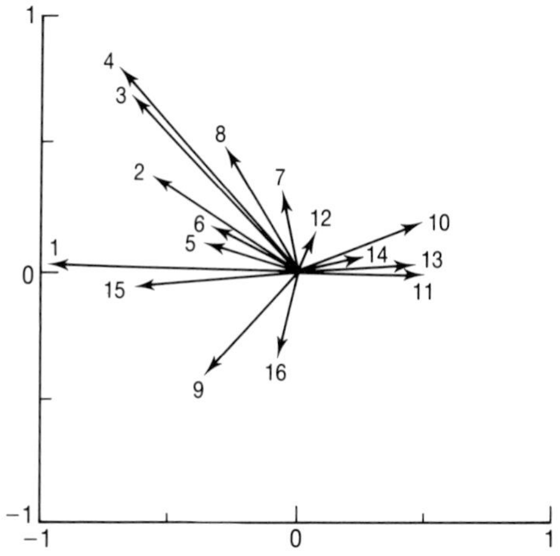

Figure 8.7 Canonical loadings for the ordinal solution. Reproduced with permission from Gifi (1990).

with the transformed original variables). In the numerical solution the transformations essentially took the discretised variables back to their original numerical values, while in the ordinal solution the transformations had rank order restrictions in force. The canonical loadings for variables 1–16 are plotted in Fig. 8.6 for the numerical solution and in Fig. 8.7 for the ordinal solution. There is a fair degree of similarity in the two diagrams, with essentially four groups of variables being identified. The first group consists of the size variables, with variables 10–14 being particularly important; the second group consists of variables 3, 4, 8 (radioactivity of gill-covers, fins and scales), the third contains variables

1 and 2 (radioactivity of eyes and gills) and the fourth has variables 5, 6 and 9 (radioactivity of liver, gullet and muscles). These results agree well with the previous analyses reported above.

Distance approach

8.20 All descriptive methods of multivariate analysis share the same basic premise and general objectives: the original data can be viewed as a collection of n points in some high (p-)dimensional space, the points corresponding to sample individuals and the dimensions to measured variables, and we seek a suitable low (q-)dimensional approximation in which the points are positioned in such a way as to retain as much information as possible from the original space. Different interpretations of the phrase 'as much information as possible' lead to the different multivariate techniques described in this volume (e.g principal components, canonical variates etc).

In Chapter 5 we described a class of techniques known as multidimensional scaling, in which the starting point was a set of dissimilarities (or proximities) among n objects and the aim was to find a q-dimensional space in which the distances between the points approximated these dissimilarities as closely as possible. Again, different interpretations of the phrase 'as closely as possible' lead to different methods of scaling (e.g. classical scaling, non-metric scaling etc).

Now when dissimilarities are not given explicitly, but are derived from multivariate data as distances between points in high dimensional space, then both the above approaches share the same objectives. Indeed, the equivalences between formal principal component analysis, canonical variate analysis, correspondence analysis on the one hand and classical scaling of appropriate distance matrices on the other has already been pointed out in **5.8** and **5.19**. This correspondence between multivariate analysis and classical multidimensional scaling has been formalised by Meulman (1986), who showed that this multidimensional scaling method could be characterised by a particular loss function to be optimised and each multivariate analysis method corresponded to a special case of the appropriate loss function. This formalisation enables unification and extension to be obtained for all the scaling methods described in Chapter 5, and also permits nonlinear generalisations to be obtained readily. We now sketch out the main ideas in this approach.

8.21 Suppose that the $(n \times p)$ multivariate data matrix $\boldsymbol{Z}$ defines the high-dimensional space in which the ith individual is represented by the point with coordinates given by the elements of the ith row $\boldsymbol{z}_i'$ of $\boldsymbol{Z}$, and we seek the $(n \times q)$ matrix $\boldsymbol{X}$ whose rows $\boldsymbol{x}_i'$ contain the coordinates of the corresponding points in the approximating low-dimensional space. To keep formulae simple, we will assume that variables are always measured about their means. Suppose further that the squared dissimilarity between the ith and jth rows of $\boldsymbol{Z}$ can be written

$$\delta_{Z,ij}^2 = (\boldsymbol{z}_i - \boldsymbol{z}_j)'\boldsymbol{W}(\boldsymbol{z}_i - \boldsymbol{z}_j), \tag{8.23}$$

where $\boldsymbol{W}$ is a positive-definite weight matrix. $\delta^2_{Z,ij}$ can thus also be viewed as the squared distance between points i and j in the high-dimensional space. Different choices of $\boldsymbol{W}$ lead to different dissimilarity/distance measures. For example, $\boldsymbol{W} = \boldsymbol{I}$ yields ordinary Euclidean distances, $\boldsymbol{W} = (\boldsymbol{Z}'\boldsymbol{Z})^{-1}$ yields Mahalanobis distances, and so on. For ease of interpretation we require the approximating low-dimensional space to be Euclidean, so that the squared distance between the ith and jth points in this space is given by

$$d^2_{X,ij} = (\boldsymbol{x}_i - \boldsymbol{x}_j)'(\boldsymbol{x}_i - \boldsymbol{x}_j). \qquad (8.24)$$

Denote by $\boldsymbol{\Delta}_Z$ the $(n \times n)$ matrix with elements $\delta_{Z,ij}$, and by $\boldsymbol{D}_X$ the $(n \times n)$ matrix with elements $d_{X,ij}$. It will also be convenient to write $\boldsymbol{\Delta}_Z{}^2$ for the $(n \times n)$ matrix with elements $\delta^2_{Z,ij}$, and $\boldsymbol{D}_X{}^2$ for the $(n \times n)$ matrix with elements $d^2_{X,ij}$.

Obtaining the low-dimensional space $\boldsymbol{X}$ by classical scaling has been described in **5.6–5.8**, and it has been shown in **5.8** that the solution is the projection of the original points in which criterion (5.5), ie $\psi = \sum_i \sum_j (\delta^2_{Z,ij} - d^2_{X,ij})$, is minimum. Meulman (1986) explicitly formalises the problem as being that of finding the projection $\boldsymbol{X}$ that minimises this criterion, and establishes that the criterion can be written equivalently as either

$$\text{STRAIN} = (\boldsymbol{Q} - \boldsymbol{X}\boldsymbol{X}')'(\boldsymbol{Q} - \boldsymbol{X}\boldsymbol{X}'), \qquad (8.25)$$

where $\boldsymbol{Q} = -\frac{1}{2}\boldsymbol{J}\boldsymbol{\Delta}_Z{}^2\boldsymbol{J}$ for $\boldsymbol{J} = (\boldsymbol{I} - \boldsymbol{1}\boldsymbol{1}'/n)$ (see **5.6**), or

$$\text{STRAIN} = \frac{1}{4}\text{tr}[\boldsymbol{J}(\boldsymbol{\Delta}_Z{}^2 - \boldsymbol{D}_X{}^2)'\boldsymbol{J}(\boldsymbol{\Delta}_Z{}^2 - \boldsymbol{D}_X{}^2)\boldsymbol{J}]. \qquad (8.26)$$

She then goes on to establish that familiar multivariate techniques such as principal component analysis, canonical variate and correlation analysis, homogeneity analysis (i.e. multiple correspondence analysis) and analysis of asymmetry can all be obtained by applying this approach to an appropriate distance matrix $\boldsymbol{\Delta}_Z$.

8.22 Apart from formalising the connection between classical multidimensional scaling and other multivariate techniques, the advantage of the distance approach is that it opens up the possibility of yet another means of generalising linear multivariate techniques to nonlinear ones. Consider transforming each variable by means of some nonlinear transformation. This will generate a new data matrix $\boldsymbol{Z}_*$ from $\boldsymbol{Z}$, and hence a new distance matrix $\boldsymbol{\Delta}_{Z*}$ which can be inserted into (8.26). Minimising the result over $\boldsymbol{X}$ will yield the best approximate space for this *particular* set of transformations. Allowing a further (outer) minimisation over all possible nonlinear transformations (subject to suitable constraints to ensure a non-trivial solution) will thus fully generalise the technique to the nonlinear case, and Meulman (1986) provides the appropriate loss functions for nonlinear principal components and nonlinear canonical variates obtained by this means.

8.23 However, the STRAIN loss function defined above has two special features which perhaps make it less than ideal. First, it is the *squared* distances in one space that are approximated by the *squared* distances in the other space (thus yielding a *quadratic* approximation). Secondly, the approximation is *from below*, because $d^2_{X,ij} \leqslant \delta^2_{Z,ij}$ for each i, j pair (see **5.8**). This is a consequence of classical scaling being a *projection* technique. It has already been suggested in Chapter 5 that alternative procedures might therefore be deemed preferable in some circumstances; Meulman puts the case even more strongly for nonlinear analysis, and recommends using STRESS (**5.10**) rather than STRAIN as the loss function. Thus we require to find the configuration $\boldsymbol{X}$ minimising

$$\text{STRESS} = \text{tr}[(\boldsymbol{\Delta}_Z - \boldsymbol{D}_X)'(\boldsymbol{\Delta}_Z - \boldsymbol{D}_X)]. \tag{8.27}$$

Comparing this expression with STRAIN of (8.26) we see that both the centring operator $\boldsymbol{J}$ and the squares have been removed, which implies that the dissimilarities $\delta_{Z,ij}$ are now approximated in a least squares sense and *from both sides* by the distances $d_{X,ij}$. Removal of the centring operator only would leave a least squares loss function on the *squared* distances, i.e. SSTRESS of Takane *et al* (1977) (see **5.10**). However, Meulman concentrates on results for STRESS.

8.24 STRESS can be minimised using the majorisation approach developed by De Leeuw and Heiser (1980). Let the elements a_{ij} of the matrix $\boldsymbol{A}$ be defined by $a_{ij} = \delta_{Z,ij}/d_{X,ij}$ for $i \neq j$, with $a_{ij} = 0$ if $d_{X,ij} = 0$. Also, let $\boldsymbol{B}$ be a diagonal matrix with the elements of $\boldsymbol{1}'\boldsymbol{A}$ on the diagonal, and let $\boldsymbol{C} = \boldsymbol{B}-\boldsymbol{A}$. Then a convergent series of configurations is given by the algorithm $\boldsymbol{X}_i = n^{-1}\boldsymbol{C}\boldsymbol{X}_{i-1}$, from any arbitrary starting configuration $\boldsymbol{X}_0$. In practice the iterations would continue until differences between successive configurations were less than a preset level of tolerance.

Given any particular structure on the high-dimensional space $\boldsymbol{Z}$, or specific objectives of analysis, the dissimilarities $\delta_{Z,ij}$ can be obtained in appropriate manner. For example, unstructured quantitative data would suggest the use of Euclidean distances, quantitative data partitioned into groups would suggest Mahalanobis distances, while qualitative incidence data would suggest chi-squared distances; Meulman (1986) gives the appropriate versions of (8.27) for each of these choices. Of course, the change in loss function from STRAIN to STRESS means that these analyses are no longer the duals of principal component analysis, canonical variate analysis or correspondence analysis respectively. However, they will clearly have close connections with these techniques. Moreover, nonlinear generalisations can be obtained in exactly the same way as for the same special cases of STRAIN, by permitting initial nonlinear transformation of $\boldsymbol{Z}$ to $\boldsymbol{Z}_*$ and minimising STRESS over all nonlinear transformations as well as over $\boldsymbol{X}$. Meulman (1986) restricts the search for optimal nonlinear transformations to the class of general monotonic transformations, and gives full details of the necessary algorithms for the special forms of STRESS arising from particular dissimilarity measures. The ones considered in detail can be described as nonlinear versions of principal component analysis, canonical variate analysis, homogeneity analysis and redundancy analysis.

As a final point, it is worth emphasising the distinction between this version of nonlinear distance analysis and nonmetric multidimensional scaling (**5.12**). Use of the same loss function STRESS and focus on monotonic transformations in both cases might imply a close connection between the two sets of

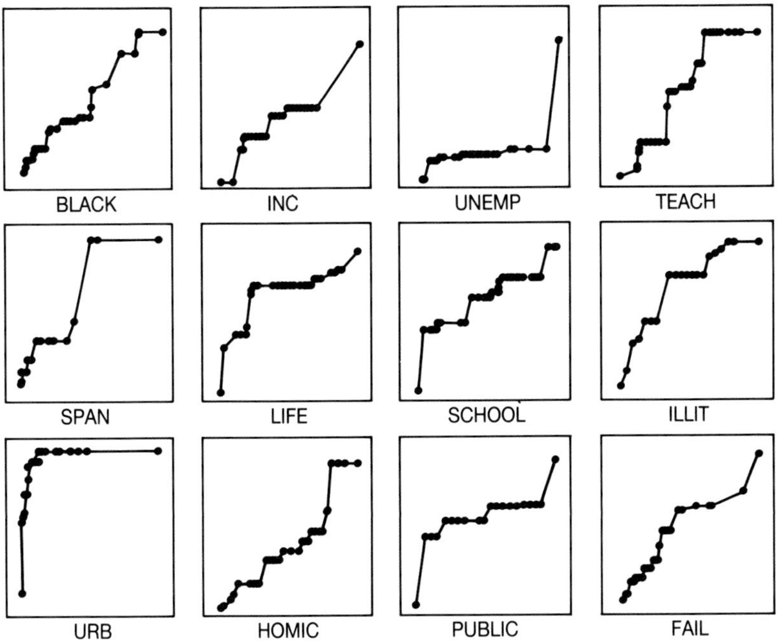

Figure 8.8 Transformations of variables in nonlinear canonical correlation analysis. Reproduced from Meulman (1986).

techniques. However, there is a very fundamental distinction which makes them very different. The monotonic transformations relate to the *distances* $d_{X,ij}$ in multidimensional scaling, but to the *data* in nonlinear distance analysis. Consequently, STRESS is used in nonmetric fashion in the former case but in a fully metric fashion in the latter, and different results will certainly be obtained for any particular set of data in the two cases.

Example 8.4
Meulman (1986, pp50–51) gives data on 12 variables for each of 50 States in America. The variables are as follows.

(1) BLACK: percentage of population that is of the black race;
(2) SPAN: percentage of population that is of Spanish origin;
(3) URB: ratio of urban to rural;
(4) INC: per capita income in dollars;
(5) LIFE: life expectancy in years;
(6) HOMIC: 1976 homicide and non-negligent manslaughter rate;
(7) UNEMP: 1975 unemployment rate;
(8) SCHOOL: percentage of population who are high school graduates;
(9) PUBLIC: percentage of public school enrollment;
(10) TEACH: ratio of public shool pupils to teachers;
(11) ILLIT: illiteracy rate as percent of population;
(12) FAIL: failure rate on the Selective Service mental ability test.

She gives various analyses of this data set including a nonlinear canonical

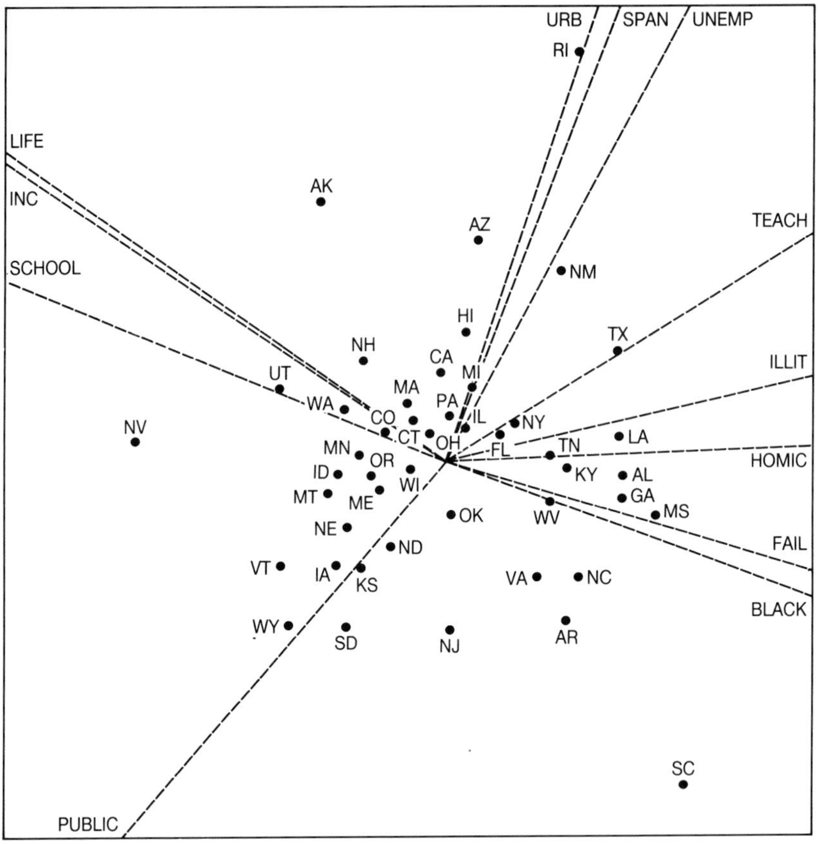

Figure 8.9 States plotted as points in the canonical common space, with transformed variables fitted into the same space and shown as vectors. Reproduced from Meulman (1986).

correlation analysis using STRESS, for which the 12 variables were divided into three sets (variables 1–7 in the first set, variables 8–10 in the second, and variables 11–12 in the third). Fig. 8.8 shows the optimal monotonic transformations achieved for each variable (original values on horizontal scales and transformed values on vertical scales), while Fig. 8.9 shows the 50 States plotted in the nonlinear canonical space derived in the analysis. The transformed variables have been fitted into the canonical space and are shown as vectors in Fig. 8.9. Correlations of these variables with the canonical space are as follows: 0.94 (SCHOOL), 0.92 (ILLIT), 0.88 (FAIL), 0.82 (BLACK), 0.65 (HOMIC), 0.63 (UNEMP), 0.59 (PUBLIC), 0.59 (INC), 0.53 (LIFE), 0.47 (URB), 0.43 (SPAN) and 0.42 (TEACH), giving an idea of how well the variables fit into this space. Interpretation of Fig. 8.9 follows the lines of interpretation of similar analyses, such as in Example 8.3. The overall plot in Fig. 8.9 shows the relative similarities among all the states, while identification of particular subsets of states with individual variables shows how these states are distinguished with respect to this variable. Also, points 'near' a variable show states with high scores on that variable. Turning to Fig. 8.8, variables showing a relatively smooth transformation (e.g. BLACK) are those for which most of the information has been used in the analysis, and are generally those that fit well into the space, while variables showing just a few large 'steps' (e.g. SPAN, URB) are ones for which little information has contributed to the analysis, and are generally those whose fit into the space is worst.

8.25 Some further work relating to the material in this chapter is described by Heiser (1986) and Van Buuren and Heiser (1989). Also, in a recent paper, Meulman (1992) has extended the distance analysis described above, first by allowing the distances to come from a set of separate distance matrices (rather than from just a single matrix) and second by allowing differential weighting of variables.

As a final comment, it is worth noting that all attempts so far at nonlinear generalisations have been directed at *descriptive* rather than *inferential* multivariate techniques. This testifies not only to the difficulty of obtaining nonlinear distributional results in general, but also to the enormous scope for further development of the subject.

Exercises

8.1 In the context of **8.4**, show that if the straight line $l(\lambda) = \boldsymbol{u}_0 + \lambda \boldsymbol{v}_0$ is self-consistent then it is a principal component.

(Hastie and Stuetzle, 1989)

8.2 Suppose that the $(n \times p)$ matrix $\boldsymbol{X}$ contains in its rows $\boldsymbol{x}_i$ the coordinates of n points in p dimensions. In the terminology of **8.9**, consider a notional sample P_r concentrated in the rth variable (so that its coordinates are given by $\rho_r \boldsymbol{e}_r$ where $\boldsymbol{e}_r$ is the rth column of the identity matrix). Assume that squared distance in this space is defined in such a way that the different variables contribute independently, i.e. $d_{ij}^2 = \sum_{k=1}^{p} f(x_{ik}, x_{jk})$ for some suitable function $f(.)$. Suppose that an $(n+1)$th point P_{n+1} has coordinates given by $\boldsymbol{\rho}' = (\rho_1, \ldots, \rho_p)$. By writing $\boldsymbol{\rho} = \sum_{r=1}^{p} \rho_r \boldsymbol{e}_r$, or otherwise, show that the squared distance from $\boldsymbol{x}_i$ to P_{n+1} can be expressed as $\sum_{r=1}^{p} d_{ir}^2 - (p-1)\delta_{ii}^2$, where d_{ir}^2 is the squared distance from $\boldsymbol{x}_i$ to P_r while δ_{ii}^2 is the squared distance of $\boldsymbol{x}_i$ from zero.

Use this result to show how sample points not on trajectories can be interpreted in nonlinear biplots.

(Gower and Harding, 1988)

A

Normal Theory Sampling Distributions

Multivariate generalisation of Student's *t*

A.1 The problem of testing the difference in means between two groups, in which $\boldsymbol{x}$ is supposed to follow a multivariate normal distribution with the same unknown dispersion matrix $\boldsymbol{\Sigma}$, is a multivariate generalisation of the univariate two-sample t-test. Related problems are concerned with inference about the parameters of the discriminant function, and confidence regions for means.

The two populations are denoted by Π_1 and Π_2, and the subscripts 1 and 2 refer to these populations.

The group means $\boldsymbol{\mu}_1$ and $\boldsymbol{\mu}_2$ are estimated by $\overline{\boldsymbol{x}}_1$ and $\overline{\boldsymbol{x}}_2$, and the elements of $\boldsymbol{\Sigma}$ have unbiased estimates w_{ij} based on $n_1 + n_2 - 2$ degrees of freedom calculated in the same way as the within-group variance in the t-test. The estimated within-group covariance matrix $\boldsymbol{W} = (w_{ij})$ is then an estimate of $\boldsymbol{\Sigma}$, with elements given by

$$w_{ij} = \frac{w_{ij}^*}{n_1 + n_2 - 2}, \tag{A.1}$$

where

$$w_{ij}^* = \sum_{x_i, x_j \in \Pi_1} (x_i - \bar{x}_{i1})(x_j - \bar{x}_{j1}) + \sum_{x_i, x_j \in \Pi_2} (x_i - \bar{x}_{i2})(x_j - \bar{x}_{j2}). \tag{A.2}$$

Now there are several ways of proceeding, apparently distinct but in fact equivalent.

(i) The Mahalanobis distance between the populations is defined as

$$\Delta^2 = (\boldsymbol{\mu}_1 - \boldsymbol{\mu}_2)' \boldsymbol{\Sigma}^{-1} (\boldsymbol{\mu}_1 - \boldsymbol{\mu}_2) \tag{A.3}$$

and the obvious 'plug-in' estimator

$$D^2 = (\overline{\boldsymbol{x}}_1 - \overline{\boldsymbol{x}}_2)' \boldsymbol{W}^{-1} (\overline{\boldsymbol{x}}_1 - \overline{\boldsymbol{x}}_2) \tag{A.4}$$

is a natural estimator of the dissimilarity, or lack of overlap, between the populations. The distribution of D^2 on the null hypothesis $\Delta^2 = 0$ provides an appropriate test (see equation A.12).

(ii) Hotelling introduced the statistic

$$T^2 = \frac{n_1 n_2}{n_1 + n_2}(\bar{\boldsymbol{x}}_1 - \bar{\boldsymbol{x}}_2)' \boldsymbol{W}^{-1}(\bar{\boldsymbol{x}}_1 - \bar{\boldsymbol{x}}_2) \tag{A.5}$$

as a natural analogue of the t statistic, equal to t^2 in the univariate case. Thus

$$T^2 = \frac{n_1 n_2}{n_1 + n_2} D^2$$

which immediately gives the distribution of T^2 under the null hypothesis $\boldsymbol{\mu}_1 = \boldsymbol{\mu}_2$.

(iii) The likelihood ratio statistic

$$L = \frac{|\boldsymbol{W}^*|}{|\boldsymbol{T}^*|} \tag{A.6}$$

was studied by Wilks and is known as Wilks' criterion. It is the ratio of the determinants of the within-group and total matrices of sums of squares and products, so that

$$\boldsymbol{T}^* = \boldsymbol{W}^* + \frac{n_1 n_2}{n_1 + n_2}(\bar{\boldsymbol{x}}_1 - \bar{\boldsymbol{x}}_2)(\bar{\boldsymbol{x}}_1 - \bar{\boldsymbol{x}}_2)'. \tag{A.7}$$

The criterion extends naturally to the general multivariate analysis of variance with $q + 1$ groups, and the general theory of likelihood ratio tests shows that

$$-n \log L \sim \chi^2_{[pq]}. \tag{A.8}$$

(iv) Define a variable y taking the values 0 and 1 for groups 1 and 2 respectively. Consider the regression of y on $\boldsymbol{x}$. It is easily verified that the sum of squares of y about the mean is $n_1 n_2/(n_1 + n_2)$, and the sums of products with $\boldsymbol{x}$ are given by

$$\frac{n_1 n_2}{n_1 + n_2}(\bar{\boldsymbol{x}}_1 - \bar{\boldsymbol{x}}_2).$$

Writing $c = n_1 n_2/(n_1 + n_2)$, $\boldsymbol{d} = (\bar{\boldsymbol{x}}_1 - \bar{\boldsymbol{x}}_2)$, $k = n_1 + n_2 - 2$, the normal equations take the form

$$\boldsymbol{T}^* \hat{\boldsymbol{\beta}} = c\boldsymbol{d}. \tag{A.9}$$

The regression sum of squares is then, using Bartlett's identity (Bartlett, 1951),

$$\begin{aligned} \hat{\boldsymbol{\beta}}' c\boldsymbol{d} &= c\boldsymbol{d}'(\boldsymbol{W}^* + c\boldsymbol{d}\boldsymbol{d}')c\boldsymbol{d} && \text{(A.10)} \\ &= c^2 \boldsymbol{d}' \boldsymbol{W}^{*-1} \boldsymbol{d} - \frac{c^3(\boldsymbol{d}' \boldsymbol{W}^{*-1} \boldsymbol{d})^2}{1 + c\boldsymbol{d}' \boldsymbol{W}^{*-1} \boldsymbol{d}}. && \text{(A.11)} \end{aligned}$$

The residual sum of squares is $c - \hat{\boldsymbol{\beta}}' c\boldsymbol{d}$, and the standard significance test for the regression is based on the statistic $\frac{cD^2}{kp}(k - p + 1)$, which is distributed as a variance ratio with p and $k - p + 1$ degrees of freedom,

$$F_{(p,k-p+1)} = \frac{cD^2}{kp}(k - p + 1), \tag{A.12}$$

or for the T^2 statistic

$$F_{(p,k-p+1)} = \frac{T^2}{kp}(k - p + 1). \tag{A.13}$$

This regression approach to the problem was given by Hotelling (1931).

These distributions apply also to comparisons of pairs of groups when there are more than two, and $\boldsymbol{W}$ is the estimated within-group dispersion matrix with k degrees of freedom.

Further, since $|\boldsymbol{T}^*| = |\boldsymbol{W}^*|(1 + c\boldsymbol{d}'\boldsymbol{W}^{*-1}\boldsymbol{d})$,

$$\frac{1-L}{L} = \frac{cD^2}{k} \tag{A.14}$$

and

$$F_{(p,k-p+1)} = \frac{1-L}{pL}(k - p + 1). \tag{A.15}$$

This result gives the exact distribution of L for the case of two groups.

An exact test is also available for the case of three groups; see Mardia *et al* (1979, p83). In this case

$$F_{(2p,2(k-p+1))} = \frac{1-\sqrt{L}}{p\sqrt{L}}(k - p + 1). \tag{A.16}$$

This test is also available for g groups, when $p = 2$, replacing p in equation (A.16) by $g - 1$.

$$F_{(2(g-1),2(k-g+2))} = \frac{1-\sqrt{L}}{(g-1)\sqrt{L}}(k - g + 2). \tag{A.17}$$

These results were first given by Wilks (1935).

Further properties of the Mahalanobis distance

A.2 Of the statistics discussed, only D^2 is an estimate of a population parameter. When $\Delta^2 = 0$, the distribution of cD^2/k is that of the ratio of two χ^2 variables. When $\Delta^2 \neq 0$, the numerator is replaced by a non-central χ^2, and the resulting test statistic is a non-central F.

$$\frac{k-p+1}{p}\frac{cD^2}{k} \sim F(p, k-p+1; c\Delta^2/k). \tag{A.18}$$

This result makes it possible, in theory, to find confidence intervals for Δ^2. Unfortunately, the non-central F distribution is extremely intractable. Various approximations have been suggested; for a description and comparisons see Tiku (1966). Tables in Pearson and Hartley (1951), and elsewhere, are primarily intended for power calculations in analysis of variance, and are not really suited to this problem. An algorithm by Lenth (1987) (see also modifications by Frick, 1990) gives non-central Beta probabilities, and it is easy to derive probabilities for the non-central F from them. If

$$F' \sim F(\nu_1/2, \nu_2/2; \lambda)$$

then

$$\Pr(F' \leqslant f) = I_x(\nu_1/2, \nu_2/2; \lambda)$$

in Lenth's notation, where $x = \nu_1 f/(\nu_1 f + \nu_2)$.

The NESI environment in S-Plus 3.0 includes a non-central F function.

A much more straightforward problem is that of testing whether the Mahalanobis distance based on a subset of r of the original p variables is equal to that based on the full set. This is equivalent to testing whether the remaining $p - r$ variables contribute significantly to the regression of y on $\boldsymbol{x}$. This is a standard problem, and it is easy to show that

$$\frac{k-p+1}{p-r}\frac{D_p^2 - D_r^2}{k + D_r^2} \sim F_{(p-r, k-p+1)} \qquad \text{(A.19)}$$

where D_p^2, D_r^2 are the Mahalanobis distances based on p and r variables, respectively.

This result is valuable in discriminant analysis, but selection of subsets of variables raises problems of multiple comparisons, just as in multiple regression. For a full discussion, see Miller (1990).

The Wishart distribution

A.3 Suppose $\boldsymbol{S}$ is a $p \times p$ matrix of sums of squares and products, $\boldsymbol{S} = \boldsymbol{X}'\boldsymbol{X}$, based on n independent observations of a $N(\boldsymbol{0}, \boldsymbol{\Sigma})$ variable. $\boldsymbol{S}$ is then said to have a Wishart distribution, generally written $\boldsymbol{S} \sim W_p(n, \boldsymbol{\Sigma})$. The joint distribution of the $\frac{1}{2}p(p+1)$ elements of $\boldsymbol{S}$ was first given by Wishart (1928). When $p = 1$, the distribution is, of course, χ^2; otherwise, it is a multivariate generalisation of the χ^2 distribution, and many of the properties of the χ^2 distribution apply also to the Wishart distribution.

(i) Degrees of freedom.

The parameter n is the degrees of freedom of the distribution. If each of the p variables is subject to r linear constraints, the distribution is $W_p(n - r, \boldsymbol{\Sigma})$. Thus, if the variables are deviations from the sample mean, $r = 1$. If the data are divided into s groups and the sample mean of each group is fitted, then $r = s$. If each variable has been adjusted by regression on s other variables, then again $r = s$.

A particular case is the *Bartlett decomposition* (Bartlett, 1933). Suppose $\boldsymbol{S} \sim W_p(n, \boldsymbol{\Sigma})$, and $\boldsymbol{S}$ and $\boldsymbol{\Sigma}$ are conformally partitioned into $\boldsymbol{S}_{11}, \boldsymbol{S}_{12}, \boldsymbol{S}_{22}$ and $\boldsymbol{\Sigma}_{11}, \boldsymbol{\Sigma}_{12}, \boldsymbol{\Sigma}_{22}$ (with $\boldsymbol{S}_{21} = \boldsymbol{S}_{12}, \boldsymbol{\Sigma}_{21} = \boldsymbol{\Sigma}_{12}$), where $\boldsymbol{S}_{11}, \boldsymbol{\Sigma}_{11}$ are $q \times q$, $q < p$. Now elimination of the $(p - q)$ variables corresponding to $\boldsymbol{\Sigma}_{22}$ gives

$$\boldsymbol{S}_{11} - \boldsymbol{S}_{12}\boldsymbol{S}_{22}^{-1}\boldsymbol{S}_{21} \sim W_q(n - p + q, \boldsymbol{\Sigma}_{11} - \boldsymbol{\Sigma}_{12}\boldsymbol{\Sigma}_{22}^{-1}\boldsymbol{\Sigma}_{21}). \qquad \text{(A.20)}$$

(ii) Additivity.

If $\boldsymbol{S} \sim W_p(n_1, \boldsymbol{\Sigma})$, $\boldsymbol{T} \sim W_p(n_2, \boldsymbol{\Sigma})$ independently,

$$\boldsymbol{S} + \boldsymbol{T} \sim W_p(n_1 + n_2, \boldsymbol{\Sigma}).$$

(iii) Scaling.
If $\boldsymbol{S} \sim W_p(n, \boldsymbol{\Sigma})$ and $\boldsymbol{A}$ is a fixed $p \times q$ matrix,

$$\boldsymbol{A}'\boldsymbol{S}\boldsymbol{A} \sim W_q(n, \boldsymbol{A}'\boldsymbol{\Sigma}\boldsymbol{A}).$$

This result follows at once because linear combinations of multivariate normal variables are multivariate normal. Of course, if the rank of $\boldsymbol{A}$ is less than q, the distribution is degenerate.

A.4 If $\boldsymbol{S} \sim W_p(n, \boldsymbol{\Sigma})$

$$f(\boldsymbol{S}) = \frac{|\boldsymbol{S}|^{(n-p-1)/2} \exp(-\frac{1}{2}\mathrm{tr}\Sigma^{-1}\boldsymbol{S})}{2^{np/2}\pi^{p(p-1)/4}|\Sigma|^{n/2}\prod_{i=1}^{p}\Gamma\frac{1}{2}(n+1-i)}. \qquad \text{(A.21)}$$

This result was proved by Wishart (1928) using the geometrical argument developed by Fisher – in fact, Fisher (1915) had given the result for the special case $p = 2$. There are several different approaches to deriving the result. Wishart (1948) gives an account of published methods up to that date. The account that follows is based on Arnold (1981), who attributes it to Stein (1969).

The method proceeds by induction on p.
(i) Consider the case $\boldsymbol{\Sigma} = \boldsymbol{I}$.
(ii) Assume the distribution is true for $p - 1$.
(iii) By partitioning the matrix $\boldsymbol{S}$ into a $(p-1) \times (p-1)$ matrix bordered by a row and a column, derive the distribution for p.
(iv) Complete the proof by noting that $\boldsymbol{\Sigma} = \boldsymbol{I}$, $p = 1$ is a standard χ^2 distribution.
(v) Generalise by considering the transformation $\boldsymbol{XT}$, where $\boldsymbol{T}$ is a Gramian square root of $\boldsymbol{\Sigma}$.

Now consider the transformation from $\boldsymbol{S} = s_{11}, \boldsymbol{S}_{12}, \boldsymbol{S}_{22}$, where $q = 1$, s_{11} is a single element, $\boldsymbol{S}_{12}$ is $1 \times (p-1)$, and $\boldsymbol{S}_{22}$ is $(p-1) \times (p-1)$, to $s_{11} - \boldsymbol{S}_{12}\boldsymbol{S}_{22}^{-1}\boldsymbol{S}_{21}, \boldsymbol{S}_{12}\boldsymbol{S}_{22}^{-1}, \boldsymbol{S}_{22}$. The Jacobian of the transformation is $|\boldsymbol{S}_{22}|^{-1}$, and we may write

$$f(\boldsymbol{S}) = |\boldsymbol{S}_{22}|^{-1} f(\boldsymbol{S}_{22}) f(\boldsymbol{S}_{12}\boldsymbol{S}_{22}^{-1}|\boldsymbol{S}_{22}) f(s_{11} - \boldsymbol{S}_{12}\boldsymbol{S}_{22}^{-1}\boldsymbol{S}_{21}). \qquad \text{(A.22)}$$

The first component is $W_{p-1}(n, \boldsymbol{I})$, which has, by hypothesis, the form given above with $\boldsymbol{\Sigma} = \boldsymbol{I}$. The second component, conditional on $\boldsymbol{S}_{22}$, is $(p-1)$-variate normal, with zero mean and covariance matrix $\boldsymbol{S}_{22}^{-1}$. The third component is χ^2 with $n - p + 1$ degrees of freedom.

Combining these terms, noting that $(s_{11} - \boldsymbol{S}_{12}\boldsymbol{S}_{22}^{-1}\boldsymbol{S}_{21})|\boldsymbol{S}_{22}| = |\boldsymbol{S}|$, gives, with some heavy algebra, $W_p(n, \boldsymbol{I})$ in the form already shown.

Finally, suppose $\boldsymbol{TT}' = \boldsymbol{\Sigma}$, where $\boldsymbol{T}$ is upper triangular (the Cholesky decomposition). Then if $\boldsymbol{S} \sim W_p(n, \boldsymbol{I})$, $\boldsymbol{S}^* = \boldsymbol{TST}'$, $\boldsymbol{S}^* \sim W_p(n, \boldsymbol{\Sigma})$ and since $\boldsymbol{S} = (\boldsymbol{T}')^{-1}\boldsymbol{ST}^{-1}$, the Jacobian is $|\boldsymbol{T}^{-1}|^{p+1}$.

Related distributions

A.5 The non-central Wishart distribution is the distribution of a matrix $\boldsymbol{X}'\boldsymbol{X}$, where $\boldsymbol{X}$ is a $n \times p$ matrix of independent observations from a p-variate normal distribution, with non-zero mean $\boldsymbol{\mu}$. The non-centrality parameter is the matrix

$\mu\mu'$. The distribution is the multivariate generalisation of the non-central chi-squared distribution, and has potentially the same sort of applications. It is not possible to express the distribution in closed form, and it is only of theoretical interest.

The inverted Wishart distribution is the distribution of the inverse of a Wishart matrix. If $S \sim W_p(n, \Sigma)$ and $U = S^{-1}$, U has an inverted Wishart distribution

$$f(U) = \frac{|U|^{-(n+p+1)/2} \exp(-\frac{1}{2}\mathrm{tr}\Sigma^{-1}U^{-1})}{2^{np/2}\pi^{p(p+1)/4}|\Sigma|^{n/2}\prod_{i=1}^{p}\Gamma\frac{1}{2}(n+1-i)}. \quad \text{(A.23)}$$

See Siskind (1972); Mardia *et al* (1979). The distribution is easily derived from the Wishart distribution by noting that the Jacobian of the transformation $U = S^{-1}$ is $|S|^{-2p}$. The expectation of U is given by

$$E(U) = \Sigma^{-1}/(n-p-1). \quad \text{(A.24)}$$

In Bayesian statistics, the inverted Wishart distribution is a conjugate prior for a covariance matrix.

Likelihood ratio tests

A.6 Many of the classical tests in multivariate analysis are likelihood ratio tests. The general theory is fully discussed in Stuart and Ord (1991, Chapters 21–25), or see Lehmann (1986). Suppose the null hypothesis imposes a constraint on the parameters, say $\theta = \theta_0$ where θ is a set of d parameters. In general, there will be other (nuisance) parameters ψ. The likelihood ratio test statistic is based on the ratio of (A) the likelihood maximised over (θ, ψ) to (B) the likelihood maximised over ψ, with $\theta = \theta_0$.

Write $l(\hat{\theta}, \hat{\psi})$ for the log likelihood of the sample when $\hat{\theta}, \hat{\psi}$ are unconstrained maximum likelihood estimates, and $l(\theta_0, \hat{\psi}_0)$ for the log likelihood when $\theta = \theta_0$ and $\hat{\psi}_0$ is the maximum likelihood estimate of ψ conditional on $\theta = \theta_0$. Then, under regularity conditions,

$$\omega = 2l(\hat{\theta}, \hat{\psi}) - 2l(\theta_0, \hat{\psi}_0) \sim \chi^2_{[d]} \quad \text{(A.25)}$$

asymptotically, as the sample size tends to infinity.

The regularity conditions are given in full in the texts already cited. The most important is that the null hypothesis must be expressible in the form of d constraints. Silvey (1959) describes the general test as the 'Lagrange multiplier test'; the d constraints imply maximising $l(\theta, \psi)$ subject to constraints that involve d Lagrange multipliers. This condition breaks down when θ_0 is 'on the edge of the parameter space', that is, when constraining some elements of θ implies that others cannot be estimated.

Two examples illustrate the point.

Example A.1

Consider the (univariate) two-phase regression problem

$$\begin{aligned} E(y) &= a + b_1(x - X), \qquad x \leqslant X \quad &\text{(A.26)} \\ &= a + b_2(x - X), \qquad x > X \quad &\text{(A.27)} \end{aligned}$$

where a, b_1, b_2, X are unknown. If the residuals are normally distributed, the maximum likelihood estimates are obtained by least squares. The minimisation does not lead to explicit expressions for the parameters, but is easily solved by iterating on X. Now the null hypothesis that the regression is linear, with no break point, involves two parameters instead of four, and it is tempting to construct an analysis of variance to test the hypothesis by a standard F-test. This analysis uses the likelihood ratio statistic discussed above, but the test is not valid. The F statistic does not follow a variance ratio distribution, and it is not even true that $2F$ has a chi-squared distribution with two degrees of freedom asymptotically as the sample size increases. The null hypothesis implies $b_1 = b_2$, but if this is true no estimate of X is possible; or if X is outside the range of the sample, one of the coefficients cannot be estimated. The null hypothesis cannot be expressed as a constraint on the four parameters involving two Lagrange multipliers.

Example A.2
The problem of estimating the parameters of a distribution mixture

$$\alpha_1 f(\boldsymbol{x}, \boldsymbol{\theta}_1) + \alpha_2 f(\boldsymbol{x}, \boldsymbol{\theta}_2) + \dots$$

where $\sum_{i=1}^{k} \alpha_i = 1$ can be solved by maximum likelihood, when $f(\cdot)$ is specified, for any given value of k. The changes in the maximised likelihood as k increases surely give an indication of the number of components in the mixture, but the distribution of the likelihood ratio statistic is unknown, even asymptotically. The null hypothesis may be expressed as $\alpha_k = 0$, or as $\theta_k = \theta_{k-1}$, but either constraint implies that the other parameter is unidentifiable.

When the regularity conditions apply, the exact distribution of the likelihood ratio statistic is sometimes known. This is true, for example, of the distribution of T^2 discussed above. In other cases, the distribution has been tabulated, so that exact significance tests are possible, at least for certain significance levels. Sometimes, however, the exact distribution is intractable and tables are not available. The asymptotic form is known, but for moderate samples – particularly for multivariate problems – tests based upon it may be seriously misleading.

Several authors have tried to find modifications that give better sub-asymptotic properties. Bartlett (1937), studying the test for homogeneity of normal variances, modified the likelihood ratio test by (a) conditioning on the means, and so using variance estimates with the appropriate degrees of freedom as divisors, and (b) multiplying by a factor to make the mean, to order $1/n$, equal to the mean of the chi-squared distribution – the appropriate degrees of freedom for the test.

This calculation gave the now well-known modification of the likelihood ratio test (Stuart and Ord, 1991, 23.9) known as Bartlett's test.

The method is quite generally applicable. It is usually true that

$$E(\omega^*) = d\{1 + \frac{b}{n} + O(n^{-3/2})\}$$

where ω^* is the criterion ω, possibly using modified maximum likelihood estimators. If b can be calculated – usually a straightforward, but complex, procedure – it is reasonable to hope that $(1 + b/n)^{-1}\omega^*$ will be approximated by the chi-squared distribution better than ω. In fact, this simple adjustment works extraordinarily well; in many cases, for moderate values of n, the probabilities given by the crude likelihood ratio test are quite misleading, and are dramatically improved by the modification. Lawley (1956b) showed that the adjustment based on the mean ensures that *all* the cumulants of $(1 + b/n)^{-1}\omega^*$ differ from those of $\chi^2_{[d]}$ by $O(n^{-3/2})$. For a full discussion, see Barndorff-Neilsen and Cox (1984) and Cordeiro (1983).

Bartlett (1954) gives a list of factors for use in likelihood ratio tests suggested by him up to that date. Lawley (1956a) gives the test used in maximum likelihood factor analysis. Pearson and Hartley (1972) give tables of the further adjustment needed, in the form of a factor (dependent on n, p and q) multiplying Bartlett's approximation, to the test of Wilks' criterion. These are based on tables by Schatzoff (1966) and Pillai and Gupta (1969). They confirm the remarkable accuracy of the approximation for moderate samples.

Box (1949) derived an asymptotic expansion for the distribution of likelihood ratio test statistics. The expressions given by the expansion are too cumbersome for general use in practical statistics, but can be used to derive Bartlett's adjustment factors. Box also suggested a further refinement; if $c \log \omega^* \sim F(v_1, v_2)$ approximately, where v_1 is the appropriate degrees of freedom for the standard asymptotic χ^2 and cv_1 is approximately 1, c and v_2 can be chosen to give an approximation of $O(n^{-2})$ to a variance-ratio distribution. (Here v_2 is not necessarily an integer). The F approximations are used to calculate P-values in some statistical packages, including SPSS. They can be regarded as effectively exact for any sensible sample size, but of course are based on the assumption of multivariate normality. Refinement of standard tests based on this assumption is of less importance than examination of their robustness.

Union-intersection tests

A.7 Any null hypothesis involving d constraints, where $d > 1$, can be regarded as the union of an infinite set of simpler hypotheses. For example, $\boldsymbol{\theta} = \boldsymbol{\theta}_o$ implies $\boldsymbol{a}'\boldsymbol{\theta} = \boldsymbol{a}'\boldsymbol{\theta}_o$ for any vector $\boldsymbol{a}$. An analysis of variance leads to an F test of equality of means; any particular contrast can be tested by a t-test, and one particular contrast (with $\boldsymbol{a}$ defined up to a multiplying factor) gives a maximum value to t. Choosing this contrast and testing it—making due allowance for the fact that the contrast has been chosen to give maximum value to t—is one possible approach to a test of the composite null hypothesis.

This approach to tests of significance was developed by Roy, and such tests are known as *union-intersection tests*. In the example above, it is well known that the t value given by the maximising contrast is $\sqrt{F}$, the square root of the overall variance ratio test; the union-intersection and the likelihood ratio approach give the same statistic and the same test. This is usually true of univariate tests, but in multivariate statistics the union-intersection method often suggests test statistics that are not likelihood ratio statistics. (Note that there is not necessarily a unique union-intersection test).

The general multivariate linear model is concerned with linear relationships between $\boldsymbol{y}$ and $\boldsymbol{x}$. Any linear combination $\boldsymbol{a}'\boldsymbol{y}$ can be regressed on $\boldsymbol{x}$ to give $\boldsymbol{a}'\boldsymbol{y} = \boldsymbol{b}'\boldsymbol{x}+e$ and, assuming e is normally distributed, tested by F. One particular choice of $\boldsymbol{a}$ gives a maximum F and a maximum multiple correlation. Then $\boldsymbol{a}'\boldsymbol{y}$, $\boldsymbol{b}'\boldsymbol{x}$ are the first pair of canonical variables, and the union-intersection principle suggests a test based on the first canonical correlation – the correlation that gives the largest possible F. This correlation, squared, is the largest eigenvalue of a matrix derived from a partitioned Wishart matrix; the likelihood ratio test is based on the determinant of the same matrix. The two tests are different, and are powerful against different alternatives. It is intuitively clear that if there is only one non-zero population eigenvalue, a test of the greatest sample eigenvalue is likely to have good power properties, while if all the population eigenvalues are non-zero a test statistic based on all the sample eigenvalues will be better. This point is discussed in more detail later.

Testing linear models

A.8 In univariate statistics, the variance ratio or F test has three main applications. The corresponding multivariate problems are concerned with testing the hypotheses:

(a) that two Wishart matrices are based on the same unknown covariance matrix;

(b) that the variables $\boldsymbol{x} = (x_1, \ldots, x_p)'$ and $\boldsymbol{y} = (y_1, \ldots, y_q)'$ are uncorrelated, where it is assumed that the residuals in any linear relationship follow a multivariate normal distribution;

(c) that the variables $\boldsymbol{x} = (x_1, \ldots, x_p)'$, assumed to have a multivariate normal distribution with a common covariance matrix in $k = q + 1$ groups, have the same mean in all groups.

These three problems are analogous to the use of the F test in (a) comparing two variance estimates, (b) multiple regression, and (c) one-way analysis of variance. The multivariate problems can all be defined in terms of a product $\boldsymbol{W}_1\boldsymbol{W}_2^{-1}$ where $\boldsymbol{W}_1$ and $\boldsymbol{W}_2$ are Wishart matrices, and the invariant statistics are the eigenvalues of this product. Problems (b) and (c) are formally identical; as in the univariate case, dummy variables $\boldsymbol{y} = (y_1, \ldots, y_q)'$ may be defined to represent the groups. Now in (b) we can, without loss of generality, specify $p \leqslant q$, and, in the same way, in (c) there is a symmetry between p and q, so that if there are more groups than variables the values p and q can be interchanged.

Problem (a) is the least important from the practical point of view. Often, as in (c), covariance matrices are assumed equal, and if this assumption is seriously wrong false conclusions may be reached. The data should be examined and if necessary transformed or edited by the removal of outliers, or robust methods may replace the traditional approach (see Chapter 3). A formal significance test, however, has limited value. A non-significant result does not justify the blind acceptance of the null hypothesis. On the other hand, tests of (a) are critically dependent on the assumption of normality, so that a significant result does not mean that the assumption of homogeneity is seriously misleading. Scheffé (1959, Chapter 10) remarks (of the corresponding univariate problem) 'If the variances are equal but the data are nonnormal with $\gamma_2 > 0$, the preliminary test is then likely to reject the hypothesis of equality of variance and the user will accordingly refrain from applying the analysis of variance of the means in a case where it is dependable'. The same point applies in the multivariate situation.

The likelihood ratio test of (a) is a special case of the test for k covariance matrices. This is a generalisation of Bartlett's test for homogeneity of variances. It was first derived by Wilks (1932). The test with Bartlett adjustments was given by Box (1949).

Suppose $\boldsymbol{S}_i$ is the estimated covariance matrix for group i, where each sum of squares or products is divided by the appropriate degrees of freedom ν_i (where $\nu_i = n_i - 1$, in the simplest case where there have been no adjustments for covariates). Suppose $\boldsymbol{S}$ is the pooled covariance matrix based on $N = \sum_{i=1}^{k} \nu_i$ degrees of freedom. Then

$$M = N \log |\boldsymbol{S}| - \sum_{i=1}^{k} \nu_i \log |\boldsymbol{S}_i| \tag{A.28}$$

is the test statistic, asymptotically distributed as χ^2 with $f_1 = \frac{1}{2}p(p+1)(k-1)$ degrees of freedom.

The adjusted test is

$$M \sim \chi^2_{[f_1]}/(1 - D_1) \tag{A.29}$$

where

$$D_1 = \frac{2p^2 + 3p - 1}{6(p+1)(k-1)} \left(\sum_{i=1}^{k} \frac{1}{\nu_i} - \frac{1}{N} \right).$$

A more accurate approximation (Box, 1949) is given by

$$M \sim bF(f_1, f_2) \tag{A.30}$$

where

$$\begin{aligned} f_2 &= \frac{f_1 + 2}{D_2 - D_1^2}, \\ D_2 &= \frac{(p-1)(p+2)}{6(k-1)} \left\{ \sum_{i=1}^{k} \frac{1}{\nu_i^2} - \frac{1}{N^2} \right\}, \\ b &= \frac{F_1}{1 - D_1 - f_1/f_2}, \end{aligned}$$

where, as usual, f_2 is not, in general an integer. Korin (1969) gives a table of values based on the Box expansion for the case when all matrices are based on equal degrees of freedom, $\nu_i = \nu_0$. This table is given in Pearson and Hartley (1972), who also quote comparisons made by Pearson (1969) between Korin's values and those given by the two approximate tests. These confirm that, for reasonable values of ν_0, the χ^2 approximation is excellent and the F

approximation even better. Lee *et al* (1977) give rather more extensive tables, reproduced in Seber (1984).

The union-intersection approach to problem (a) suggests a test based on the largest and smallest eigenvalues of $\boldsymbol{S}_1\boldsymbol{S}_2^{-1}$. The test is discussed by Seber (1984, p.105). Schurrmann *et al* (1973a,b) give some tables, and Pearson and Hartley (1972) give corresponding tables for testing whether a sample covariance matrix agrees with a known matrix ($v_2 \rightarrow \infty$). This type of test has no obvious advantages over the likelihood ratio test, and does not easily generalise to $k > 2$.

Problems (b) and (c) may be expressed in terms of Wishart matrices $\boldsymbol{H}$ and $\boldsymbol{E}$, for hypothesis and error. Here, $\boldsymbol{H}$ is a $p \times p$ sum of squares and products matrix based on q degrees of freedom representing the difference between the $p \times p$ matrix $\boldsymbol{E} + \boldsymbol{H}$ calculated assuming the null hypothesis, with v degrees of freedom, and $\boldsymbol{E}$, the residual matrix with $v - q$ degrees of freedom after fitting the full set of parameters by maximum likelihood. Thus in (b), if $\boldsymbol{V}$ is the sum of squares and products matrix for $\boldsymbol{x}$ and $\boldsymbol{y}$ partitioned into $\boldsymbol{V}_{11}$, $\boldsymbol{V}_{12}$ and $\boldsymbol{V}_{22}$, $\boldsymbol{E} + \boldsymbol{H} = \boldsymbol{V}_{11}$, $\boldsymbol{E} = \boldsymbol{V}_{11} - \boldsymbol{V}_{12}\boldsymbol{V}_{22}^{-1}\boldsymbol{V}_{21}$. In (c), $\boldsymbol{E} + \boldsymbol{H}$ is calculated from deviations from the overall mean, $\boldsymbol{E}$ from deviations from the group means.

The invariant statistics are the eigenvalues $l_1, \ldots, l_p$ of $\boldsymbol{E}(\boldsymbol{H} + \boldsymbol{E})^{-1}$, or equivalently $c_1, \ldots, c_p$, the eigenvalues of $\boldsymbol{H}\boldsymbol{E}^{-1}$, where

$$l_i = c_i/(1 + c_i).$$

Various test statistics have been proposed; the most important are:

(i) The likelihood ratio statistic, known as Wilks' criterion

$$W = \prod_{i=1}^{p}(1 - l_i) = |\boldsymbol{E}|/|\boldsymbol{H} + \boldsymbol{E}|. \tag{A.31}$$

The distribution is given by

$$-[v - \tfrac{1}{2}(p + q + 1)]\log(W) \sim C\chi^2_{[pq]} \tag{A.32}$$

where C is a multiplier tabulated by Schatzoff (1966a) and Pillai and Gupta (1969) and reproduced in Pearson and Hartley (1972). As v increases, C tends to 1 very rapidly. It is always greater than 1, so that the Bartlett χ^2 test gives a false positive rate slightly higher than the nominal significance level.

(ii) Roy's maximum root test

$$L = l_1. \tag{A.33}$$

Tables are given by Foster (1957, 1958), Foster and Rees (1957), Pillai (1960) and charts by Heck (1960). They are reproduced in many standard textbooks (Pearson and Hartley, 1972; Roy, 1957; Seber, 1984; Harris, 1975). There seems to be no simple approximation in terms of standard distributions.

(iii) The Lawley–Hotelling trace

$$H = \sum_{i=1}^{p} c_i = \mathrm{tr}\boldsymbol{H}\boldsymbol{E}^{-1}. \tag{A.34}$$

This criterion was considered by Lawley (1938), Bartlett (1939) and Hsu (1940) and discussed in detail by Hotelling (1944,1947, 1951). It is a union-intersection statistic (Mudholkar *et al*, 1974a). An approximate test, based on the first four moments, was proposed by Pillai:

$$F_{(pq,v^*)} = \frac{v^*}{pq}\frac{H}{p} \tag{A.35}$$

where $v^* = p(v - p - q - 1) + 2$.

(iv) The Pillai trace

$$D = \sum_{i=1}^{p} l_i = \text{tr}\boldsymbol{H}(\boldsymbol{H} + \boldsymbol{E})^{-1}. \tag{A.36}$$

The statistic was studied by Pillai, who proposed the approximate test:

$$F_{(pq,v^*)} = \frac{v^*}{pq}\frac{D}{p - D} \tag{A.37}$$

where $v^* = p(v - q)$.

Choice of test statistic

A.9 The test criteria discussed above, as well as others that have been proposed from time to time, differ in their power against different alternatives, and probably in robustness against non-normality and heterogeneity of covariance matrices. The non-null distribution of the eigenvalues (see **A.11**) is extremely complex, and little is known about their distribution when the assumptions of normality and homoscedasticity break down. Theoretical study of the properties of the statistics has achieved little, and the main conclusions rest on simulation.

Simulation results are inevitably limited in their applicability. Most studies have been restricted to moderate values of p and q, but even for fixed values of p, q and n the properties of the statistics depend critically on the size and pattern of the population eigenvalues. These studies give some interesting insights, but should be treated with some caution. The extreme cases are (i) when there is a single non-zero eigenvalue, and (ii) when all the eigenvalues are equal. In (c), these correspond to (i) all the group means on a single line—which may be approximately true in cases where the groups are obviously ordered—and (ii) all pairs of group means with the same Mahalanobis distance, so that they lie at the vertices of a regular $(q - 1)$-dimensional simplex in the space defined by Mahalanobis distance.

The first simulation studies were those of Schatzoff (1967) and Pillai and Jayachandran (1967). Since then, there have been many more, mainly by Pillai and collaborators. Pillai (1977) gives a very complete bibliography up to that date.

The main conclusion from the simulations is that Roy's maximum root statistic has quite different properties from the other three. When there are several non-zero population eigenvalues, its power is much less; not unexpectedly, criteria that take account of all the sample eigenvalues perform better. When there is a single non-zero eigenvalue, Roy's test has greater power, *provided that* the power is fairly large. In the study by Pillai and Jayachandran,

Roy's test performed badly when there was a single non-zero eigenvalue because the power was low, and the first sample eigenvector generally bore little relationship to the single population eigenvector. In these circumstances, the other tests were more powerful.

Comparisons among the other statistics are less clear. They are asymptotically equivalent, and for small samples comparisons depend on the exact structure of the population eigenvalues. It is easy to see that when W or H is fixed, D is a maximum when the sample eigenvalues are all equal; it is therefore reasonable to expect Pillai's trace to be most powerful against an alternative in which all the population eigenvalues are equal, whereas the other two may perform better when there are some zero eigenvalues.

On robustness against non-normality, Pillai and Hsu (1979) report that the Pillai trace was consistently most robust in all the situations they considered.

A test of dimensionality

A.10 A problem first investigated by Bartlett (1947a) is that of determining the minimum number of non-zero eigenvalues, say r, consistent with the data. This amounts to testing the null hypothesis $\lambda_{r+1} = 0$, assuming $\lambda_r > 0$. Bartlett dealt with the problem using the likelihood ratio test

$$-[v - \frac{1}{2}(p+q+1)] \sum_{i=1}^{p} \log(1 - l_i) \sim \chi^2_{[pq]}. \qquad \text{(A.38)}$$

Now a significant value in this test shows that $\lambda_1 \neq 0$. Then to test $\lambda_2 = 0$ it is reasonable to eliminate the first pair of canonical variables, and then test for a relationship. The elimination of a pair of canonical variables is equivalent to reducing each set of variables by 1, and so

$$-[v - \frac{1}{2}(p+q+1)] \sum_{i=2}^{p} \log(1 - l_i) \sim \chi^2_{[(p-1)(q-1)]}. \qquad \text{(A.39)}$$

This process can be continued, at each step reducing each of the factors in the degrees of freedom by unity, until the test gives a non-significant result.

The procedure is asymptotically valid, but for moderate samples should be interpreted with caution. There is an implicit assumption that the first sample eigenvector coincides approximately with the first population eigenvector. This assumption is probably true if the test gives a highly significant result, but it is not clear how the subsequent tests are affected if the sample vector is not close to the population direction.

Bartlett presents the procedure as a 'partitioning of χ^2', with $p+q-1$ degrees of freedom associated with l_1, $p+q-3$ with l_2 and so on as long as results are significant. It should be emphasised that this is purely formal; the test of the null hypothesis after eliminating the first canonical variables is legitimate, but the procedure does not give a test for the first eigenvalue. Misinterpreting the results in this way can be wildly misleading, as Harris (1975), for example, points out.

The likelihood ratio criterion is traditionally used in this test, but there is no reason why other statistics should not be tested in the same way. If l_1 is obviously significant, a test of l_2, looking up the value in tables of the largest eigenvalue with $p-1$ and $q-1$ replacing p and q is reasonable, subject to the same caveats as for the likelihood ratio test.

Example A.3

Bartlett (1947a) studied a set of data, now famous, first published by Barnard (1935). The data studied consisted of four measurements on four series of ancient Egyptian skulls. A total of 398 skulls were included in the study, so that $p = 3$ (the degrees of freedom between series), $q = 4$, and $\nu = 397$. The dates of the four series were approximately known, and one hypothesis of interest was that the changes in the means might be predominantly time related, giving a single dominant eigenvector, possibly with the spacing of the means related to the time intervals between the series.

The eigenvalues were calculated as

$$\begin{aligned} 1 - l_1 &= 0.8902 \\ 1 - l_2 &= 0.9404 \\ 1 - l_3 &= 0.9813 \end{aligned}$$

The likelihood ratio criterion gives

$$\begin{aligned} \chi^2_{[12]} &= 393 \sum_{i=1}^{3} \log(1 - l_i) \\ &= 77.30 \end{aligned}$$

The means clearly differ significantly. The Lawley–Hotelling trace and the Pillai trace lead to similar conclusions. For the former,

$$\begin{aligned} c_1 &= 0.1233 \\ c_2 &= 0.0634 \\ c_3 &= 0.0191 \end{aligned}$$

and $\nu^*/p = 389.67$. Then the F statistic given above, multiplied by pq, is approximately distributed as χ^2, and has the value 80.19. The Pillai trace is 0.1881, with $\nu^*/p = 393$, and the corresponding χ^2 value is 78.87.

The three values are very similar, and lead to the same conclusions. The value of l_1 is also highly significant—well above any critical values in the published tables—but cannot be compared with the other statistics by calculating a χ^2 value.

Bartlett gave the following partitioning of the likelihood ratio χ^2 test:

	χ^2	Degrees of freedom
l_1	45.72	6
l_2	24.16	4
l_3	7.42	2
	77.30	12

The interpretation of this table is:
(i) The likelihood ratio χ^2 value, 77.30 with 12 degrees of freedom, is highly significant; there are real differences among the series.
(ii) Elimination of the first pair of canonical variables leaves a χ^2 value of 31.58 with 6 degrees of freedom. Again, the result is highly significant, and the series means are not collinear.
(iii) Elimination of the first two pairs of canonical variables leaves a χ^2 value of 7.42 with 2 degrees of freedom. This value is still significant ($P \approx 0.025$), and there is some evidence that a two-dimensional plot of the first two canonical variables does not fully represent the differences among the series.
A similar analysis could be carried out using either of the trace criteria or the separate eigenvalues. The same conclusion would be reached in step (ii), and in step (iii) the tests (when the reduced $p = 1$) are exactly the same.

Eigenvalue distributions

A.11 The squared sample canonical correlations are the eigenvalues $c_1, \ldots, c_p$ of $\boldsymbol{HE}^{-1}$, where $\boldsymbol{H}$ and $\boldsymbol{E}$ are independent Wishart matrices corresponding to the 'hypothesis' and 'error' terms in an analysis of variance. The distribution of the test statistics discussed in **A.8** depends on the joint distribution of these eigenvalues.

The null distribution, when the population eigenvalues are zero, was given independently by Fisher (1939), Hsu (1939b) and Roy (1939). It has the form

$$f(\boldsymbol{c}) = C \prod_{i=1}^{p} \left\{ c_i^{\frac{1}{2}(q-p-1)} (1 - c_i)^{\frac{1}{2}(n-q-p-1)} \prod_{j=i+1}^{p} (c_i - c_j) \right\} \tag{A.40}$$

where the constant C is given by

$$\pi^{\frac{1}{2}p} \prod_{i=0}^{p-1} \left\{ \Gamma\left[\frac{1}{2}(n-i)\right] \Big/ \left(\Gamma\left[\frac{1}{2}(p-i)\right] \Gamma\left[\frac{1}{2}(q-i)\right] \Gamma\left[\frac{1}{2}(n-q-i)\right] \right) \right\}.$$

Here, p and q are the number of hypothesis degrees of freedom and the number of variables. They are interchangeable, and it is assumed that $p \leqslant q$, without loss of generality. The eigenvalues $c_1, \ldots, c_p$ are ordered, $c_1 < c_2 < \ldots < c_p$. Equal sample eigenvalues have zero probability.

This distribution underlies the distribution of the test statistics discussed above. It is a rather intractable expression, which reduces to a polynomial when both the indices $\frac{1}{2}(q - p - 1)$ and $\frac{1}{2}(n - q - p - 1)$ are integers.

The general distribution, when the population eigenvalues are not zero, is much more complicated. Bartlett (1947b) first studied the joint distribution of the canonical correlations and gave formal expressions for the general distribution in terms of hypergeometric functions. James (1960) gave the distribution of the eigenvalues of the general Wishart matrix, and Constantine

(1963) discussed the non-central Wishart distribution and the distribution of the canonical correlations.

James (1964) gives a comprehensive survey of these and other non-central multivariate distributions. They are expressed in terms of hypergeometric functions of matrix argument. These functions are defined as sums of multiples of the *zonal polynomials* of the matrices involved. The general results are rather complex, although they simplify considerably in special cases, for example when there is a single non-zero population canonical correlation. Muirhead (1982) reviews the theory and the asymptotic results.

References

Aitchison, J. (1982). The statistical analysis of compositional data (with discussion). *Journal of the Royal Statistical Society, Series B*, **44**, 139–177.

Aitchison, J. (1986). *The Statistical Analysis of Compositional Data*. Chapman and Hall, London, England.

Aitchison, J. and Shen, S. M. (1980). Logistic-normal distributions; some properties and uses. *Biometrika*, **67**, 261–272.

Aitkin, M. A. (1974). Simultaneous inference and the choice of variable subsets in multiple regression. *Technometrics*, **16**, 221–227.

Anderson, E. (1957). A semigraphical method for the analysis of complex problems. *Proceedings of the National Academy of Science*, **13**, 923–927. (Reprinted, with an appended note, in *Technometrics*, 1960, **2**, 387–391.)

Anderson, T. W. (1984). *An Introduction to Multivariate Statistical Analysis*, 2nd ed. Wiley, New York, U.S.A.

Andrews, D. F. (1971). A note on the selection of data transformations. *Biometrika*, **58**, 249–254.

Andrews, D. F. (1972). Plots of high-dimensional data. *Biometrics*, **28**, 125–136.

Andrews, D. F., Gnanadesikan, R. and Warner, J. L. (1971). Transformations of multivariate data. *Biometrics*, **27**, 825–840.

Andrews, D. F., Gnanadesikan, R. and Warner, J. L. (1973). Methods for assessing multivariate normality. In *Multivariate Analysis III* (ed P. R. Krishnaiah), pp. 95–116. Academic Press, New York, U.S.A.

Arabie, P. (1978). Random versus rational strategies for initial configurations in non-metric multidimensional scaling. *Psychometrika*, **43**, 111–113.

Armitage, P. (1966). The chi-square test for heterogeneity of proportions, after adjustment for stratification. *Journal of the Royal Statistical Society, Series B*, **28**, 150–163. (Addendum: **29**, 197).

Armitage, P., McPherson, C. K. and Copas, J. C. (1969). Statistical studies of prognosis in advanced breast cancer. *Journal of Chronic Diseases*, **22**, 343–360.

Arnold, G. M. and Collins, A. J. (1993). Interpretation of transformed axes in multivariate analysis. *Applied Statistics*, **42**, 381–400.

Arnold, H. J. (1964). Permutation support for multivariate techniques. *Biometrika*, **51**, 65–70.

Arnold, S. F. (1981). *The Theory of Linear Models and Multivariate Analysis.* Wiley, New York, U.S.A.

Ashton, E. H., Healy, M. J. R. and Lipton, S. (1957). The descriptive use of discriminant functions in physical anthropology. *Proceedings of the Royal Society, Series B*, **146**, 552–572.

Asimov, D. (1985). The grand tour; a tool for viewing multidimensional data. *SIAM Journal on Scientific and Statistical Computing*, **6**, 128–143.

Atkinson, A.C. (1985). *Plots, Transformations, and Regression.* Clarendon Press, Oxford, England.

Atkinson, A. C. and Mulira, H.-M. (1993). The stalactite plot for the detection of multivariate outliers. *Statistics and Computing*, **3**, 27–35.

Aykroyd, R. G. and Green, P. J. (1991). Global and local priors, and the location of lesions using gamma-camera imagery. *Philosophical Transactions of the Royal Society, London*, **337**, 323–342.

Banfield, J. D. and Raftery, A. E. (1992). Ice floe identification in satellite images using mathematical morphology and clustering about principal curves. *Journal of the American Statistical Association*, **87**, 7–15.

Barlow, R. E., Bartholomew, D. J., Bremner, J. M. and Brunk, H. M. (1972). *Statistical Inference Under Order Restrictions.* J. Wiley, London, England.

Barnard, M. M. (1935). The secular variations of skull characters in four series of Egyptian skulls. *Annals of Eugenics*, **6**, 352–371.

Barndorff-Neilson, O. E. and Cox, D. R. (1984). The effect of sampling rules on likelihood statistics. *International Statistical Review*, **52**, 309–326.

Barnett, V. (1974). *Elements of Sampling Theory.* English Universities Press, London, England.

Barnett, V. (1976). The ordering of multivariate data (with discussion). *Journal of the Royal Statistical Society, Series A*, **139**, 318–355.

Barnett, V. and Lewis, T. (1978). *Outliers in Statistical Data.* Wiley, Chichester, England.

Barry, D. (1986). Nonparametric Bayesian regression. *Annals of Statistics*, **14**, 934–953.

Bartlett, M. S. (1933). On the theory of statistical regression. *Proceedings of the Royal Society of Edinburgh*, **53**, 260–283.

Bartlett, M. S. (1937). Properties of sufficiency and statistical tests. *Proceedings of the Royal Society, Series A*, **168**, 268–282.

Bartlett, M. S. (1939). A note on tests of significance in multivariate analysis. *Proceedings of the Cambridge Philosophical Society*, **35**, 180–185.

Bartlett, M. S. (1947a). Multivariate analysis (with discussion). *Supplement to the Journal of the Royal Statistical Society*, **9**, 176–197.

Bartlett, M. S. (1947b). The general canonical correlation distribution. *Annals of Mathematical Statistics*, **18**, 1–17.

Bartlett, M. S. (1950). Tests of significance in factor analysis. *British Journal of Psychology, Statistical Section*, **3**, 77–85.

Bartlett, M. S. (1951). An inverse matrix adjustment arising in discriminant analysis. *Annals of Mathematical Statistics*, **22**, 107–111.

Bartlett, M. S. (1954). A note on the multiplying factors for various χ^2 approximations. *Journal of the Royal Statistical Society, Series B*, **16**, 296–298.

Beale, E. M. L. and Little, R. J. A. (1975). Missing values in multivariate analysis. *Journal of the Royal Statistical Society, Series B*, **37**, 129–145.

Becker, R. A., Chambers, J. M. and Wilks, A. R. (1988). *The New S Language*. Wadsworth, New York, U.S.A.

Becker, R. A., Cleveland, W. S. and Wilks, A. R. (1987). Dynamic graphics for data analysis. *Statistical Science*, **2**, 355–383.

Bekker, P. and De Leeuw, J. (1988). Relations between variants of nonlinear principal component analysis. In *Component and Correspondence Analysis* (eds J. L. A. Van Rijckevorsel and J. De Leeuw), pp. 1–31. Wiley, Chichester, England.

Bennett, B. M. (1951). Note on a solution of the generalized Behrens–Fisher problem. *Annals of the Institute of Statistical Mathematics*, **2**, 87–90.

Bergström, H. (1952). On some expansions of stable distributions. *Arkiv för Matematik*, **22**, 375–378.

Bertier, P. and Bouroche, J-M. (1975). *Analyse des Données Multidimensionelles*. Presses Universitaires de France, Paris, France.

Bhattacharyya, A. (1946). On a measure of divergence between two multinomial populations. *Sankhyā*, **7**, 401–406.

Bickel, P. J. and Doksum, K. A. (1981). An analysis of transformations revisited. *Journal of the American Statistical Association*, **76**, 145–168.

Bloomfield, P. (1974). Transformations for multivariate binary data. *Biometrics*, **30**, 609–617.

Bloxom, B. (1974). An alternative method of fitting a model of individual differences in multidimensional scaling. *Psychometrika*, **39**, 365–367.

Bollen, K. A. (1989). *Structural Equations with Latent Variables*. Wiley, New York, U.S.A.

Boneva, L. I. (1971). A new approach to a problem of archaeological seriation associated with the works of Plato. In *Mathematics in the Archaeological and Historical Sciences* (eds F. R. Hodson, D. G. Kendall and P. Tautu), pp. 173–185, Edinburgh University Press, Edinburgh, Scotland.

Bookstein, F. L. (1986). Size and shape spaces for landmark data in two dimensions (with discussion). *Statistical Science*, **1**, 181–242.

Borg, I. and Lingoes, J. C. (1980). *Multidimensional Similarity Structure Analysis*. Springer-Verlag, Heidelberg, Germany.

Bouroche, J.-M. and Saporta, G. (1980). *L'Analyse des Données*. Presses Universitaires de France, Paris, France.

Bowman, K. O. and Shenton, L. R. (1973a). Notes on the distribution of $\sqrt{b_1}$ in sampling from Pearson distributions. *Biometrika*, **60**, 155–167.

Bowman, K. O. and Shenton, L. R. (1973b). Remarks on the distribution of $\sqrt{b_1}$ in sampling from a normal mixture and normal Type A distribution. *Journal of the American Statistical Association*, **68**, 998–1003.

Bowman, K. O. and Shenton, L. R. (1975). Omnibus test contours for departures from normality based on $\sqrt{b_1}$ and b_2. *Biometrika*, **62**, 243–249.

Box, G. E. P. (1949). A general distribution theory for a class of likelihood criteria. *Biometrika*, **36**, 317–346.

Box, G. E. P. (1950). Problems in the analysis of growth and wear curves. *Biometrics*, **6**, 362–389.

Box, G. E. P. and Cox, D. R. (1964). An analysis of transformations. *Journal of the Royal Statistical Society, Series B*, **26**, 211–252.

Box, G. E. P. and Cox, D. R. (1982). An analysis of transformations revisited, rebutted. *Journal of the American Statistical Association*, **77**, 209–210.

Box, G. E. P. and Muller, M. E. (1958). A note on the generation of random normal deviates. *Annals of Mathematical Statistics*, **29**, 610–611.

Box, G. E. P. and Tiao, G. C. (1965). Multiparameter problems from a Bayesian point of view. *Annals of Mathematical Statistics*, **36**, 1468–1482.

Box, G. E. P. and Tiao, G. C. (1973). *Bayesian Inference in Statistical Analysis.* Addison-Wesley, Reading, Massachusetts, U.S.A.

Box, G. E. P. and Watson, G. S. (1962). Robustness to nonnormality of regression tests. *Biometrika*, **49**, 93–106. Correction *Biometrika*, **52**, 669.

Bradu, D. D. and Gabriel, K. R. (1976). The biplot as a diagnostic tool for models of two-way tables. *Technometrics*, **20**, 47–68.

Brady, H. E. (1985). Statistical consistency and hypothesis testing for nonmetric multidimensional scaling. *Psychometrika*, **50**, 509–537.

Breiman, L., Friedman, J. H., Olshen, R. A. and Stone, C. J. (1984). *Classification and Regression Trees.* Wadsworth, Belmont, California, U.S.A.

Brothwell, D. R. and Krzanowski, W. J. (1974). Evidence of biological differences between early British populations from Neolithic to Medieval times, as revealed by eleven commonly available cranial vault measurements. *Journal of Archaeological Science*, **1**, 249–260.

Brown, P. J. (1982). Multivariate calibration (with discussion). *Journal of the Royal Statistical Society, Series B*, **44**, 287–321.

Brown, P. J., Spiegelman, C. H. and Denham, M. C. (1991). Chemometrics and spectral frequency selection. *Philosophical Transactions of the Royal Society, London*, **337**, 311–322.

Buck, S. F. (1960). A method of estimation of missing values in multivariate data suitable for use with an electronic computer. *Journal of the Royal Statistical Society, Series B*, **22**, 302–306.

Cailliez, F. (1983). The analytical solution to the additive constant problem. *Psychometrika*, **48**, 305–308.

Cailliez, F. and Pagès, J. P. (1976). *Introduction à l'Analyse des Données.* SMASH, Paris, France.

Campbell, N. A. (1980). Robust procedures in multivariate analysis. I. Robust covariance estimation. *Applied Statistics*, **29**, 231–237.

Campbell, N. A. (1984). Canonical variate analysis with unequal covariance matrices. Generalizations of the usual solution. *Mathematical Geology*, **16**, 109–124.

Carroll, J. D. (1968). Generalization of canonical correlation analysis to three or more sets of variables. *Proceedings of the 76th Annual Convention of the American Psychological Association*, 227–228.

Carroll, J. D. (1969). Polynomial factor analysis. *Proceedings of the 77th Annual Convention of the American Psychological Association*, **4**, 103–104.

Carroll, J. D. and Arabie, P. (1980). Multidimensional scaling. *Annual Reviews in Psychology*, **31**, 607–649.

Carroll, J. D. and Chang, J. J. (1970). Analysis of individual differences in multidimensional scaling via an *N*-way generalisation of the 'Eckart–Young' decomposition. *Psychometrika*, **35**, 283–319.

Casella, G. and George, E. I. (1992). Explaining the Gibbs sampler. *The American Statistician*, **46**, 167–174.

Cattell, R. B. (1966). The scree test for the number of factors. *Multivariate Behavioral Research*, **1**, 245–276.
Chambers, J. M., Cleveland, W. S., Kleiner, B. and Tukey, P. A. (1983). *Graphical Methods for Data Analysis*. Wadsworth, Belmont, California, U.S.A.
Chambers, J. M., Mallows, C. L. and Stuck, B. W. (1976). A method for simulating stable random variables. *Journal of the American Statistical Association*, **71**, 340–344.
Chatfield, C., Ehrenberg, A. S. C. and Goodhardt, G. J. (1966). Progress on a simplified model of stationery purchasing behaviour. *Journal of the Royal Statistical Society, Series A*, **129**, 317–367.
Chauhan, J, Harper, R., and Krzanowski, W. J. (1983). Comparison between direct similarity assessments and descriptive profiles of certain soft drinks. In *Sensory Quality in Foods and Beverages; its Definition, Measurement and Control* (eds A. A. Williams and R. K. Aitken), pp 297–309. Ellis Horwood, Chichester, England.
Chen, C. F. (1979). Bayesian inference for a normal dispersion matrix and its applications to stochastic multiple regression analysis. *Journal of the Royal Statistical Society, Series B*, **41**, 235–248.
Chen, H. (1991). Estimation of a projection-pursuit regression model. *Annals of Statistics*, **19**, 142–157.
Chernoff, H. (1973). Using faces to represent points in k-dimensional space graphically. *Journal of the American Statistical Association*, **68**, 361–368.
Chernoff, H. and Rizvi, M. H. (1975). Effect on classification error of random permutations of features in representing multivariate data by faces. *Journal of the American Statistical Association*, **70**, 548–554.
Chew, V. (1977). *Comparisons among Treatment Means in an Analysis of Variance*. Agricultural Research Service of United States Department of Agriculture. Washington, U.S.A.
Clark, C. E. (1961). The greatest of a finite set of random variables. *Operations Research*, **9**, 145–162.
Cleveland, W. S. (1979). Robust locally weighted regression and smoothing scatterplots. *Journal of the American Statistical Association*, **74**, 829–836.
Cleveland, W. S. and Kleiner, B. (1974). The analysis of air pollution data from New Jersey and New York. Paper presented at the annual meeting of the American Statistical Association, St. Louis, Missouri, U.S.A., August 1974.
Cliff, N. (1966). Orthogonal rotation to congruence. *Psychometrika*, **31**, 33–42.
Cliff, N. (1968). The 'idealised individual' interpretation of individual differences in multidimensional scaling. *Psychometrika*, **33**, 225–232.
Cohen, A. M., Cutts, J. F., Fielder, R., Jones, D. E., Ribbans, J. and Stuart, E. (1973). *Numerical Analysis*. Halsted Press, New York, U.S.A.
Connor, R. J. and Mosimann, J. E. (1969). Concepts of independence for proportions with a generalization of the Dirichlet distribution. *Journal of the American Statistical Association*, **64**, 194–206.
Constantine, A. G. (1963). Some non-central distribution problems in multivariate analysis. *Annals of Mathematical Statistics*, **34**, 1270–1285.
Constantine, A. G. and Gower, J. C. (1978). Graphical representation of asymmetric matrices. *Applied Statistics*, **27**, 297–304.
Cook, R. D. and Hawkins, D. M. (1990). Comment on Rousseeuw and van

Zomeren (1990). *Journal of the American Statistical Association*, **85**, 640–644.

Corbet, G. B., Cummins, J., Hedges, S. R. and Krzanowski, W. J. (1970). The taxonomic status of British water voles, genus *Arvicola*. *Journal of Zoology*, **161**, 301–316.

Cordeiro G. M. (1983). Improved likelihood ratio statistics for generalized linear models. *Journal of the Royal Statistical Society, Series B*, **45**, 404–413.

Cormack, R. M. (1971). A review of classification (with discussion). *Journal of the Royal Statistical Society, Series A*, **134**, 321–367.

Cornish E. A. (1954). The multivariate t-distribution associated with a set of normal sample deviates. *Australian Journal of Physics*, **7**, 531–542.

Cox, D. R. (1968). Notes on some aspects of regression analysis. *Journal of the Royal Statistical Society, Series A*, **131**, 265–279.

Cox, D. R. and Small, N. J. H. (1978). Testing multivariate normality. *Biometrika*, **65**, 263–272.

Cox, D. R. and Wermuth N. (1992). Response models for mixed binary and quantitative variables. *Biometrika*, **79**, 441–461.

Critchley, F. (1985). Influence in principal component analysis. *Biometrika*, **72**, 627–636.

Crowder, M. J. (1994). Least squares with simulated means for a problem in fibre strength testing. *Applied Statistics*, **43**, 109–115.

D'Agostino, R. B. (1971). An omnibus test of normality for moderate and large sample sizes. *Biometrika*, **58**, 341–348.

D'Agostino, R. B. (1972). Small sample probability points for the D test of normality. *Biometrika*, **59**, 219–221.

D'Agostino, R. B. (1986). Tests for the normal distribution. In *Goodness-of-fit Techniques*, (eds R. B. D'Agostino and M. A. Stephens) pp 367–419, Dekker, New York, U.S.A.

Das Gupta, S. (1971). Nonsingularity of the sample covariance matrix. *Sankhyā A*, **33**, 475–478.

Das Gupta, S. and Perlman, M. D. (1974). Power of the non-central F-test: effect of additional variables on Hotelling's T^2 test. *Journal of the American Statistical Association*, **69**, 174–180.

Davis, A. W. (1978). On the asymptotic distribution of Gower's m^2 goodness of fit criterion in a particular case. *Annals of the Institute of Statistical Mathematics*, **30**, 71–79.

Davison, A. C., Hinkley, D. V., and Schechtman, E. (1986). Efficient bootstrap simulation. *Biometrika*, **73**, 555–566.

De Boor, C. (1978). *A Practical Guide to Splines*. Springer, New York, U.S.A.

De Bruijn, N. G. (1961). *Asymptotic Methods in Analysis*. North-Holland, Amsterdam, The Netherlands.

De Leeuw, J. (1984). The Gifi system of nonlinear multivariate analysis. In *Data Analysis and Informatics, Vol. 3* (eds E. Diday, M. Jambu, L. Lebart, J. Pagès and R. Tomassone), pp. 415–424. North-Holland, Amsterdam, The Netherlands.

De Leeuw, J. and Heiser, W. J. (1980). Multidimensional scaling with restrictions on the configuration. In *Multivariate Analysis V* (ed P. R. Krishnaiah), pp. 501–522, North-Holland, Amsterdam, The Netherlands.

De Leeuw, J. and Meulman, J. (1986). A special jack-knife for multidimensional scaling. *Journal of Classification*, **3**, 97–112.
Dempster, A. P. (1972). Covariance selection. *Biometrics*, **28**, 157–175.
Dempster, A. P., Laird, N. M. and Rubin, D. B. (1977). Maximum likelihood from incomplete data via the EM algorithm (with discussion). *Journal of the Royal Statistical Society, Series B*, **39**, 1–38.
Denham, M. C. and Brown, P. J. (1993). Calibration with many variables. *Applied Statistics*, **42**, 515–528.
Devlin, S. J., Gnanadesikan, R. and Kettenring, J. R. (1975). Robust estimation and outlier detection with correlation coefficients. *Biometrika*, **62**, 531–545.
Devlin, S. J., Gnanadesikan, R. and Kettenring, J. R. (1981). Robust estimation of dispersion matrices and principal components. *Journal of the American Statistical Association*, **76**, 354–362.
De Waal, D. J. (1985). Matrix valued distributions. In *Encyclopedia of Statistical Sciences, Volume 5* (eds S. Kotz and N. L. Johnson), pp. 326–333. Wiley, New York, U.S.A.
DiCiccio, T. J. and Romano, J. P. (1988). A review of bootstrap confidence intervals (with discussion). *Journal of the Royal Statistical Society, Series B*, **50**, 338–370.
Dickey, J. M., Lindley, D. V. and Press, S. J. (1985). Bayesian estimation of the dispersion matrix of a multivariate normal distribution. *Communications in Statistics, Theory and Methods*, **14**, 1019–1034.
Diggle, P. J. and Gratton, R. J. (1984). Monte Carlo methods of inference for implicit statistical models (with discussion). *Journal of the Royal Statistical Society, Series B*, **46**, 193–227.
Draper, N. R. and Cox, D. R. (1969). On distributions and their transformations to normality. *Journal of the Royal Statistical Society, Series B*, **31**, 472–476.
Draper, N. R. and Hunter, W. G. (1969). Transformations: some examples revisited. *Technometrics*, **11**, 23–40.
Duncan, D. B. (1965). A Bayesian approach to multiple comparisons. *Technometrics*, **7**, 171–222.
Duncan, D. B. (1975). *t* tests and intervals for comparisons suggested by the data. *Biometrics*, **31**, 339–359.
Dunnett, C. W. (1989). Algorithm AS 251: Multivariate normal probability integrals with product correlation structure. *Applied Statistics*, **38**, 564–579.
Dyer, A. R. (1974). Comparison of tests for normality with a cautionary note. *Biometrika*, **61**, 185–189.
Dykstra, R. L. (1970). Establishing the positive definiteness of the sample covariance matrix. *Annals of Mathematical Statistics*, **41**, 2153–2154.
Eastment, H. T. and Krzanowski, W. J. (1982). Cross-validatory choice of the number of components from a principal component analysis. *Technometrics*, **24**, 73–78.
Eaton, M. L. and Perlman, M. D. (1973). The non-singularity of generalised sample covariance matrices. *Annals of Statistics*, **1**, 710–717.
Eckart, C. and Young, G. (1936). The approximation of one matrix by another of lower rank. *Psychometrika*, **1**, 211–218.
Edwards, A. W. F. (1971). Distances between populations on the basis of gene frequencies. *Biometrics*, **27**, 873–881.

Edwards, A. W. F. and Cavalli-Sforza, L. L. (1964). Reconstruction of evolutionary trees. Phenetic and phylogenetic classification. *The Systematics Association, London, Publication number 6*, 67–76.

Edwards, D. (1987). *A guide to MIM.* Research Report 87/1. Statistical Research Unit, University of Copenhagen, Denmark.

Edwards, D. (1990). Hierarchical interaction models. *Journal of the Royal Statistical Society, Series B*, **52**, 3–20.

Edwards, D. (1992). *Graphical Modelling with MIM (version 2.0).* Hypergraph Software, Copenhagen, Denmark.

Efron, B. (1979). Bootstrap methods: another look at the jackknife. *Annals of Statistics*, **7**, 1–26.

Efron, B. (1982). *The Jackknife, the Bootstrap, and Other Resampling Plans.* Monograph No. 38, Society for Industrial and Applied Mathematics, Philadelphia, U.S.A.

Efron, B. (1987). Better bootstrap confidence intervals and bootstrap approximations. *Journal of the American Statistical Association*, **82**, 171–200.

Efron, B. (1990). More efficient bootstrap computations. *Journal of the American Statistical Association*, **85**, 79–89.

Efron, B. (1992). Jackknife-after-bootstrap standard errors and influence functions (with discussion). *Journal of the Royal Statistical Society, Series B*, **54**, 83–127.

Efron, B. and Gong, G. (1983). A leisurely look at the bootstrap, the jackknife, and cross-validation. *The American Statistician*, **37**, 36–48.

Efron, B. and Tibshirani, R. (1986). Bootstrap methods for standard errors, confidence intervals and other measures of statistical accuracy. *Statistical Science*, **1**, 54–77.

Embrechts, P. and Herzberg, A. M. (1991). Variations of Andrews' plots. *International Statistical Institute Review*, **59**, 175–194.

Eslava-Gómez, G. (1989). *Projection Pursuit and Other Graphical Methods for Multivariate Data.* Unpublished D. Phil. Thesis, University of Oxford, U.K.

Etezadi-Amoli, J. and McDonald, R. P. (1983). A second generation nonlinear factor analysis. *Psychometrika*, **48**, 315–342.

Evans, I. G. (1965). Bayesian estimation of parameters of a multivariate normal distribution. *Journal of the Royal Statistical Society, Series B*, **27**, 279–283.

Everitt, B. S. (1979). A Monte Carlo investigation of the robustness of Hotelling's one- and two-sample T^2 statistic. *Journal of the American Statistical Association*, **74**, 48–51.

Everitt, B. S. and Dunn, G. (1991). *Applied Multivariate Data Analysis.* Edward Arnold, London, England.

Fang, K-T. and Zhang, Y-T. (1990). *Generalized Multivariate Analysis.* Science Press, Beijing, China and Springer-Verlag, Berlin, Germany.

Fang, K-T., Kotz, S. and Ng, K-W. (1990). *Symmetric Multivariate and Related Distributions.* Chapman and Hall, London, England.

Fauquet, C., Desbois, D., Fargette, D. and Vidal, G. (1988). Classification of furoviruses based upon the amino acid composition of their coat proteins. In *Viruses with Fungal Vectors* (eds J. I. Cooper and M. J. C. Asher), pp. 19–36. Association of Applied Biologists, Edinburgh, Scotland.

Feller, W. (1966). *An Introduction to Probability Theory and its Applications.* Wiley, New York, U.S.A.

Fenlon, J. S. and Beever, D. E. (1976). An examination of the net changes in amino-acid composition within the rumen of mature wether sheep using canonical variate analysis. *Journal of Agricultural Science*, **87**, 255–268.

Ferguson, T. S. (1961). On the rejection of outliers. *Proceedings of the Fourth Berkeley Symposium on Mathematical Statistics and Probability*, 253–287.

Fernandez de la Reguera, P. A. (1983). *Statistical Analysis of Genetic Variation of Pines in Central America.* Unpublished D. Phil. Thesis, University of Oxford, England.

Fernandez de la Reguera, P. A., Marriott, F. H. C. and Burley, J. (1988). Multiple-set canonical analysis: an application to forestry genetics. *Biometrics*, **44**, 875–880.

Fienberg, S. E. (1979). Graphical methods in statistics. *The American Statistician*, **33**, 165–178.

Fisher, R. A. (1915). Frequency distribution of the values of the correlation coefficient in samples from an indefinitely large population. *Biometrika*, **10**, 507–521.

Fisher, R. A. (1939). The sampling distribution of some statistics obtained from non-linear equations. *Annals of Eugenics*, **9**, 238–249.

Fisher, R. A. (1940). The precision of discriminant functions. *Annals of Eugenics*, **10**, 422–429.

Fleishman, E. A. and Hempel, W. E. (1954). Changes in factor structure of a complex psychomotor test as a function of practice. *Psychometrika*, **19**, 239–252.

Flury, B. (1984). Common principal components in k groups. *Journal of the American Statistical Association*, **79**, 892–898.

Flury, B. (1986). Asymptotic theory for common principal component analysis. *Annals of Statistics*, **14**, 418–430.

Flury, B. (1987). Two generalizations of the common principal component model. *Biometrika*, **74**, 59–69.

Flury, B. (1988). *Common Principal Components and Related Models.* Wiley, New York, U.S.A.

Flury, B. (1994). Developments in principal component analysis: a review. In *Descriptive Multivariate Analysis* (ed W. J. Krzanowski). Clarendon Press, Oxford, England.

Flury, B. and Riedwyl, H. (1981). Graphical representation of multivariate data by means of asymmetrical faces. *Journal of the American Statistical Association*, **76**, 757–765.

Flury, B. and Riedwyl, H. (1988). *Multivariate Statistics, a Practical Approach.* Chapman and Hall, London, England.

Foster, F. G. (1957). Upper percentage points of the generalized Beta distribution. II. *Biometrika*, **44**, 441–453.

Foster, F. G. (1958). Upper percentage points of the generalized Beta distribution. III. *Biometrika*, **45**, 492–502.

Foster, F. G. and Rees, D. H. (1957). Upper percentage points of the generalized Beta distribution. I. *Biometrika*, **44**, 237–247.

Freund, J. E. (1961). A bivariate extension of the exponential distribution. *Journal of the American Statistical Association*, **56**, 971–977.

Frick, H. (1990). Algorithm AS R84. A remark on Algorithm AS 226: Computing non-central Beta probabilities. *Applied Statistics*, **39**, 311–312.

Friedman, J. H. (1987). Exploratory projection pursuit. *Journal of the American Statistical Association*, **82**, 249–266.

Friedman, J. H. (1991). Multivariate adaptive regression splines (with discussion). *Annals of Statistics*, **19**, 1–141.

Friedman, J. H. and Stuetzle, W. (1981). Projection pursuit regression. *Journal of the American Statistical Association*, **76**, 817–823.

Friedman, J. H., Stuetzle, W. and Schroeder, A. (1984). Projection pursuit density estimation. *Journal of the American Statistical Association*, **79**, 599–608.

Friedman, J. H. and Tukey, J. W. (1974). A projection pursuit algorithm for exploratory data analysis. *IEEE Transactions on Computers*, **23**, 881–889.

Gabriel, K. R. (1966). Simultaneous test procedures for multiple comparisons on categorical data. *Journal of the American Statistical Association*, **61**, 1081–1096.

Gabriel, K. R. (1968). Simultaneous test procedures in multivariate analysis of variance. *Biometrika*, **55**, 489–504.

Gabriel, K. R. (1969). Simultaneous test procedures—some theory of multiple comparisons. *Annals of Mathematical Statistics*, **40**, 224–250.

Gabriel, K. R. (1971). The biplot – graphic display of matrices with application to principal component analysis. *Biometrika*, **58**, 453–467.

Gabriel, K. R. (1981). Biplot display of multivariate matrices for inspection of data and diagnosis. In *Interpreting Multivariate Data* (ed. V. Barnett), pp. 147–174. Wiley, Chichester, England.

Gains, N., Krzanowski, W. J. and Thomson, D. M. H. (1988). A comparison of variable reduction techniques in an attitudinal investigation of meat products. *Journal of Sensory Studies*, **3**, 37–48.

Galambos, J. (1985). Multivariate stable distributions. In *Encyclopedia of Statistical Sciences, Volume 6* (eds S. Kotz and N. L. Johnson), pp. 125–129. Wiley, New York, U.S.A.

Gelfand, A. E. and Smith, A. F. M. (1990). Sampling-based approaches to calculating marginal densities. *Journal of the American Statistical Association*, **85**, 398–409.

Geman, S. and Geman, D. (1984). Stochastic relaxation, Gibbs distributions and the Bayesian restoration of images. *IEEE Transactions on Pattern Analysis and Machine Intelligence*, **6**, 721–741.

Geweke, J. (1988). Antithetic acceleration of Monte Carlo integration in Bayesian inference. *Journal of Econometrics*, **38**, 73–90.

Geweke, J. (1989). Bayesian inference in econometric models using Monte Carlo integration. *Econometrika*, **57**, 1317–1339.

Gifi, A. (1990). *Nonlinear Multivariate Analysis.* Wiley, New York, U.S.A.

Giri, N. C. (1977). *Multivariate Statistical Inference.* Academic Press, New York, U.S.A.

Gittens, R. (1985). *Canonical Analysis. A Review with Applications in Ecology.* Springer-Verlag, Berlin, Germany.

Gnanadesikan, R. (1977). *Methods for Statistical Data Analysis of Multivariate Observations.* Wiley, New York, U.S.A.

Gnanadesikan, R. and Kettenring, J. R. (1972). Robust estimates, residuals

and outlier detection with multiresponse data. *Biometrics*, **28**, 81–124.
Gnanadesikan, R. and Wilk, M. B. (1969). Data analytic methods in multivariate statistical analysis. In *Multivariate Analysis II* (ed P. R. Krishnaiah), pp. 593–638. Academic Press, New York, U.S.A.
Goodall, C. R. (1991). Procrustes methods in the statistical analysis of shape (with discussion). *Journal of the Royal Statistical Society, Series B*, **53**, 285–339.
Goodchild, N. A. and Vijayan, K. (1974). Significance tests in plots of multidimensional data in two dimensions. *Biometrics*, **30**, 209–210.
Goodman, L. A. (1964). Simultaneous confidence intervals for contrasts among multinomial populations. *Annals of Mathematical Statistics*, **35**, 716–725.
Goodman, L. A. (1981). Association models and canonical correlation in the analysis of cross-classifications having ordered categories. *Journal of the American Statistical Association*, **76**, 320–334.
Goodman, L. A. (1985). The analysis of cross-classified data having ordered and/or unordered categories: association models, correlation models, and asymmetry models for contingency tables with or without missing entries. *Annals of Statistics*, **13**, 10–69.
Gordon, A. D. (1981). *Classification.* Chapman and Hall, London, England.
Gower, J. C. (1966a). Some distance properties of latent root and vector methods used in multivariate analysis. *Biometrika*, **53**, 325–338.
Gower, J. C. (1966b). A *Q*-technique for the calculation of canonical variates. *Biometrika*, **53**, 588–589.
Gower, J. C. (1967). Multivariate analysis and multidimensional geometry. *The Statistician*, **17**, 13–25.
Gower, J. C. (1968). Adding a point to vector diagrams in multivariate analysis. *Biometrika*, **55**, 582–585.
Gower, J. C. (1971a). A general coefficient of similarity and some of its properties. *Biometrics*, **27**, 857–872.
Gower, J. C. (1971b). Statistical methods of comparing different multivariate analyses of the same data. In *Mathematics in the Archaeological and Historical Sciences* (eds F. R. Hodson, D. G. Kendall and P. Tautu), pp. 138–149, Edinburgh University Press, Edinburgh, Scotland.
Gower, J. C. (1975). Generalized Procrustes analysis. *Psychometrika*, **40**, 33–50.
Gower J. C. (1982). Euclidean distance geometry. *Mathematical Scientist*, **7**, 1–14.
Gower J. C. (1984). Distance matrices and their Euclidean approximation. In *Data Analysis and Informatics 3* (eds E. Diday, M. Jambu, L. Lebart, J. Pagès and R. Tomassone), pp. 3–21, North-Holland, Amsterdam, The Netherlands.
Gower, J. C. (1987). Comments in Jones, M. C. and Sibson, R. (1987). What is projection pursuit? (with discussion). *Journal of the Royal Statistical Society, Series A*, **150**, 1–36.
Gower, J. C. (1990a). Three-dimensional biplots. *Biometrika*, **77**, 773–785.
Gower, J. C. (1990b). The generalised biplot: software potential. *Compstat 1990*, 151–156. Physica-Verlag, Heidelberg, Germany.
Gower, J. C. (1993). Biplot geometry. *Submitted for publication.*
Gower, J. C. and Harding, S. A. (1988). Non-linear biplots. *Biometrika*, **73**, 445–455.

Gower, J. C. and Legendre, P. (1986). Metric and Euclidean properties of dissimilarity coefficients. *Journal of Classification*, **3**, 5–48.

Green, B. F. (1952). The orthogonal approximation of an oblique structure in factor analysis. *Psychometrika*, **17**, 429–440.

Greenacre, M. J. (1984). *Theory and Applications of Correspondence Analysis.* Academic Press, London, England.

Greenacre, M. J. (1988a). Clustering the rows and columns of a contingency table. *Journal of Classification*, **5**, 39–51.

Greenacre, M. J. (1988b). Correspondence analysis of multivariate categorical data by weighted least squares. *Biometrika*, **75**, 457–467.

Greenacre, M. J. (1993). *Correspondence Analysis in Practice.* Academic Press, London, England.

Gruvaeus, G. T. (1970). A general approach to Procrustes pattern rotation. *Psychometrika*, **35**, 493–505.

Guttman, L. (1941). The quantification of a class of attributes: a theory and method of scale construction. In *The Prediction of Personal Adjustment* (ed P. Horst), pp. 319–348. Social Science Research Council, New York, U.S.A.

Guttman, L. (1968). A general non-metric technique for finding the smallest coordinate space for a configuration of points. *Psychometrika*, **33**, 469–506.

Hadi, A. S. (1992). Identifying multiple outliers in multivariate data. *Journal of the Royal Statistical Society, Series B*, **54**, 761–771.

Hall, P. (1988). Theoretical comparison of bootstrap confidence intervals (with discussion). *Annals of Statistics*, **16**, 927–985.

Hall, P. (1992) *The Bootstrap and Edgeworth Expansions.* Springer-Verlag, New York, U.S.A.

Hand, D. J. (1982). *Kernel Discriminant Analysis.* Research Studies Press, Letchworth, England.

Harary, F. (1969). *Graph Theory.* Addison-Wesley, Reading, Massachussetts, U.S.A.

Härdle, W. (1990). *Applied Nonparametric Regression.* Cambridge University Press, Cambridge, England.

Harris R. J. (1975). *A Primer of Multivariate Analysis.* Academic Press, New York, U.S.A.

Harshman, R. A., Ladefoged, P. and Goldstein, L. (1977). Factor analysis of tongue shapes. *Journal of the Acoustical Society of America*, **62**, 738–750.

Hartigan, J. A. (1975a). *Clustering Algorithms.* Wiley, New York, U.S.A.

Hartigan, J. A. (1975b). Printer graphics for clustering. *Journal of Statistical Computation and Simulation*, **4**, 187–213.

Hastie, T. and Stuetzle, W. (1989). Principal curves. *Journal of the American Statistical Association*, **84**, 502–516.

Hastie, T. and Tibshirani, R. (1990). *Generalized Additive Models.* Chapman and Hall, London, England.

Hastings, W. K. (1970). Monte Carlo simulation methods using Markov Chains and their applications. *Biometrika*, **57**, 97–109.

Hawkins, D. M. (1980). *Identification of Outliers.* Chapman and Hall, London, England.

Healy, M. J. R. (1968). Multivariate normal plotting. *Applied Statistics*, **17**, 157–161.

Heck, D. L. (1960). Charts of some upper percentage points of the distribution of the largest characteristic root. *Annals of Mathematical Statistics*, **31**, 625–642.

Heiser, W. J. (1986). Undesired nonlinearities in nonlinear multivariate analysis. In *Data Analysis and Informatics IV* (eds E. Diday *et al*), pp. 455–469. North-Holland, Amsterdam, The Netherlands.

Heiser, W. J. (1987). Correspondence analysis with least absolute residuals. *Computational Statistics and Data Analysis*, **5**, 337–356.

Heiser, W. J. and Meulman, J. J. (1993). Homogeneity analysis: exploring the distribution of variables and their nonlinear relationships. In *Correspondence Analysis in the Social Sciences: Recent Developments and Applications* (eds M. J. Greenacre, J. Blasius and W. Kristof), in press.

Hensler, G. L., Mehrotra, K. G. and Michalek, J. E. (1977). A goodness of fit test for multivariate normality. *Communications in Statistics, Theory and Methods*, **6**, 33–41.

Hernandez, F. and Johnson, R. A. (1980). The large-sample behaviour of transformations to normality. *Journal of the American Statistical Association*, **75**, 855–861.

Heyde, C. C. and Johnstone, I. M. (1979) On asymptotic posterior normality for stochastic processes. *Journal of the Royal Statistical Society, Series B*, **41**, 184–189.

Higham, C. F. W., Kijngam, A. and Manly, B. F. J. (1980). An analysis of prehistoric canid remains from Thailand. *Journal of Archaeological Science*, **7**, 149–165.

Hill, M. O. (1973). Reciprocal averaging: an eigenvector method of ordination. *Journal of Ecology*, **61**, 237–251.

Hill, M. O. (1982). Correspondence analysis. In *Encyclopedia of Statistical Sciences, Vol 2* (eds S. Kotz and N. L. Johnson), pp. 204–210. Wiley, New York, U.S.A.

Hinkley, D. V. (1975). On power transformations to symmetry. *Biometrika*, **62**, 101–111.

Hinkley, D. V. (1988). Bootstrap methods (with discussion). *Journal of the Royal Statistical Society, Series B*, **50**, 321–337 and 355–370.

Hirotsu, C. (1983). Defining the pattern of association in two-way contingency tables. *Biometrika*, **70**, 579–589.

Hogg, R. V. (1979). An introduction to robust estimation. In *Robustness in Statistics* (eds R. L. Launer and G. N. Wilkinson), pp. 1–17. Academic Press, New York, U.S.A.

Holgate, P. (1966). Bivariate generalizations of Neyman's Type A distribution. *Biometrika*, **53**, 241–245.

Holtsmark, J. (1919). Über die Vebreitering von Spektrallinier. *Annalen der Physik*, **58**, 577–630.

Hong, Z.-Q. and Yang, J.-Y. (1991). Optimal discriminant plane for a small number of samples and design method of classifier on the plane. *Pattern Recognition*, **24**, 317–324.

Horan, C. B. (1969). Multidimensional scaling: combining observations when individuals have different perceptual structures. *Psychometrika*, **34**, 139–165.

Horst, P. (1965). *Factor Analysis of Data Matrices*. Holt, Rinehart and Winston,

New York, U.S.A.

Hotelling, H. (1931). The generalization of Student's ratio. *Annals of Mathematical Statistics*, **2**, 360–378.

Hotelling, H. (1933). Analysis of a complex of statistical variables into principal components. *Journal of Educational Psychology*, **24**, 417–441.

Hotelling, H. (1944). Some improvements in weighing and other experimental techniques. *Annals of Mathematical Statistics*, **15**, 297–306.

Hotelling, H. (1947). A generalized T measure of multivariate dispersion. (Abstract). *Annals of Mathematical Statistics*, **18**, 298.

Hotelling, H. (1951). A generalized T test and measure of multivariate dispersion. *Proceedings of the 2nd Berkeley Symposium in Mathematical Statistics and Probability*, 23–41.

Hsu, P. L. (1939a). A new proof of the joint product moment distribution. *Proceedings of the Cambridge Philosophical Society*, **35**, 336–338.

Hsu, P. L. (1939b). On the distribution of the roots of certain determinantal equations. *Annals of Eugenics*, **9**, 250–258.

Hsu, P. L. (1940). On generalised analysis of variance. *Biometrika*, **31**, 221–237.

Huber, P. J. (1981). *Robust Statistics*. Wiley, New York, U.S.A.

Hudson, W. N. and Mason, J. D. (1981). Operator-stable distribution on R^2 with multiple exponents. *The Annals of Probability*, **9**, 482–489.

Hurley, J. R. and Cattell, R. B. (1962). The Procrustes program: producing direct rotation to test a hypothesised factor structure. *Behavioural Science*, **7**, 258–262.

Ito, K. (1969). On the effect of heteroscedasticity and nonnormality upon some multivariate test procedures. In *Multivariate Analysis*, Vol II (ed P. R. Krishnaiah), pp. 87–120. Academic Press, New York, U.S.A.

Ito, K. and Schull, W. J. (1964). On the robustness of the T_0^2 test in multivariate analysis of variance when variance-covariance matrices are not equal. *Biometrika*, **51**, 71–82.

Izenman, A. J. (1991). Recent developments in non-parametric density estimation. *Journal of the American Statistical Association*, **86**, 205–224.

Jackson, J. E. (1959). Some multivariate statistical techniques used in colour matching data. *Journal of the Optical Society of America*, **49**, 585–592.

Jackson, J. E. (1962). Some multivariate statistical techniques used in colour matching data—addenda and errata. *Journal of the Optical Society of America*, **52**, 835–836.

Jackson, J. E. (1991). *A User's Guide to Principal Components*. Wiley, New York, U.S.A.

Jacob, R. J. K. (1983). Investigating the space of Chernoff faces. In *Recent Advances in Statistics* (eds M. H. Rizvi, J. Rustagi, and D. Siegemund), pp. 449–468. Academic Press, New York, U.S.A.

Jambu, M. (1991). *Exploratory and Multivariate Data Analysis*. Academic Press, Boston, U.S.A.

James, A. T. (1960). The distribution of the latent roots of the covariance matrix. *Annals of Mathematical Statistics*, **31**, 151–158.

James, A. T. (1964). Distributions of matrix variates and latent roots derived from normal samples. *Annals of Mathematical Statistics*, **35**, 475–501.

James, G. S. (1954). Tests of linear hypotheses in univariate and multivariate analysis when the ratios of the population variances are unknown. *Biometrika*, **41**, 19–43.

James, W. and Stein, C. (1961). Estimation with quadratic loss. *Proceedings of the Fourth Berkeley Symposium in Mathematical Statistics and Probability*, **1**, 361–379. University of California Press, Berkeley, U.S.A.

Jee, R. (1985). *A Study on Projection Pursuit Methods.* Unpublished Ph.D. Thesis, Rice University, U.S.A.

Jeffers, J. N. R. (1967). Two case studies on the application of principal component analysis. *Applied Statistics*, **16**, 225–236.

Jeffreys, H. (1939). *Theory of Probability.* Clarendon Press, Oxford, England.

John, J. A. and Draper, N. R. (1980). An alternative family of transformations. *Applied Statistics*, **29**, 190–197.

Johnson, N. L. and Kotz, S. (1969). *Distributions in Statistics; Discrete Distributions.* Wiley, New York, U.S.A.

Johnson, N. L. and Kotz, S. (1972). *Distributions in Statistics; Continuous Multivariate Distributions.* Wiley, New York, U.S.A.

Johnson, R. A. and Wichern, D. W. (1982). *Applied Multivariate Statistical Analysis.* Prentice-Hall, Englewood Cliffs, New Jersey, U.S.A.

Johnson, R. M. (1973). Pairwise non-metric multidimensional scaling. *Psychometrika*, **38**, 11–18.

Jolicoeur, P. (1963). The multivariate generalization of the allometry equation. *Biometrics*, **19**, 497–499.

Jolicoeur, P. and Mosimann, J. E. (1960). Size and shape variation in the painted turtle, a principal component analysis. *Growth*, **24**, 339–354.

Jolliffe, I. T. (1972). Discarding variables in principal component analysis. I: Artificial data. *Applied Statistics*, **21**, 160–173.

Jolliffe, I. T. (1973). Discarding variables in principal component analysis. II: Real data. *Applied Statistics*, **22**, 21–31.

Jolliffe, I. T. (1986). *Principal Component Analysis.* Springer-Verlag, New York, U.S.A.

Jones, M. C. and Sibson, R. (1987). What is projection pursuit? (with discussion). *Journal of the Royal Statistical Society, Series A*, **150**, 1–36.

Juang, B. H. and Rabiner, L. R. (1991). Hidden Markov models for speech recognition. *Technometrics*, **33**, 251–272.

Kaiser, H. F. (1958). The varimax criterion for analytic rotation in factor analysis. *Psychometrika*, **23**, 187–200.

Kendall, D. G. (1971). Seriation from abundance matrices. In *Mathematics in the Archaeological and Historical Sciences* (eds F. R. Hodson, D. G. Kendall and P. Tautu), pp. 215–252, Edinburgh University Press, Edinburgh, Scotland.

Kendall, D. G. (1989). A survey of the statistical theory of shape (with discussion). *Statistical Science*, **4**, 87–120.

Kendall, D. G. and Kendall, W. S. (1980). Internal alignments in random two-dimensional sets of points. *Advances in Applied Probability*, **12**, 384–424.

Kendall, M. G. (1980). *Multivariate Analysis, 2nd Edition.* Charles Griffin & Co., London, England.

Kettenring, J. R. (1971). Canonical analysis of several sets of variables. *Biometrika*, **58**, 433–451.

Khatri, C. G. and Pillai, K. C. S. (1965). Some results on the non-central multivariate beta distribution and moments of traces of two matrices. *Annals of Mathematical Statistics*, **36**, 1511–1520.

Kim, H. (1992). Measures of influence in correspondence analysis. *Journal of Statistical Computation and Simulation*, **40**, 201–218.

Kirkpatrick, S., Gellatt, C. D. and Vecchi, M. P. (1983). Optimization by simulated annealing. *Science*, **220**, 671–680.

Kleiner, B. and Hartigan, J. A. (1981). Representing points in many dimensions by trees and castles. *Journal of the American Statistical Association*, **76**, 260–269.

Korin, B. P. (1968). On the distribution of a statistic used for testing a covariance matrix. *Biometrika*, **55**, 171–178.

Korin, B. P. (1969). On testing the equality of k covariance matrices. *Biometrika*, **56**, 216–218.

Korin, B. P. and Stevens, E. H. (1973). Some approximations for the distribution of a multivariate likelihood ratio criterion. *Journal of the Royal Statistical Society, Series B*, **35**, 24–27.

Kotz, S. (1975). Multivariate distributions at a cross road. In *Statistical Distributions in Scientific Work, I* (eds G. P. Patil and J. K. Ord), pp. 247–270. Reidel, Dordrecht, The Netherlands.

Kotz, S. and Johnson, N. L. (1985). *Encyclopedia of Statistical Sciencs, Volume 6*. Wiley, New York, U.S.A.

Koutras, M. (1986). On the generalized non-central chi-squared distribution induced by an elliptical Gamma law. *Biometrika*, **73**, 528–532.

Krishnaiah, P. R. and Lee, J. C. (1980). Likelihood ratio tests for mean vectors and covariance matrices. In *Handbook of Statistics*, Vol 1 (ed P. R. Krishnaiah), pp. 513–570. North-Holland, Amsterdam, The Netherlands.

Kristof, W. and Wingersky, B. (1971). Generalization of the orthogonal Procrustes rotation procedure to more than two matrices. In *Proceedings of the 79th annual convention, American Psychological Association*, 89–90.

Krusińska, E. (1991). Suitable location model selection in the terminology of graphical models. *Biometrical Journal*, **32**, 817–826.

Krusińska, E. (1992). Discriminant analysis in graphical and hierarchical and graphical interaction models. In *Statistical Modelling* (eds P. G. M. van der Heijden, W. Jansen, B. Francis and G. U. H. Seeber). Elsevier Science, Amsterdam, The Netherlands.

Kruskal, J. B. (1964a). Multidimensional scaling by optimising goodness-of-fit to a nonmetric hypothesis. *Psychometrika*, **29**, 1–27.

Kruskal, J. B. (1964b). Nonmetric multidimensional scaling: a numerical method. *Psychometrika*, **29**, 115–129.

Kruskal, J. B. (1969). Towards a practical method which helps uncover the structure of a set of multivariate observations by finding the linear transformation which optimizes a new 'index of condensation'. In *Statistical Computation* (eds. R. C. Milton and J. A. Nelder), pp. 427–441. Academic Press, London. England.

Kruskal, J. B. (1972). Linear transformation of multivariate data to reveal clustering. In *Multidimensional Scaling; Theory and Applications in the Behavioural Sciences*, Vol. I (eds R. N. Shepard, A. K. Romney and S. B. Nerlove), pp. 179–191. Seminar Press, London, England.

Kruskal, J. B. (1977). Multidimensional scaling and other methods for discovering structure. In *Statistical Methods for Digital Computers, Vol 3*, (eds K. Enslein, A. Ralston and H. S. Wilf), pp. 296–339, Wiley, New York, U.S.A.

Kruskal, J. B. and Wish, M. (1978). *Multidimensional Scaling*. Sage, Beverley Hills, California, U.S.A.

Krzanowski, W. J. (1971). A comparison of some distance measures applicable to multinomial data, using a rotational fit technique. *Biometrics*, **27**, 1062–1068.

Krzanowski, W. J. (1979). Between-groups comparison of principal components. *Journal of the American Statistical Association*, **74**, 703–707, (correction **76**, 1022).

Krzanowski, W. J. (1983). Cross-validatory choice in principal component analysis; some sampling results. *Journal of Statistical Computation and Simulation*, **18**, 299–314.

Krzanowski, W. J. (1984). Sensitivity of principal components. *Journal of the Royal Statistical Society, Series B*, **46**, 558–563.

Krzanowski, W. J. (1987a). Selection of variables to preserve multivariate data structure, using principal components. *Applied Statistics*, **36**, 22–33.

Krzanowski, W. J. (1987b). Cross-validation in principal component analysis. *Biometrics*, **43**, 575–584.

Krzanowski, W. J. (1988a). *Principles of Multivariate Analysis: a User's Perspective*. Clarendon Press, Oxford, England.

Krzanowski, W. J. (1988b). Missing value imputation in multivariate data using the singular value decomposition. *Biometrical Letters*, **25**, 31–39.

Krzanowski, W. J. (1993a). Attribute selection in correspondence analysis of incidence matrices. *Applied Statistics*, **42**, 529–541.

Krzanowski, W. J. (1993b). Permutational tests for correlation matrices. *Statistics and Computing*, **3**, 37–44.

Krzanowski, W. J. and Radley, D. (1989). Nonparametric confidence and tolerance regions in canonical variate analysis. *Biometrics*, **45**, 1163–1173.

Langron, S. P. and Collins, A. J. (1985). Perturbation theory for generalized Procrustes analysis. *Journal of the Royal Statistical Society, Series B*, **47**, 277–284.

Lawley, D. N. (1938). Generalization of Fisher's z-test. *Biometrika*, **30**, 180–187, (correction: **30**, 467–469).

Lawley, D. N. (1956a). Tests of significance for the latent roots of covariance and correlation matrices. *Biometrika*, **43**, 128–136.

Lawley, D. N. (1956b). A general method of approximating to the distribution of likelihood ratio criteria. *Biometrika*, **43**, 295–303.

Lawley, D. N. (1959). Tests of significance in canonical analysis. *Biometrika*, **46**, 59–66.

Lawley, D. N. (1963). On testing a set of correlation coefficients for equality. *Annals of Mathematical Statistics*, **34**, 149–151.

Layard, M. W. J. (1972). Large sample tests for the equality of two covariance matrices. *Annals of Mathematical Statistics* , **43**, 123–141.

Layard, M. W. J. (1974). A Monte Carlo comparison of tests for equality of covariance matrices. *Biometrika*, **61**, 461–465.

Le Cam, L. (1956). On the asymptotic theory of estimation and testing hypotheses. *Proceedings of the Third Berkeley Symposium on Mathematical*

Statistics and Probability, **1**, 129–156.

Lee, J. C., Chang, T. C. and Krishnaiah, P. R. (1977). Approximations to the distributions of the likelihood ratio statistics for testing certain structures on the covariance matrices of real multivariate normal populations. In *Multivariate Analysis*, Vol IV (ed P. R. Krishnaiah), pp. 105–118. North-Holland, Amsterdam, The Netherlands.

Lee, P. (1989). *Bayesian Statistics: an Introduction.* Edward Arnold, London, U.K.

Leech, F. B. and Healy, M. J. R. (1959). The analysis of experiments on growth rate. *Biometrics*, **15**, 98–106 (correction: **15**, 631).

Lehmann, E. H. (1986) *Testing Statistical Hypotheses*, 2nd. ed. John Wiley, New York, U.S.A.

Lenth, R. V. (1987). Algorithm AS 226. Computing non-central Beta probabilities. *Applied Statistics*, **36**, 241–244.

Leonard, T. and Hsu, J. S. J. (1992). Bayesian inference for a covariance matrix. *Annals of Statistics*, **20**, 1669–1696.

Leurgans, S. and Ross, R. T. (1992). Multilinear models: applications in spectroscopy (with discussion). *Statistical Science*, **7**, 289–319.

Lévy, P. (1925). *Calcul des Probabilités.* Gauthier-Villars, Paris, France.

Lévy, P. (1937). *Théorie de l'Addition des Variables Aléatoires.* Gauthier-Villars, Paris, France.

Li, H. W., Meng, C. J. and Lin, T. N. (1936). Field results in a millet breeding experiment. *Journal of the American Society of Agronomy*, **28**, 1–15.

Lindley, D. V. (1965). *Introduction to Probability and Statistics. Vol. 2 — Inference.* Cambridge University Press, Cambridge, England.

Lindley, D. V. (1980). Approximate Bayesian methods. In *Bayesian Statistics* (eds J. M. Bernardo, M. H. De Groot, D. V. Lindley and A. F. M. Smith), pp. 223–245. Valencia Press, Valencia, Spain.

Lindsey, J. K. (1975). The role of transformations to normality. *Biometrics*, **31**, 274–279.

Lingoes, J. C. (1968). The multivariate analysis of qualitative data. *Multivariate Behavioral Research*, **3**, 61–94.

Lingoes, J. C. (1971). Some boundary conditions for a monotone analysis of symmetric matrices. *Psychometrika*, **36**, 195–203.

Lingoes, J. C. and Roskam, E. E. (1973). A mathematical and empirical study of two multidimensional scaling algorithms. *Psychometrika*, **38**, monograph supplement no. 19.

Linnet, K. (1988). Testing normality of transformed data. *Applied Statistics*, **37**, 180–186.

Little, R. J. A. and Rubin, D. B. (1987). *Statistical Analysis with Missing Data.* Wiley, New York, U.S.A.

Lohr, S. L. (1993). Algorithm AS 285: Multivariate normal probabilities of star-shaped regions. *Applied Statistics*, **42**, 576–582.

Lubischew, A. A. (1962). On the use of discriminant functions in taxonomy. *Biometrics*, **18**, 455–477.

Lukacs, E. (1960). *Characteristic Functions.* Griffin, London, England.

Malkovich, J. F. and Afifi, A. A. (1973). On tests for multivariate normality. *Journal of the American Statistical Association*, **68**, 176–179.

Mallows, C. L. (1973). Some comments on C_p. *Technometrics*, **15**, 661–675.

Mandelbrot, B. (1963). The variation of certain speculative prices. *Journal of Business*, **36**, 394–419.
Manly, B. F. J. (1976). Exponential data transformations. *The Statistician*, **25**, 37–42.
Manly, B. F. J. (1986). *Multivariate Statistical Methods, a Primer*. Chapman and Hall, London, England.
Manly, B. F. J. (1991). *Randomization and Monte Carlo Methods in Biology*. Chapman and Hall, London, England.
Manly, B. F. J. and Rayner, J. C. W. (1987). The comparison of sample covariance matrices using likelihood ratio tests. *Biometrika*, **74**, 841–847.
Mardia, K. V. (1970). Measures of multivariate skewness and kurtosis with applications. *Biometrika*, **57**, 519–520.
Mardia, K. V. (1971). The effect of nonnormality on some multivariate tests and robustness to nonnormality in the linear model. *Biometrika*, **58**, 105–121.
Mardia, K. V. (1974). Applications of some measures of multivariate skewness and kurtosis for testing normality and robustness studies. *Sankhyā B*, **36**, 115–128.
Mardia, K. V. (1975). Assessment of multinormality and the robustness of Hotelling's T^2 test. *Applied Statistics*, **24**, 163–171.
Mardia, K. V. (1978). Some properties of classical multidimensional scaling. *Communications in Statistics — Theory and Methods*, **A7**, 1233–1241.
Mardia, K. V., Kent, J. T. and Bibby, J. M. (1979). *Multivariate Analysis*. Academic Press, London, England.
Mark, H. L. and Tunnell, D. (1985). Qualitative near-infrared reflectance analysis using Mahalanobis distances. *Analytical Chemistry*, **57**, 1449–1456.
Maronna, R. A. (1976). Robust *M*-estimators of multivariate location and scatter. *Annals of Statistics*, **4**, 51–67.
Marriott, F. H. C. (1982). Optimization methods of cluster analysis. *Biometrika*, **69**, 417–422.
Marriott, F. H. C. (1987). Comments in Jones, M. C. and Sibson, R. (1987). What is projection pursuit? (with discussion). *Journal of the Royal Statistical Society, Series A*, **150**, 1–36.
Marshall, A. W. and Olkin, I. (1967). A multivariate exponential distribution. *Journal of the American Statistical Association*, **62**, 30–44.
Mathai, A. M. and Katiyar, R. S. (1979). The distribution and the exact percentage points for Wilks' L_{mvc} criterion. *Annals of the Institute of Statistical Mathematics*, **31**, 215–224.
Maung, K. (1941). Measurement of association in a contingency table with special reference to the pigmentation of hair and eye colours of Scottish school children. *Annals of Eugenics*, **11**, 189–205.
McCabe, G. P. (1982). *Principal Variables*. Technical Report No. 82–83, Department of Statistics, Purdue University, U.S.A.
McCabe, G. P. (1984). Principal variables. *Technometrics*, **26**, 137–144.
McCullagh, P. and Nelder, J. A. (1990). *Generalized Linear Models*, 2nd ed. Chapman and Hall, London, England.
McCulloch, W. W. and Pitts, W. (1943). A logical calculus of the ideas immanent in nervous activity. *Bulletin of Mathematical Biophysics*, **5**, 115–133.
McGee, V. E. (1968). Multidimensional scaling of *n* sets of similarity measures:

a non-metric individual differences approach. *Multivariate Behavioral Research*, **3**, 233–248.

McKay, R. J. (1977). Variable selection in multivariate regression: an application of simultaneous test procedures. *Journal of the Royal Statistical Society, Series B*, **39**, 371–380.

McKay, R. J. (1979). The adequacy of variable subsets in multivariate regression. *Technometrics*, **21**, 475–479.

McReynolds, W. O. (1970). Characterization of some liquid phases. *Journal of Chromatographic Science*, **8**, 685–691.

Mead, A. (1992). Review of the development of multidimensional scaling methods. *The Statistician*, **41**, 27–39.

Metropolis, N., Rosenbluth, A. W., Rosenbluth, M. N., Teller, A. H. and Teller, E. (1953). Equations of state calculations by fast computing machines. *Journal of Chemical Physics*, **21**, 1087–1092.

Meulman, J. J. (1986). *A Distance Approach to Nonlinear Multivariate Analysis.* DSWO Press, Leiden, The Netherlands.

Meulman, J. J. (1992). The integration of multidimensional scaling and multivariate analysis with optimal transformations. *Psychometrika*, **54**, 539–565.

Meulman, J. J. and Heiser, W. J. (1993). Nonlinear biplots for nonlinear mappings. In *Studies in Classification, Data Analysis and Knowledge Organization* (eds O. Opitz, B. Lansen and R. Klar). Springer-Verlag, Heidelberg, Germany.

Michaelewicz, Z. and Janikow, C.Z. (1991). Genetic algorithms for numerical optimization. *Statistics and Computing*, **1**, 75–91.

Miller, A. J. (1990). *Subset Selection in Regression.* Chapman and Hall, London, England.

Minsky, M. L. and Papert, S. (1969). *Perceptrons.* MIT Press, Cambridge, U.S.A.

Minsky, M. L. and Papert, S. (1988). *Perceptrons. Expanded Edition.* MIT Press, Cambridge, U.S.A.

Mitchell, A. F. S. and Krzanowski, W. J. (1985). The Mahalanobis distance and elliptical distributions. *Biometrika*, **72**, 464–467.

Modarres, R. and Jernigan, R. W. (1992). Testing the equality of correlation matrices. *Communications in Statistics, Theory and Methods*, **21**, 2107–2125.

Moonen, M., van Dooren, P. and Vandewalle, J. (1992). A singular value decomposition updating algorithm for subspace tracking. *SIAM Journal on Matrix Analysis and Applications*, **13**, 1015–1038.

Moran, P. A. P. (1967). Testing for serial correlation with exponentially distributed variates. *Biometrika*, **54**, 395–401.

Morrison, D. F. (1976). *Multivariate Statistical Methods*, 2nd ed. McGraw-Hill, New York, U.S.A.

Mosier, C. I. (1939). Determining a simple structure when loadings for certain tests are known. *Psychometrika*, **4**, 149–162.

Mosimann, J. E. (1970). Size allometry; size and shape variables with characterizations of the lognormal and gamma distributions. *Journal of the American Statistical Association*, **65**, 930–945.

Moss, M. L., Pucciarelli, H. M., Moss-Salentijn, L., Skalak, R., Bose, A., Goodall, C. R. and Sen, K. (1987). Effects of pre-weaning undernutrition on 21 day-old male rat skull form as described by the finite element method. *Gegenbaurs Morphologisches Jahrbuch*, **133**, 837–868.

Mudholkar, G. S., Davidson, M. L. and Subbaiah, P. (1974a). A note on the union-intersection character of some MANOVA procedures. *Journal of Multivariate Analysis*, **4**, 486–493.

Mudholkar, G. S., Davidson, M. L. and Subbaiah, P. (1974b). Extended linear hypotheses and simultaneous tests in multivariate analysis of variance. *Biometrika*, **61**, 467–477.

Mudholkar, G. S., McDermott, M. and Srivastava, D. K. (1992). A test of *p*-variate normality. *Biometrika*, **79**, 850–854.

Mudholkar, G. S., Trivedi, M. C. and Lin, C. T. (1982). An approximation to the distribution of the likelihood ratio test statistic for testing complete independence. *Technometrics*, **24**, 139–143.

Muirhead, R. J. (1982). *Aspects of Multivariate Statistical Theory*. Wiley, New York, U.S.A.

Muirhead, R. J. and Waternaux, C. M. (1980). Asymptotic distributions in canonical correlation analysis and other multivariate procedures for non-normal populations. *Biometrika*, **67**, 31–43.

Nagarsenker, B. N. (1978). Nonnull distributions of some statistics associated with testing for the equality of two covariance matrices. *Journal of Multivariate Analysis*, **8**, 396–404.

Nagarsenker, B. N. and Pillai, K. C. S. (1973a). The distribution of the sphericity test criterion. *Journal of Multivariate Analysis*, **3**, 226–235.

Nagarsenker, B. N. and Pillai, K. C. S. (1973b). Distribution of the likelihood ratio criterion for testing a hypothesis specifying a covariance matrix. *Biometrika*, **60**, 359–364.

Naylor, J. C. and Smith, A. F. M. (1982). Applications of a method for the efficient computation of posterior distributions. *Applied Statistics*, **31**, 214–225.

Naylor, J. C. and Smith, A. F. M. (1983). A contamination model in clinical chemistry. In *Practical Bayesian Statistics* (eds A. P. Dawid and A. F. M. Smith), Longman, Harlow, England.

Nishisato, S. (1980). *Analysis of Categorical Data: Dual Scaling and its Applications*. University of Toronto Press, Toronto, Canada.

Obenchain, R. L. (1970). *Simplex Distributions Generated by Transformations*. Bell Telephone Laboratories Technical Report, Murray Hill, U.S.A.

O'Hagan, A. (1994). *Kendall's Advanced Theory of Statistics – Bayesian Inference*. Edward Arnold, London, U.K.

Olkin, I. and Siotani, M. (1976). Asymptotic distribution of functions of a correlation matrix. In *Essays in Probability and Statistics*, (eds S. Ikeda *et al*), pp. 235–251. Shinko Tsusho, Tokyo, Japan.

Olkin, I. and Tomsky, T. L. (1975). A new class of multivariate tests based on the union-intersection principle. *Bulletin of the International Statistical Institute*, **46**, 202–204.

Olshen, R. A., Biden, E. N., Wyatt, M. P. and Sutherland, D. H. (1989). Gait analysis and the bootstrap. *Annals of Statistics*, **17**, 1419–1440.

Pack, P. and Jolliffe, I. T. (1992). Influence in correspondence analysis. *Applied Statistics*, **41**, 365–380.

Parker, D. B. (1982). *Learning-logic*. Invention Report S81–64, File 1, Office of Technology Licensing, Stanford University, U.S.A.

Pearson, E. S. (1969). Some comments on the accuracy of Box's approximation to the distribution of *M*. *Biometrika*, **56**, 219–220.

Pearson, E. S. and Hartley, H. O. (1951). Charts of the power function for analysis of variance tests derived from the non-central *F*-distribution. *Biometrika*, **38**, 112–130.

Pearson, E. S. and Hartley, H. O. (1972). *Biometrika Tables for Statisticians*, Vol. 2. Cambridge University Press, Cambridge, England.

Pearson, K. (1898). Mathematical contributions to the theory of evolution. *V*. On the reconstruction of the stature of prehistoric races. *Philosophical Transactions of the Royal Society of London, Series A*, **192**, 169–244.

Pearson, K. (1901). On lines and planes of closest fit to systems of points in space. *The London, Edinburgh and Dublin Philosophical Magazine and Journal of Science, Sixth Series*, **2**, 559–572.

Peay, E. R. (1988). Multidimensional rotation and scaling of configurations to optimal agreement. *Psychometrika*, **53**, 199–208.

Penrose, L. S. (1947). Some notes on discrimination. *Annals of Eugenics*, **13**, 228–237.

Pickett, R. and White, B. W. (1966). Constructing data pictures. *Proceedings of the 7th National Symposium of Information Display*, 75–81.

Pillai, K. C. S. (1955). Some new criteria in multivariate analysis. *Annals of Mathematical Statistics*, **26**, 117–121.

Pillai, K. C. S. (1960). *Statistical Tables for Tests of Multivariate Hypotheses*. Statistical Center, University of the Phillipines, Manila, Phillipines.

Pillai, K. C. S. (1977). Distributions of characteristic roots in multivariate analysis. Part II: Non-null distributions. *Canadian Journal of Statistics, Series A and B*, **5**, 1–62.

Pillai, K. C. S. and Gupta, A. K. (1969). On the exact distribution of Wilks' criterion. *Biometrika*, **51**, 109–118.

Pillai, K. C. S. and Hsu, Y. S. (1979). Exact robustness studies of the test of independence based on four multivariate criteria and their distribution problems under violations. *Annals of the Institute of Statistical Mathematics*, **31**, 85–101.

Pillai, K. C. S. and Jayachandran, K. (1967). Power comparison of tests of two multivariate hypotheses based on four criteria. *Biometrika*, **55**, 195–210.

Pitman, E. J. G. (1937a). Significance tests which may be applied to any population. *Supplement to the Journal of the Royal Statistical Society*, **4**, 119–130.

Pitman, E. J. G. (1937b). Significance tests which may be applied to any population. II. The correlation coefficient test. *Supplement to the Journal of the Royal Statistical Society*, **4**, 225–232.

Pitman, E. J. G. (1938). Significance tests which may be applied to any population. III. The analysis of variance test. *Biometrika*, **29**, 322–335.

Press, S. J. (1972a). *Applied Multivariate Analysis*. Holt, Rinehart and Winston, New York, U.S.A.

Press, S. J. (1972b). Estimation in univariate and multivariate stable distributions. *Journal of the American Statistical Association*, **67**, 842–846.

Press, S. J. (1989). *Bayesian Statistics: Principles, Models and Applications*. Wiley, New York, U.S.A.

Press, W. H., Flannery, B. P., Teukolsky, S. A. and Vetterling, W. T. (1989). *Nu-*

merical Recipes (FORTRAN Version). Cambridge University Press, England.

Puri, M. L. and Sen, P. K. (1971). *Non-parametric Methods in Multivariate Analysis*. Wiley, New York, U.S.A.

Ramsay, J. O. (1977). Maximum likelihood estimation in multidimensional scaling. *Psychometrika*, **42**, 241–266.

Ramsay, J. O. (1978). Confidence regions for multidimensional scaling analysis. *Psychometrika*, **43**, 145–160.

Ramsay, J. O. (1982). Some statistical approaches to multidimensional scaling data (with discussion). *Journal of the Royal Statistical Society, Series A*, **145**, 285–312.

Rao, C. R. (1948). Tests of significance in multivariate analysis. *Biometrika*, **35**, 58–79.

Rao, C. R. (1964). The use and interpretation of principal components in applied research. *Sankhyā Series A*, **26**, 329–358.

Rao, C. R. (1965). The theory of least squares when the parameters are stochastic and its application to the analysis of growth curves. *Biometrika*, **52**, 447–458.

Rao, C. R. (1966). Covariance adjustment and related problems in multivariate analysis. In *Multivariate Analysis I*, (ed. P.R.Krishnaiah), pp. 87–103. Academic Press, New York, U.S.A.

Rao, C. R. (1980). Matrix approximations and reduction of dimensionality in multivariate statistical analysis. In *Multivariate Analysis V* (ed P. R. Krishnaiah), pp. 3–22, North-Holland, Amsterdam, The Netherlands.

Rayner, J. C. W. , Manly, B. F. J. and Liddell, G. F. (1990). Hierarchic likelihood ratio tests for equality of covariance matrices. *Journal of Statistical Computation and Simulation*, **35**, 91–99.

Reinsch, C. (1967). Smoothing by spline functions. *Numerische Mathematik*, **10**, 177–183.

Rice, J. A. and Silverman, B. W. (1991). Estimating the mean and covariance structure nonparametrically when the data are curves. *Journal of the Royal Statistical Society, Series B*, **53**, 233–243.

Ripley, B. D. and Sutherland, A. I. (1990). Finding spiral structures in images of galaxies. *Philosophical Transactions of the Royal Society, London*, **332**, 477–485.

Robert, P. and Escoufier, Y. (1976). A unifying tool for linear statistical methods: the *RV*-coefficient. *Applied Statistics*, **25**, 257–265.

Rohlf, F. J. (1975). Generalisation of the gap test for the detection of multivariate outliers. *Biometrics*, **31**, 93–101.

Rollet, E. (1889). *De la Mensuration des Os Longs des Membres*. Lyon, France.

Romesburg, H. C. (1984). *Cluster Analysis for Researchers*. Lifetime Learning Publications, Belmont, California, U.S.A.

Rosenblatt, F. (1962). *Principles of Neurodynamics*, Spartan Books, New York, U.S.A.

Ross, J. (1966). A remark on Tucker and Messick's 'points of view' analysis. *Psychometrika*, **31**, 27–32.

Rothkopf, E. Z. (1957). A measure of stimulus similarity and errors in some paired-associate learning tasks. *Journal of Experimental Psychology*, **53**, 94–101.

Rousseeuw, P. J. and van Zomeren, B. C. (1990). Unmasking multivariate outliers and leverage points. *Journal of the American Statistical Association*, **85**, 633–639.

Roy, S. N. (1939). *p*-statistics, or some generalizations in analysis of variance appropriate to multivariate problems. *Sankhyā*, **4**, 381–396.

Roy, S. N. (1953). On a heuristic method of test construction and its use in multivariate analysis. *Annals of Mathematical Statistics*, **29**, 1177–1187.

Roy, S. N. (1957). *Some Aspects of Multivariate Analysis.* Wiley, New York, U.S.A.

Roy, S. N., Gnanadesikan, R. and Srivastava, J. N. (1971). *Analysis and Design of Certain Quantitative Multiresponse Experiments.* Pergamon Press, Oxford, England.

Rudeforth, C. C. and Bradley, R. I. (1972). *Soils, Land Classification and Land Use of West and Central Pembrokeshire. Special Survey No. 6.* Soil Survey of England and Wales, Harpenden, U.K.

Rumelhart, D. E., Hinton, G. E. and Williams, R. J. (1986). Learning internal representations by error propagation. In *Neural Information Processing Systems*, ed. D. Z. Anderson, pp. 602–611. American Institute of Physics, New York, U.S.A.

Ryan, B. F., Joiner, B. L. and Ryan, T. A. (1985). *MINITAB Handbook.* PWS-Kent Publishing Company, Boston, U. S. A.

Sammon, J. W. (1969). A non-linear mapping for data structure analysis. *IEEE Transactions in Computing*, **C-18**, 401–409.

Sanghvi, L. D. (1966). Genetic adaptability in man. In *The Biology of Human Adaptability* (eds P. T. Baker and J. S. Weiner), pp. 305–328, Clarendon Press, Oxford, England.

Schatzoff, M. (1966a). Exact distribution of Wilks's likelihood ratio criterion. *Biometrika*, **53**, 347–358.

Schatzoff, M. (1966b). Sensitivity comparisons among tests of the general linear hypothesis. *Journal of the American Statistical Association*, **61**, 415–435.

Scheffé, H. (1943). On solution of the Behrens–Fisher problem based on the *t*-distribution. *Annals of Mathematical Statistics*, **14**, 35–44.

Scheffé, H. (1953). A method for judging all contrasts in the analysis of variance. *Biometrika*, **40**, 87–104.

Scheffé, H. (1959). *The Analysis of Variance.* Wiley, New York, U.S.A.

Schervish, M. J. (1984). Algorithm AS 195. Multivariate normal probabilities with error bound. *Applied Statistics*, **33**, 81–87.

Schoenberg, I. J. (1935). Remarks to Maurice Fréchet's article 'Sur la définition axiomatique d'une classe d'espaces vectoriels distanciés applicable vectoriellement sur l'espace de Hilbert. *Annals of Mathematics*, **36**, 724–732.

Schönemann, P. H. (1966). A generalised solution of the orthogonal Procrustes problem. *Psychometrika*, **31**, 1–10.

Schönemann, P. H. (1968). On two-sided orthogonal Procrustes problems. *Psychometrika*, **33**, 19–33.

Schönemann, P. H. (1970). On metric multidimensional unfolding. *Psychometrika*, **35**, 349–365.

Schönemann, P. H. and Carroll, R. M. (1970). Fitting one matrix to another under choice of a central dilation and rigid motion. *Psychometrika*, **35**, 245–255.

Schurrmann, F. J., Waikar, V. B. and Krishnaiah, P. R. (1973a). Percentage points of the joint distribution of the extreme roots of the random matrix $(S_1 + S_2)^{-1}$. *Journal of Statistical Computation and Simulation*, **2**, 17–38.

Schurrmann, F. J., Waikar, V. B. and Chattopadhyay, A. K. (1973b). On the distributions of the ratios of the extreme roots to the trace of the Wishart matrix. *Journal of Multivariate Analysis*, **3**, 445–453.

Schwerteman, N. C. and Allen, D. M. (1981). Smoothing an indefinite variance-covariance matrix. *Journal of Statistical Computation and Simulation*, **9**, 183–194.

Seal, H. (1964). *Multivariate Statistical Analysis for Biologists*. Methuen, London, U.K.

Seber, G. A. F. (1984). *Multivariate Observations*. Wiley, New York, U.S.A.

Shapiro, S. S. and Wilk, M. B. (1965). An analysis-of-variance test for normality (complete samples). *Biometrika*, **52**, 591–611.

Shenton, L. R. and Bowman, K. O. (1977). A bivariate model for the distribution of $\sqrt{b_1}$ and b_2. *Journal of the American Statistical Association*, **72**, 206–211.

Shepard, R. N. (1962a). The analysis of proximities: multidimensional scaling with an unknown distance function I. *Psychometrika*, **27**, 125–140.

Shepard, R. N. (1962b). The analysis of proximities: multidimensional scaling with an unknown distance function II. *Psychometrika*, **27**, 219–246.

Shepard, R. N. (1966). Metric structures in ordinal data. *Journal of Mathematical Psychology*, **3**, 287–315.

Shepard, R. N. and Carroll, J. D. (1966). Parametric representations of non-linear data structures. In *Multivariate Analysis* (ed P. R. Krishnaiah), pp. 561–592. Academic Press, New York, U.S.A.

Sheppard, W. F. (1898). On the geometric treatment of the 'normal curve' of statistics, with special reference to correlation and the theory of errors. *Proceedings of the Royal Society of London*, **62**, 170–173.

Shumway, R. H. (1982). Discriminant analysis for time series. In *Handbook of Statistics, 2* (eds P. R. Krishnaiah and L. Kanal), pp. 1–46. North-Holland, Amsterdam, The Netherlands.

Sibson, R. (1972). Order invariance methods for data analysis (with discussion). *Journal of the Royal Statistical Society, Series B*, **34**, 311–349.

Sibson, R. (1978). Studies in the robustness of multidimensional scaling: Procrustes statistics. *Journal of the Royal Statistical Society, Series B*, **40**, 234–238.

Sibson, R. (1979). Studies in the robustness of multidimensional scaling: perturbation analysis of classical scaling. *Journal of the Royal Statistical Society, Series B*, **41**, 217–229.

Siegel, A. F. and Benson, R. H. (1982). A robust comparison of biological shapes. *Biometrics*, **28**, 341–350.

Siegel, J. H., Goldwyn, R. M. and Friedman, H. P. (1971). Pattern and process of the evolution of human septic shock. *Surgery*, **70**, 232–245.

Silverman, B. W. (1985). Some aspects of spline smoothing approaches to non-parametric regression curve fitting (with discussion). *Journal of the Royal Statistical Society, Series B*, **47**, 1–52.

Silverman, B. W. (1986). *Density Estimation in Statistics and Data Analysis*. Chapman and Hall, London, England.

Silvey, S. D. (1959). The Lagrangian multiplier test. *Annals of Mathematical Statistics*, **30**, 389–407.

Siotani, M. (1959). The extreme value of the generalised distances of the individual points in the multivariate normal sample. *Annals of the Institute of Statistical Mathematics, Tokyo*, **10**, 183–208.

Siskind, V. (1972). Second moments of inverse Wishart-matrix elements. *Biometrika*, **59**, 691–692.

Smith, A. F. M. (1991). Bayesian computational methods. *Philosophical transactions of the Royal Society of London, Series A*, **337**, 369–386.

Smith, A. F. M. and Roberts, G. O. (1993). Bayesian computation via the Gibbs sampler and related Markov Chain Monte Carlo methods. *Journal of the Royal Statistical Society, Series B*, **55**, 3–23.

Smith, A. F. M., Skene, A. M., Shaw, J. E. H., Naylor, J. C. and Dransfield, M. (1985). The implementation of the Bayesian paradigm. *Communications in Statistics, Theory and Methods*, **14**, 1079–1102.

Smith, R. L. and Naylor, J. C. (1984). A comparison of maximum likelihood and Bayesian estimators for the three parameter Weibull distribution. Technical Report, Imperial College, London.

Snedecor, G. W. (1946). *Statistical methods*, 4th ed. Iowa State College, Ames, U.S.A.

Southwell, R. V. (1946). *Relaxation Methods in Theoretical Physics*. Oxford University Press, England.

Spearman, C. (1904a). The proof and measurement of association between two things. *American Journal of Psychology*, **15**, 88–103.

Spearman, C. (1904b). 'General intelligence' objectively determined and measured. *American Journal of Psychology*, **15**, 201–293.

Speed, T. P. (1978). *Graph-theoretic Methods in the Analysis of Interaction*. Lecture Notes, Institute of Mathematical Statistics, University of Copenhagen, Denmark.

Spence, I. and Young, F. W. (1978). Monte Carlo studies in non-metric scaling. *Psychometrika*, **43**, 115–117.

SPSS (1990). *SPSS Categories, User's Manual*. SPSS Inc., Chicago, U.S.A.

Srivastava, M. S. and Awan, H. M. (1982). On the robustness of Hotelling's T^2-test and distribution of linear and quadratic forms in sampling from a mixture of two multivariate normal populations. *Communications in Statistics, Theory and Methods A*, **11**, 81–107.

Srivastava, M. S. and Carter, E. M. (1983). *An Introduction to Applied Multivariate Statistics*. North-Holland, New York, U.S.A.

Steel, R. G. D. (1951). Minimum generalised variance for a net of linear functions. *Annals of Mathematical Statistics*, **22**, 456–460.

Stein, C. (1956). Inadmissibility of the usual estimator for the mean of a multivariate normal distribution. *Proceedings of the Third Berkeley Symposium in Mathematical Statistics and Probability*, **1**, 197–206. University of California Press, Berkeley, U.S.A.

Stein, C. (1969). *Multivariate Analysis I. (notes by M.L.Eaton)*. Technical Report no. 42, Stanford University, U.S.A.

Stewart, D. and Love, W. (1968). A general canonical correlation index. *Psychological Bulletin*, **70**, 160–163.

Stigler, S. M. (1990). The 1988 Neyman memorial lecture: A Galtonian perspective on shrinkage estimators. *Statistical Science*, **5**, 147–155.

Stoyanov, J. M. (1987). *Counterexamples in Probability*. Wiley, New York, U.S.A.

Stuart, A. and Ord, J. K. (1987). *Kendall's Advanced Theory of Statistics, Vol I*, 5th ed. Charles Griffin & Co., London, England.

Stuart, A. and Ord, J. K. (1991). *Kendall's Advanced Theory of Statistics, Vol II*, 5th ed. Edward Arnold, London, England.

Subrahmaniam, K. and Subrahmaniam, K. (1973). On the multivariate Behrens–Fisher problem. *Biometrika*, **60**, 107–111.

Subrahmaniam, K. and Subrahmaniam, K. (1975). On the confidence region comparison of some solutions for the multivariate Behrens–Fisher problem. *Communications in Statistics*, **4**, 57–67.

Sundberg, R. and Brown, P. J. (1989). Multivariate calibration with more variables than observations. *Technometrics*, **31**, 365–371.

Sutradher, B. C. (1990). Discrimination of observations into one of two *t* populations. *Biometrics*, **46**, 827–835.

Swain, P. H. (1982). Pattern recognition techniques for remote sensing applications. In *Handbook of Statistics, 2* (eds P. R. Krishnaiah and L. Kanal), pp. 609–620. North-Holland, Amsterdam, The Netherlands.

Takane, Y. (1981). Multidimensional successive categories scaling: a maximum likelihood method. *Psychometrika*, **46**, 9–28.

Takane, Y. and Carroll, J. D. (1981). Non-metric maximum likelihood multidimensional scaling from directional rankings of similarities. *Psychometrika*, **46**, 389–405.

Takane, Y., Young, F. W. and De Leeuw, J. (1977). Nonmetric individual differences multidimensional scaling: an alternating least squares method with optimal scaling features. *Psychometrika*, **42**, 7–67.

Tanner, M. A. and Wong, W. (1987). The calculation of posterior distributions by data augmentation (with discussion). *Journal of the American Statistical Association*, **82**, 528–550.

Ten Berge, J. M. F. (1977). Orthogonal Procrustes rotation for two or more matrices. *Psychometrika*, **42**, 267–276.

Tenenhaus, M. and Young, F. W. (1985). An analysis and synthesis of multiple correspondence analysis, optimal scaling, dual scaling, homogeneity analysis, and other methods for quantifying categorical multivariate data. *Psychometrika*, **50**, 91–119.

Thompson, D. W. (1917). *On Growth and Form*, (2 volumes). Cambridge University Press, Cambridge, England.

Tiago de Oliveira, J. (1980). Bivariate extremes; foundations and statistics. In *Multivariate Analysis V* (ed P. R. Krishnaiah), pp. 349–366. North-Holland, Amsterdam, The Netherlands.

Tiao, G. C. and Guttman, I. (1965). The Inverted Dirichlet distribution with applications. *Journal of the American Statistical Association*, **60**, 793–805 (correction: **60**, 1251–1252).

Tierney, L. and Kadane, J. B. (1986). Accurate approximations for posterior moments and marginal densities. *Journal of the American Statistical Association*, **81**, 82–86.

Tierney, L., Kass, R. E. and Kadane, J. B. (1989). Approximate marginal densities of nonlinear functions. *Biometrika*, **76**, 425–434.

Tiku, M. L. (1966). Tables of the power of the F-test. *Journal of the American Statistical Association*, **61**, 709–710.

Tiku, M. L. (1967). Tables of the power of the F-test. *Journal of the American Statistical Association*, **62**, 525–539.

Tiku, M. L. (1972). More tables of the power of the F-test. *Journal of the American Statistical Association*, **67**, 709–710.

Titterington, D. M. (1979). Estimation of correlation coefficients by ellipsoidal trimming. *Applied Statistics*, **27**, 227–234.

Torgerson, W. S. (1952). Multidimensional scaling: I. Theory and method. *Psychometrika*, **17**, 401–419.

Torgerson, W. S. (1958). *Theory and Methods of Scaling.* Wiley, New York, U.S.A.

Tucker, L. R. (1966). Some mathematical notes on three-mode factor analysis. *Psychometrika*, **31**, 279–311.

Tucker, L. R. and Messick, S. (1963). An individual differences model for multidimensional scaling. *Psychometrika*, **28**, 333–367.

Tukey, J. W. (1949). Comparing individual means in the analysis of variance. *Biometrics*, **5**, 99–114.

Tukey, J. W. (1957). On the comparative anatomy of transformations. *Annals of Mathematical Statistics*, **28**, 602–632.

Tukey, J. W. (1991). The philosophy of multiple comparisons. *Statistical Science*, **6**, 100–116.

Van Bemmel, J. H. (1982). Recognition of electrocardiographic patterns. In *Handbook of Statistics, 2* (eds P. R. Krishnaiah and L. Kanal), pp. 501–526. North-Holland, Amsterdam, The Netherlands.

Van Buuren, S. and Heiser, W. J. (1989). Clustering N objects into K groups under optimal scaling of variables. *Psychometrika*, **54**, 699–706.

Van De Geer, J. P. (1984). Linear relations between k sets of variables. *Psychometrika*, **49**, 79–94.

Van den Wollenberg, A. L. (1977). Redundancy analysis: an alternative for canonical correlation analysis. *Psychometrika*, **42**, 207–219.

Van Der Burg, E., De Leeuw, J. and Verdegaal, R. (1988). Homogeneity analysis with k sets of variables: an alternating least squares method with optimal scaling features. *Psychometrika*, **53**, 173–193.

Van Der Heiden, P. G. M., De Falguerolles, A. and De Leeuw, J. (1989). A combined approach to contingency table analysis using correspondence analysis and log-linear analysis. *Applied Statistics*, **38**, 249–292.

Van Rijckevorsel, J. L. A. (1982). Canonical analysis with B-splines. In *COMPSTAT 82, Proceedings in Computational Statistics* (eds H. Caussinus, P. Ettinger and R. Tomassone), pp. 393–398. Physika Verlag, Vienna, Austria.

Verboon, P. and Heiser, W. J. (1992). Resistant orthogonal Procrustes analysis. *Journal of Classification*, **9**, 237–256.

von Neuman J. (1966). *Theory of Self-reproducing Automata*, edited and completed by A.W. Burks. University of Illinois Press, U.S.A.

Wainer, H. (1981). Comment on a paper by Kleiner and Hartigan. *Journal of the American Statistical Association*, **76**, 272–275.

Wakimoto, K. and Taguri, M. (1978). Constellation graphical method for representing multidimensional data. *Annals of the Institute of Statistical Mathematics*, **30**, 97–104.

Wasserman, P. D. (1989). *Neural Computing*, Van Nostrand Reinhold, New York, U.S.A.

Watson, G. S. (1964). Smooth regression analysis. *Sankhyā, A*, **26**, 359–372.

Webster, R. and McBratney, A. B. (1981). Soil segment overlap in character space and its implication for soil classification. *Journal of Soil Science*, **32**, 133–147.

Weihs, C. (1992). Canonical discriminant analysis: comparison of resampling methods and convex-hull approximations. Proceedings of the 16th Conference of the German Classification Society.

Weihs, C. and Schmidli, H. (1990). OMEGA: online multivariate exploratory graphical analysis: routine searching for structure (with discussion). *Statistical Science*, **5**, 175–226.

Weinberg, S. L., Carroll, J. D. and Cohen, H. S. (1984). Confidence regions for INDSCAL using the jackknife and bootstrap techniques. *Psychometrika*, **49**, 475–491.

Weinman, D. G. (1966). *A Multivariate Extension of the Exponential Distribution*. Unpublished Ph. D. Thesis, Arizona State University, U.S.A.

Welch, B. L. (1937). The significance of the difference between two means when the population variances are unequal. *Biometrika*, **29**, 350.

Welch, B. L. (1947). The generalization of 'Students' problem when several different population variances are involved. *Biometrika*, **34**, 28–35.

Werbos, P. J. (1974). *Beyond Regression: New Tools for Prediction and Analysis in the Behavioral Sciences*, Unpublished Masters Thesis, Harvard University, U.S.A.

Whittaker, J. (1990). *Graphical Models in Applied Multivariate Statistics*. Wiley, Chichester, England.

Wilk, M. B. and Gnanadesikan,R. (1968). Probability plotting methods for the analysis of data. *Biometrika*, **55**, 1–17.

Wilks, S. S. (1932). Certain generalisations in the analysis of variance. *Biometrika*, **24**, 471–494.

Wilks, S. S. (1935). On the independence of k sets of normally distributed statistical variables. *Econometrika*, **3**, 309–326.

Wilks, S. S. (1946). Sample criteria for testing equality of means, equality of variances, and equality of covariances in a normal multivariate distribution. *Annals of Mathematical Statistics*, **17**, 257–281.

Wilks, S. S. (1962). *Mathematical Statistics*. Wiley, New York, U.S.A.

Williams, A. A. and Langron, S. P. (1984). Use of free-choice profiling for evaluation of commercial ports. *Journal of Science and Food in Agriculture*, **35**, 558–568.

Williams, E. J. (1959). *Regression Analysis*. Wiley, New York, U.S.A.

Winsberg, S. (1988). Two techniques: monotone spline transformations for dimension reduction in PCA and easy-to-generate metrics for PCA of sampled functions. In *Component and Correspondence Analysis* (eds J. L. A. Van Rijckevorsel and J. De Leeuw), pp.115–135. Wiley, Chichester, England.

Winsberg, S. and Ramsay, J. O. (1980). Monotonic transformations to additivity using splines. *Biometrika*, **67**, 669–674.

Winsberg, S. and Ramsay, J. O. (1981). Analysis of pairwise preference data using integrated B-splines. *Psychometrika*, **46**, 171–186.

Winsberg, S. and Ramsay, J. O. (1982). Monotone splines: a family of transformations useful for data analysis. In *COMPSTAT 82, Proceedings in Computational Statistics* (eds H. Caussinus, P. Ettinger and R. Tomassone), pp. 451–456. Physika Verlag, Vienna, Austria.

Winsberg, S. and Ramsay, J. O. (1983). Monotone spline transformations for dimension reduction. *Psychometrika*, **48**, 575–595.

Wishart, J. (1928). The generalized product moment distribution in samples from a normal multivariate distribution. *Biometrika*, **20A**, 32–52, (correction **20A**, 424).

Wishart, J. (1938). Growth rate determinations in nutrition studies with the bacon pig and their analysis. *Biometrika*, **30**, 16–28.

Wishart, J. (1948). Proofs of the distribution law of the second order moment statistics. *Biometrika*, **35**, 55–57, (note **35**, 422).

Wold, S. (1976). Pattern recognition by means of disjoint principal components models. *Pattern Recognition*, **8**, 127–139.

Wold, S. (1978). Cross-validatory estimation of the number of components in factor and principal component analysis. *Technometrics*, **20**, 397–405.

Wright, S. (1954). The interpretation of multivariate systems. In *Statistics and Mathematics in Biology* (eds O. Kempthorne, T. A. Bancroft, J. W. Gowen and J. L. Lush), pp11–33. State University Press, Iowa, U.S.A.

Yao, Y. (1965). An approximate degrees of freedom solution to the multivariate Behrens–Fisher problem. *Biometrika*, **52**, 139–147.

Yenyukov, I. S. (1988). Detecting structure by means of projection pursuit. In *Compstat 1988* (eds D. Edwards and N. E. Raun), pp. 47–58. Physica-Verlag, Heidelburg, Germany, for IASC.

Young, D. M., Marco, V. R. and Odell, P. L. (1987). Quadratic discrimination: some results on optimal low-dimensional representation. *Journal of Statistical Planning and Inference*, **17**, 307–319.

Young, F. W. (1970). Non-metric multidimensional scaling: recovery of metric information. *Psychometrika*, **35**, 455–473.

Young, F. W. (1981). Quantitative analysis of qualitative data. *Psychometrika*, **46**, 357–388.

Young, F. W. and Null, C. H. (1978). Multidimensional scaling of nominal data: the recovery of metric information with ALSCAL. *Psychometrika*, **43**, 367–379.

Young, F. W. and Rheigans, P. (1991). Visualizing structure in high-dimensional multivariate data. *IBM Journal of Research and Development*, **35**, 97–107.

Young, F. W., De Leeuw, J. and Takane, Y. (1980). Quantifying qualitative data. In *Similarity and Choice* (eds E. D. Lantermann and H. Feger). Huber, Berne, Switzerland.

Young, G. and Householder, A. S. (1938). Discussion of a set of points in terms of their mutual distances. *Psychometrika*, **3**, 19–22.

Yule, G. U. (1907). On the theory of correlation for any number of variables treated by a new system of notation. *Proceedings of the Royal Society, Series A*, **79**, 182–193.

Yule, W., Berger, M., Butler, S., Newham, V. and Tizard, J. (1969). The WPPSI: an empirical evaluation with a British sample. *British Journal of Educational Psychology*, **39**, 1–13.

Author Index

Afifi, A. A. 58, 97, 254.
Aitchison, J. 29, 30, 31, 237,
Aitkin, M. A. 189, 191, 237.
Allen, D. M. 110, 261.
Amiard, J.-C. 211.
Anderson, E. 45, 237.
Anderson, T. W. 80, 162, 166, 182, 184, 237.
Andrews, D. F. 21, 44, 47, 48, 50, 58, 60, 61, 63, 64, 71, 237.
Arabie, P. 117, 237.
Armitage, P. 3, 36, 237.
Arnold, G. M. 9, 237.
Arnold, H. J. 173, 238.
Arnold, S. F. 225, 238.
Ashton, E. H. 47, 238.
Asimov, D. 94, 238.
Atkinson, A.C. 55, 182, 238.
Awan, H. M. 173, 262.
Aykroyd, R. G. 6, 238.

Banfield, J. D. 198, 199, 238.
Barlow, R. E. 116, 238.
Barnard, M. M. 234, 238.
Barndorf-Neilson, O. E. 228, 238,
Barnett, V. 7, 50, 160, 238.
Barry, D. 198, 238.
Bartholomew, D. J. 116, 238.
Bartlett, M. S. 41, 83, 222, 224, 227, 228, 231, 233, 234, 235, 238.
Beale, E. M. L. 17, 239.
Becker, R. A. 43, 198, 239.
Beever, D. E. 2, 245.
Bekker, P. 206, 207, 239.
Bennett, B. M. 172, 239.
Benson, R. H. 137, 261.
Berger, M. 3, 15, 266.
Bergström, H. 37, 239.
Bertier, P. 87, 239.
Bhattacharyya, A. 137, 139, 239.
Bibby, J. M. 36, 57, 83, 108, 110, 145, 157, 163, 164, 167, 175, 176, 184, 223, 226, 255.
Bickel, P. J. 61, 239.
Biden, E. N. 5, 257.
Bloomfield, P. 32, 239.
Bloxom, B. 122, 239.
Bollen, K. A. 18, 239.
Boneva, L. I. 3, 239.
Bookstein, F.L. 80, 239.
Borg, I. 117, 239.
Bose, A. 6, 256.
Bouroche, J.-M. 87, 212, 239.
Bowman, K. O. 56, 239,
Box, G. E. P. 21, 40, 60, 61, 62, 161, 167, 181, 186, 228, 230, 239, 240.
Bradley, R. I. 202, 260.
Bradu, D. D. 87, 240.
Brady, H. E. 124, 240.
Breiman, L. 198, 240.
Bremner, J. M. 116, 238.
Brothwell, D. R. 2, 240.

Brown, P. J. 5, 180, 181, 240, 243, 263.
Brunk, H. M. 116, 238.
Buck, S. F. 16, 240.
Burley, J. 91, 245.
Butler, S. 3, 15, 266.

Cailliez, F. 108, 145, 211, 240.
Campbell, N. A. 68, 69, 73, 240.
Carroll, J. D. 117, 121, 122, 124, 125, 161, 198, 210, 240, 261, 263, 265.
Carroll, R. M. 137, 260.
Carter, E. M. 172, 262.
Casella, G. 155, 240.
Cattell, R. B. 83, 137, 241, 250.
Cavalli-Sforza, L. L. 138, 244.
Chambers, J. M. 38, 43, 198, 239, 241.
Chang, J. J. 121, 122, 240.
Chang, T. C. 168, 231, 240, 254.
Chatfield, C. 35, 241.
Chattopadhyay, A. K. 231, 261.
Chauhan, J. 106, 122, 126, 241.
Chen, C. F. 151, 241.
Chen, H. 99, 241.
Chernoff, H. 3, 47, 49, 50, 241.
Chew, V. 188, 241.
Clark, C. E. 32, 241.
Cleveland, W. S. 43, 46, 198, 241.
Cliff, N. 121, 137, 241.
Cohen, A. M. 153, 241.
Cohen, H. S. 125, 161, 265.
Collins, A. J. 9, 141, 142, 237, 253.
Connor, R. J. 29, 30, 241.
Constantine, A. G. 125, 126, 146, 235, 241.
Cook, R. D. 55, 241.
Copas, J. C. 3, 237.
Corbet, G. B. 2, 114, 242.
Cordeiro G. M. 228, 242.
Cormack, R. M. 11, 242.
Cornish E. A. 27, 242.
Cox, D. R. 21, 36, 42, 52, 60, 61, 62, 228, 238, 239, 240, 242.
Critchley, F. 182, 242, 243.
Crowder, M. J. 149, 242.
Cummins, J. 2, 114, 242.
Cutts, J. F. 153, 241.

D'Agostino, R. B. 56, 242.
Das Gupta, S. 71, 164, 242.
Davidson, M. L. 189, 232, 257.
Davis, A. W. 140, 242.
Davison, A. C. 160, 242.
De Boor, C. 198, 242.
De Bruijn, N. G. 153, 242.
De Falguerolles, A. 134, 264.
De Leeuw, J. 112, 117, 122, 125, 134, 206, 207, 208, 210, 216, 239, 242, 243, 263, 264, 266.
Dempster, A. P. 17, 168, 243.
Denham, M. C. 5, 181, 240. 243.
Desbois, D. 92, 244.
Devlin, S. J. 66, 67, 243.
De Waal, D. J. 39, 243.
Diaconis, P. 156.
DiCiccio, T. J. 159, 243.
Dickey, J. M. 151, 243.
Diggle, P. J. 149, 243.
Doksum, K. A. 61, 239.
Dransfield, M. 153, 262.
Draper, N. R. 61, 243, 251.
Duncan, D. B. 161, 188, 243.
Dunn, G. 3, 244.
Dunnett, C. W. 25, 243.
Dyer, A. R. 56, 243.
Dykstra, R. L. 71, 243.

Eastment, H. T. 83, 84, 243.
Eaton, M. L. 71, 243.
Eckart, C. 87, 111, 121, 243.
Edwards, A. W. F. 138, 243, 244.
Edwards, D. 36, 191, 244.
Efron, B. 124, 159, 244.
Ehrenberg, A. S. C. 35, 241.
Embrechts, P. 49, 244.
Escoufier, Y. 137, 259.
Eslava-Gomez, G. 92, 96, 244.
Etezadi-Amoli, J. 198, 244.
Evans, I. G. 151, 244.
Everitt, B. S. 3, 173, 244.

Fang, K-T. 27, 28, 29, 149, 150, 173, 174, 244.
Fargette, D. 92, 244.
Fauquet, C. 92, 244.
Feller, W. 37, 245.
Fenlon, J. S. 2, 245.
Ferguson, T. S. 54, 245.

Fernandez de la Reguera, P. A. 76, 90, 91, 245.
Fielder, R. 153, 241.
Fienberg, S. E. 48, 50, 245.
Fisher, R. A. 129, 225, 235, 245.
Flannery, B. P. 102, 258.
Fleishman, E. A. 3, 245.
Flury, B. 47, 82, 171, 196, 245.
Foster, F. G. 231, 245.
Freund, J. E. 31, 245.
Frick, H. 223, 246.
Friedman, H. P. 46, 261.
Friedman, J. H. 94, 95, 97, 99, 100, 198, 240, 246.

Gabriel, K. R. 87, 127, 189, 200, 240, 246.
Gains, N. 142, 143, 246.
Galambos, J. 38, 246.
Gelfand, A. E. 154, 155, 246.
Gellatt, C. D. 102, 251.
Geman, D. 155, 246.
Geman, S. 155, 246.
George, E. I. 155, 240.
Geweke, J. 154, 246.
Gifi, A. 120, 203, 204, 205, 207, 208, 209, 210, 211, 246.
Giri, N. C. 167, 246.
Gittens, R. 90, 246.
Gnanadesikan, R. 21, 51, 52, 55, 57, 58, 60, 61, 63, 64, 66, 67, 72, 182, 195, 196, 237, 243, 246, 247, 260, 265.
Goldstein, L. 85, 248.
Goldwyn, R. M. 46, 261.
Gong, G. 124, 159, 244.
Goodall, C. R. 6, 80, 137, 141, 247, 256.
Goodchild, N. A. 45, 71, 247.
Goodhardt, G. J. 35, 241.
Goodman, L. A. 127, 129, 247.
Gordon, A. D. 106, 247.
Gower, J. C. 44, 86, 94, 106, 107, 108, 109, 110, 125, 126, 134, 137, 141, 142, 145, 146, 201, 202, 219, 241, 247, 248.
Gratton, R. J. 149, 243.
Green, B. F. 136, 137, 248.
Green, P. J. 6, 238.
Greenacre, M. J. 86, 127, 128, 129, 133, 134, 146, 248.
Gruvaeus, G. T. 137, 248.
Gupta, A. K. 228, 231, 258.
Guttman, I. 29, 263.
Guttman, L. 117, 209, 248.

Hadi, A. S. 55, 248.
Hall, P. 160, 161, 248.
Hand, D. J. 15, 248.
Harary, F. 114, 248.
Harding, S. A. 201, 202, 219, 247.
Härdle, W. 99, 248.
Harper, R. 106, 122, 126, 241.
Harris R. J. 231, 233, 248.
Harshman, R. A. 85, 248.
Hartigan, J. A. 3, 46, 47, 248, 252.
Hartley, H. O. 184, 223, 228, 230, 231, 258.
Hastie, T. 196, 197, 198, 217, 219, 248.
Hastings, W. K. 154, 248.
Hawkins, D. M. 50, 52, 53, 54, 55, 72, 241, 248.
Healy, M. J. R. 47, 52, 57, 187, 238, 248, 254.
Heck, D. L. 231, 249.
Hedges, S. R. 2, 114, 242.
Heiser, W. J. 117, 134, 137, 202, 204, 207, 216, 219, 242, 249, 256, 264.
Hempel, W. E. 3, 245.
Hensler, G. L. 58, 249.
Hernandez, F. 61, 249.
Herzberg, A. M. 49, 244.
Heyde, C. C. 152, 249.
Higham, C. F. W. 12, 249.
Hill, M. O. 129, 133, 249.
Hinkley, D. V. 61, 159, 160, 242, 249.
Hinton, G. E. 103, 260.
Hirotsu, C. 127, 249.
Hogg, R. V. 66, 249.
Holgate, P. 35, 249.
Holtsmark, J. 37, 249.
Hong, Z.-Q. 110, 249.
Horan, C. B. 121, 249.
Horst, P. 91, 249.
Hotelling, H. 75, 223, 231, 250.
Householder, A. S. 109, 266.
Hsu, J. S. J. 151, 254.
Hsu, P. L. 231, 235, 250.

Hsu, Y. S. 233, 258.
Huber, P. J. 66, 250.
Hudson, W. N. 38, 250.
Hunter, W. G. 61, 243.
Hurley, J. R. 137, 250.

Ito, K. 170, 173, 250.
Izenman, A. J. 100, 250.
Jackson, J. E. 82, 83, 250.
Jacob, R. J. K. 50, 250.
Jambu, M. 133, 250.
James, A. T. 235, 236, 250.
James, G. S. 172, 250.
James, W. 150, 251.
Janikow, C. Z. 103, 256.
Jayachandran, K. 186, 232, 258.
Jee, R. 96, 251.
Jeffers, J. N. R. 84, 251.
Jeffreys, H. 161, 251.
Jensen D. R. 28.
Jernigan, R. W. 172, 256.
John, J. A. 61, 251.
Johnson, N. L. 28, 29, 31, 34, 251, 252.
Johnson, R. A. 61, 157, 158, 159, 175, 249, 251.
Johnson, R. M. 117, 251.
Johnstone, I. M. 152, 249.
Joiner, B. L. 55, 260.
Jolicoeur, P. 79, 251.
Jolliffe, I. T. 82, 84, 134, 251, 257.
Jones, D. E. 153, 241.
Jones, M. C. 15, 95, 251.
Juang, B. H. 5, 251.

Kadane, J. B. 153, 263.
Kaiser, H.F. 104, 251.
Kass, R. E. 153, 263.
Katiyar, R. S. 168, 255.
Kendall, D. G. 80, 120, 251.
Kendall, M. G. 3, 251.
Kendall, W. S. 80, 251.
Kent, J. T. 36, 57, 83, 108, 110, 145, 157, 163, 164, 167, 175, 176, 184, 223, 226, 255.
Kettenring, J. R. 51, 52, 66, 67, 72, 91, 182, 210, 243, 246, 251.
Khatri, C. G. 39, 251.
Kijngam, A. 12, 249.
Kim, H. 134, 252.
Kirkpatrick, S. 102, 252.
Kleiner, B. 43, 46, 47, 241, 252.
Korin, B. P. 166, 168, 230, 252.
Kotz, S. 27, 28, 29, 31, 34, 244, 252.
Koutras, M. 27, 252.
Krishnaiah, P. R. 168, 231, 252, 254, 260.
Kristof, W. 141, 252.
Krusińska, E. 191, 252.
Kruskal, J. B. 94, 111, 116, 117, 253.
Krzanowski, W. J. 2, 17, 27, 81, 82, 83, 84, 106, 114, 122, 126, 138, 139, 142, 143, 161, 174, 175, 240, 241, 242, 243, 246, 253, 256.

Ladefoged, P. 85, 248.
Laird, N. M. 17, 243.
Langron, S. P. 141, 142, 143, 253, 265.
Lawley, D. N. 168, 228, 231, 253.
Layard, M. W. J. 173, 253.
Le Cam, L. 152, 253.
Lee, J. C. 168, 231, 252, 254.
Lee, P. 161, 254.
Leech, F. B. 187, 254.
Legendre, P. 106, 107, 108, 145, 248.
Lehman, E. H. 162, 226, 254.
Lenth, R. V. 223, 224, 254.
Leonard, T. 151, 254.
Leurgans, S. 122, 254.
Lewis, T. 50, 238.
Lévy, P. 36, 37, 254.
Li, H. W. 183, 254.
Liddell, G. F. 172, 259.
Lin, C. T. 168, 257.
Lin, T. N. 183, 254.
Lindley, D. V. 151, 152, 153, 243, 254.
Lindsey, J. K. 61, 254.
Lingoes, J. C. 108, 117, 133, 145, 239, 254.
Linnet, K. 61, 254.
Lipton, S. 47, 238.
Little, R. J. A. 17, 239, 254.
Lohr, S. L. 25, 254.
Love, W. 192, 262.
Lubischew, A. A. 172, 254.
Lukacs, E. 37, 254.

Malkovich, J. F. 58, 97, 254.
Mallows, C. L. 38, 99, 241, 254.

Mandelbrot, B. 37, 255.
Manly, B. F. J. 12, 61, 118, 172, 174, 249, 255, 259.
Marco, V. R. 266.
Mardia, K. V. 36, 57, 58, 83, 108, 110, 111, 145, 157, 163, 164, 167, 173, 174, 175, 176, 184, 186, 223, 226, 255.
Mark, H. L. 3, 255.
Maronna, R. A. 67, 255.
Marriott, F. H. C. 11, 91, 96, 245, 255.
Mason, J. D. 38, 250.
Marshall, A. W. 31, 255.
Mathai, A. M. 168, 255.
Maung, K. 129, 255.
McBratney, A. B. 3, 265.
McCabe, G. P. 84, 255.
McCullagh, P. 34, 255.
McCulloch, W. W. 102, 255.
McDermott, M. 58, 257.
McDonald, R. P. 198, 244.
McGee, V. E. 121, 255.
McKay, R. J. 190, 192, 256.
McPherson, C. K. 3, 237.
McReynolds, W. O. 3, 256.
Mead, A. 121, 256.
Mehrotra, K. G. 58, 249.
Meng, C. J. 183, 254.
Messick, S. 121, 264.
Metropolis, N. 102, 154, 256.
Meulman, J. J. 125, 202, 203, 204, 207, 214, 215, 216, 217, 219, 243, 249, 256.
Michaelewicz, Z. 103, 256.
Michalek, J. E. 58, 249.
Miller, A. J. 224, 256.
Minsky, M. L. 103, 256.
Mitchell, A. F. S. 27, 256.
Modarres, R. 172, 256.
Moonen, M. 84, 256.
Moran, P.A.P. 31, 256.
Morrison, D. F. 79, 80, 256.
Mosier, C. I. 137, 256.
Mosimann, J. E. 29, 30, 79, 80, 241, 251, 256.
Moss, M. L. 6, 256.
Moss-Salentijn, L. 6, 256.
Mudholkar, G. S. 58, 168, 189, 232, 257.
Muirhead, R. J. 150, 162, 167, 171, 173, 236, 257.
Mulira, H.-M. 55, 182, 238.
Muller, M. E. 40, 240.
Munford, A. G. 61, 62.

Nagarsenker, B. N. 168, 171, 257.
Naylor, J. C. 153, 257, 262.
Nelder, J. A. 34, 255.
Newham, V. 3, 15, 266.
Ng, K-W. 27, 28, 29, 244.
Nishisato, S. 133, 257.
Null, C. H. 117, 266.

Obenchain, R. L. 30, 257.
Odell, P. L. 266.
O'Hagan, A. 147, 257.
Olkin, I. 31, 167, 168, 255, 257.
Olshen, R. A. 5, 198, 240, 257.
Ord, J. K. 7, 19, 22, 24, 37, 65, 127, 147, 162, 177, 178, 180, 181, 226, 227, 263.

Pack, P. 134, 257.
Pagès, J. P. 211, 240.
Papert, S. 103, 256.
Parker, D. B. 103, 257.
Pearson, E. S. 184, 223, 228, 230, 231, 257, 258.
Pearson, K. 23, 75, 258.
Peay, E. R. 142, 258.
Penrose, L. S. 79, 258.
Perlman, M. D. 71, 164, 242, 243.
Pickett, R. 46, 258.
Pillai, K. C. S. 39, 168, 186, 228, 231, 232, 233, 251, 257, 258.
Pitman, E. J. G. 186, 258.
Pitts, W. 102, 255.
Press, S. J. 38, 54, 151, 153, 154, 161, 174, 243, 258.
Press, W. H. 102, 258.
Pucciarelli, H. M. 6, 256.
Puri, M. L. 148, 259.

Rabiner, L. R. 5, 251.
Radley, D. 161, 253.
Raftery, A. E. 198, 199, 238.
Ramsay, J. O. 124, 207, 259, 265, 266.
Rao, C. R. 79, 87, 165, 187, 259.

Rayner, J. C. W. 172, 255. 259.
Rees, D. H. 231, 245.
Reinsch, C. 99, 259.
Rheigans, P. 44, 266.
Ribbans, J. 153, 241.
Rice, J. A. 5, 259.
Riedwyl, H. 47, 245.
Ripley, B. D. 6, 259.
Rizvi, M. H. 50, 241.
Robert, P. 137, 154, 156, 259.
Roberts, G. O. 262.
Rohlf, F. J. 58, 259.
Rollet, E. 23, 259.
Romano, J. P. 159, 243.
Romesburg, H. C. 118, 259.
Rosenblatt, F. 103, 259.
Rosenbluth, A. W. 102, 154, 256.
Rosenbluth, M. N. 102, 154, 256.
Rosenthal, J. S. 156.
Roskam, E. E. 117, 254.
Ross, J. 121, 259.
Ross, R. T. 122, 254.
Rothkopf, E. Z. 106, 259.
Rousseeuw, P. J. 54, 260.
Roy, S. N. 64, 97, 181, 228, 231, 235, 260.
Rubin, D. B. 17, 243, 254.
Rudeforth, C. C. 202, 260.
Rumelhart, D. E. 103, 260.
Ryan, B. F. 55, 260.
Ryan, T. A. 55, 260.

Sammon, J. W. 111, 260.
Sanghvi, L. D. 137, 260.
Saporta, G. 212, 239.
Schatzoff, M. 228, 231, 232, 260.
Schechtman, E. 160, 242.
Scheffé, H. 172, 188, 189, 230, 260.
Schervish, M. J. 25, 260.
Schmidli, H. 9, 94, 265.
Schoenberg, I. J. 108, 260.
Schönemann, P. H. 125, 137, 260.
Schroeder, A. 99, 100, 246.
Schull, W. J. 170, 250.
Schurrmann, F. J. 231, 261.
Schwerteman, N. C. 110, 261.
Seal, H. 170, 261.
Seber, G. A. F. 52, 54, 55, 108, 145, 150, 173, 231, 261.
Sen, K. 6, 256.
Sen, P. K. 148, 259.
Shapiro, S. S. 56, 58, 261.
Shaw, J. E. H. 153, 262.
Shen, S. M. 30, 237.
Shenton, L. R. 56, 239, 261.
Shepard, R. N. 116, 117, 198, 261.
Sheppard, W. F. 41, 261.
Shumway, R. H. 6, 261.
Sibson, R. 15, 95, 111, 116, 117, 137, 140, 142, 146, 251, 261.
Siegel, A. F. 46, 137, 261.
Silverman, B. W. 5, 15, 95, 198, 259, 261.
Silvey, S. D. 226, 262.
Siotani, M. 51, 54, 168, 257, 262.
Siskind, V. 226, 262.
Skalak, R. 6, 256.
Skene, A. M. 153, 262.
Small, N. J. H. 58, 242.
Smith, A. F. M. 153, 154, 155, 156, 246, 257, 262.
Smith, R. L. 153, 262.
Snedecor, G. W. 183, 262.
Southwell, R. V. 102, 262.
Spearman, C. 79, 86, 262.
Speed, T. P. 23, 262.
Spence, I. 117, 262.
Spiegelman, C. H. 5, 240.
Srivastava, M. S. 58, 64, 172, 173, 257, 260, 262.
Steel, R. G. D. 91, 262.
Stein, C. 150, 225, 251, 262.
Stevens, E. H. 168, 252.
Stewart, D. 192, 262.
Stigler, S. M. 150, 262.
Stone, C. J. 198, 240.
Stoyanov, J. M. 40, 263.
Stuart, A. 7, 19, 22, 24, 37, 65, 127, 147, 162, 177, 178, 180, 181, 226, 227, 263.
Stuart, E. 153, 241.
Stuck, B. W. 38, 241.
Stuetzle, W. 97, 99, 100, 196, 197, 198, 217, 219, 246, 248.
Styles, B. T. 76.
Subbaiah, P. 189, 232, 257.
Subrahmaniam, K. 172, 263.
Sundberg, R. 181, 263.

Sutherland, A. I. 6, 259.
Sutherland, D. H. 5, 257.
Sutradher, B. C. 28, 263.
Swain, P. H. 6, 263.

Taguri, M. 47, 264.
Takane, Y. 112, 117, 122, 124, 210, 216, 263, 266.
Tanner, M. A. 155, 263.
Teller, A. H. 102, 154, 256.
Teller, E. 102, 154, 256.
Ten Berge, J. M. F. 137, 141, 142, 263.
Tenenhaus, M. 208, 209, 263.
Teukolsky, S. A. 102, 258.
Thompson, D. W. 79, 263.
Thomson, D. M. H. 142, 143, 246.
Tiago de Oliveira, J. 32, 263.
Tiao, G. C. 29, 161, 240, 263.
Tibshirani, R. 159, 198, 244, 248.
Tierney, L. 153, 263.
Tiku, M. L. 164, 223, 264.
Titterington, D. M. 160, 264.
Tizard, J. 3, 15, 266.
Tomsky, T. L. 167, 257.
Torgerson, W. S. 109, 264.
Trivedi, M. C. 168, 257.
Tucker, L. R. 85, 121, 264.
Tukey, P. A. 43, 188, 241.
Tukey, J. W. 60, 95, 97, 246, 264.
Tunnell, D. 3, 255.

Van Bemmel, J. H. 5, 264.
Van Buuren, S. 217, 219, 264.
Van De Geer, J. P. 210, 264.
Van Den Wollenberg, A. L. 193, 264.
Van Der Burg, E. 210, 264.
Van Der Heiden, P. G. M. 134, 264.
Vandewalle, J. 84, 256.
van Dooren, P. 84, 256.
Van Rijckevorsel, J. L. A. 209, 264.
van Zomeren, B. C. 54, 260.
Vecchi, M. P. 102, 251.
Verboon, P. 137, 264.
Verdegaal, R. 210, 264.
Vetterling, W.T. 102, 258.
Vidal, G. 92, 244.
Vijayan, K. 45, 71, 247.
von Neuman J. 103, 264.

Waikar, V. B. 231, 261.
Wainer, H. 47, 264.
Wakimoto, K. 47, 264.
Warner, J. L. 21, 58, 60, 63, 64, 237,
Wasserman, P. D. 103, 265.
Waternaux, C. M. 173, 257.
Watson, G. S. 186, 198, 240, 265.
Webster, R. 3, 265.
Weihs, C. 9, 94, 161, 265.
Weinberg, S. L. 125, 161, 265.
Weinman, D. G. 31, 265.
Welch, B. L. 172, 265.
Werbos, P.J. 103, 265.
Wermuth N. 36, 42, 242.
White, B. W. 46, 258.
Whittaker, J. 18, 23, 36, 168, 191, 265.
Wichern, D. W. 157, 158, 159, 175, 251.
Wilk, M. B. 55, 56, 58, 195, 196, 247, 265.
Wilks, A. R. 43, 198, 239.
Wilks, S. S. 72, 168, 223, 230, 265.
Williams, A. A. 143, 265.
Williams, E. J. 181, 265.
Williams, R. J. 103, 260.
Wingersky, B. 141, 252.
Winsberg, S. 207, 265, 266.
Wish, M. 117, 253.
Wishart, J. 187, 224, 225, 266.
Wold, S. 83, 266.
Wong, W. 155, 263.
Wright, S. 9, 266.
Wyatt, M. P. 5, 257.

Yang, J.-Y. 110, 249.
Yao, Y. 172, 266.
Yenyukov, I. S. 95, 266.
Young, D. M. 266.
Young, F. W. 44, 112, 117, 122, 208, 209, 210, 216, 262, 263, 266.
Young, G. 87, 109, 111, 121, 243, 266.
Yule, G. U. 22, 266.
Yule, W. 3, 15, 266.

Zhang, Y-T. 27, 149, 150, 173, 174, 244.

Subject Index

allometry 79
all-subsets search 140
ALSCAL 112, 117, 122
alternating least squares 112, 117, 121, 204, 207
alternative hypothesis 13, 53, 162, 166, 168, 169, 173
analysis
  of covariance 182, 187
  of variance 13
    see also MANOVA
Andrews' curves 44
angles between subspaces 81, 99
association 14
atypicality 50

backward elimination 140
Bartlett decomposition 224
barycentre 109, 129, 130, 137
Behrens-Fisher problem 172, 183
bilinear model 122
biplots 86, 200
  nonlinear 200, 219
BMDP 91, 182, 189, 190
Bonferroni inequalities 188, 190
bootstrap, bootstrapping 16, 124, 159, 174
Burt matrix 134

calibration 180
Canberra metric 70
canonical
  decomposition 125
  variables 86, 88, 182, 185, 190, 192, 194, 233
  variate analysis 14, 47, 50, 192
central limit theorem 13, 16, 24, 33, 148, 159, 175, 178
  Bayesian 152
chemometrics 3
Chernoff faces 47
chi-square
  distance 128, 130, 131, 133
  test of association 127
Cholesky decomposition 225
classical scaling 109, 130
classification 14, 17, 89, 91
cluster analysis 11, 17, 21, 114, 204
  hierarchical 11
  nearest-neighbour 12
column profile 128, 132
common principal components 81, 171
computer-intensive methods 15, 159
conditional independence 23, 24, 168, 191
confidence region 13, 33, 45, 124, 156, 189, 221
  percentile 160
  simultaneous 157
conjugate prior 151, 226
consensus configuration 141

contingency table 1, 33, 87, 126, 133, 191
convex hull 160
coordinates 7, 121, 123, 132
correlation
  canonical 84, 89, 133, 192, 210
    nonlinear 210
  matrix 14, 23, 51, 77, 78, 86, 205
  multiple 22, 191
  partial 22, 168
correspondence analysis 32, 86, 131, 146, 208
  multiple 134, 208
covariance
  matrix 21, 26, 75, 88, 168
  selection models 168
  structure modelling 18
credible region 156, 161
cross-validation 16, 83
cumulant generating function 20, 24, 34
cumulants 20, 32, 96
Czekanowski coefficient 70

data
  categorical 16, 32, 86
  clustered 95
  compositional 29
  graphical representation of 43, 106, 127, 190
  mixed binary and continuous 35, 71
  ordering 50
  qualitative 16
  resampling 124, 159
  sphering 94
  standardised 51
  see also variables
data matrix 1, 7, 17, 43, 75, 83, 87, 133
  geometrical representation of 7, 8
dendrogram 11
density estimation
  kernel 15, 95
  projection pursuit 99
descriptive profiling 122
design matrix 86
deviance 33, 168
dilation 136, 141
discriminant analysis 14, 15, 17, 36, 91, 182, 187, 212, 224
discriminant function 91, 221
dispersion matrix 14, 61, 66, 169, 171
  see also correlation matrix, covariance matrix, variance matrix
dissimilarity 10, 69, 105, 214
  matrix 86, 106, 121, 145
distance 10, 51, 69, 214
  between multinomial populations 137
  chi-square *see* chi-square distance
  Euclidean *see* Euclidean distance
  Mahalanobis *see* Mahalanobis distance
distribution mixture 227
distributions, multivariate 19
  Bessel 28
  beta 39
  Cauchy 28, 38
  conditional 20, 25, 61, 154
  conditional Gaussian 36, 191
  discrete 32-35
  Dirichlet 28-30
  elliptical 26-28, 80, 148, 173, 174, 197
  gamma 31
  hypergeometric 33
  Laplace 28
  Liouville 29
  logistic-normal 30, 35
  marginal 20, 25, 31, 61
  matrix-value 39-40, 174
  multinomial 32, 174
  negative binomial 34
  normal 15, 24, 32, 38, 40, 53, 61, 95, 148, 151, 156, 163, 174, 221, 225, 229
  Poisson 34
  posterior 149, 150, 161
  prior 149, 150, 161
  rotated Laplace 26
  spherical 25, 197
  stable 36-39
  t 27
  T^2 28
  uniform on sphere 26
  Wishart 31, 39, 156, 224
    inverted 151, 174, 226
    non-central 225

distribution function 19
distribution theory 17, 19
dual scaling 133
dynamic graphics 44

eigenvalues, eigenvectors 65, 71, 75, 80, 83, 89, 109, 118, 126, 130, 132, 166, 169, 170, 181, 184, 192, 193, 196, 229, 231, 232, 233, 235
EM algorithm 17
entropy criterion 95, 104
error matrix 169, 182, 231, 235
estimation 13, 148
  interval 156
    simultaneous 157
  point 148
    Bayesian 151
  region 156
    Bayesian 161
    simultaneous 157
  robust *see* robust estimates
Euclidean
  configuration 107
  distance 45, 70, 86, 91, 105, 110, 128, 131, 144, 200, 214
  space 7, 214
expectation 20

factor analysis 15, 18, 75, 79, 80, 83, 86, 137
Fourier curves 44
free-choice profiling 143
function optimisation 100

Gauss-Markov theorem 178
generalised
  biplots 202
  principal components 195
  Procrustes analysis 141
  variance 192
genetic algorithms 16, 103
GENSTAT 71
Gibbs sampling 150, 154
Gifi system 204
glyphs 45
goodness-of-fit function 10, 110, 141
grand tour 94
graphical
  displays 43, 75, 120
  modelling 18, 23, 168, 191
graph theory 58, 114, 191
group stimulus space 121, 123
growth curves 85, 168, 182, 187
guided tour 44

Hellinger metric 96
Hessian matrix 153
heterogeneity 128, 232
heteroscedasticity 60
HOMALS 210
homogeneity 128
  analysis 204, 209
  of dispersions 171, 183, 227, 230
horseshoe effect 120
Hotelling's generalised T^2 54, 174
  see also distributions, T^2
hypothesis
  matrix 169, 231, 235
  test 13, 45, 52, 161
    for outliers 52

image analysis 6, 18, 153
importance sampling 153
imputation 16
indicator matrix 133, 207
individual differences 117, 120
INDSCAL 122, 123, 125
inertia 128
  principal 132
inference
  Bayesian 147
  frequentist 147
  non-parametric 147
  parametric 147
influence measures
  for correspondence analysis 134
  for principal components 52, 182
information index 95
inter-point distances 10
intraclass correlation 168

Jaccard coefficient 70, 145
jackknife, jackknifing 16, 124

kernel density estimation 15, 95
Kronecker product 39
kurtosis 41, 58, 97, 172, 186

Lagrange multiplier 75, 89, 164, 226
landmarks 6, 80
Laplace method 153
latent
  root *see* eigenvalue
  variables 15, 18
Lawley-Hotelling trace 181, 184, 185, 189, 231
least squares 177, 204, 216
likelihood 60, 65
  ratio statistic 33, 79, 83, 162, 163, 168, 169, 181, 184, 222, 226, 231
linear
  combination 15, 75, 86, 175, 189, 210, 225
  contrast 79
  model 13, 177, 179, 229
log-ratio analysis 30
loss
  function 149
  of consistency 209
  of discrimination 209
  of homogeneity 205, 209

Mahalanobis distance 70, 91, 105, 110, 140, 190, 214, 216, 221, 223
majorisation 216
MANOVA 54, 85, 181, 182, 222
  simultaneous inference in 187
matching
  coefficient 70
  configurations 134, 141
maximum likelihood estimates 60, 65, 102, 124, 148, 150, 152, 163, 166, 169, 226
MDS(X) 122
mean radial distance 96
M-estimates 67, 72
metric
  inequality 106
  property of proximity matrices 107
  scaling 108, 112, 124
minimum spanning tree 58, 114
MINITAB 55, 61
Minkowski metric 70
missing values 16, 70
moment
  generating function 20
  index 95
moments 20, 32, 152
Monte Carlo methods 16, 149, 153
  Markov chain 154
multidimensional
  scaling 11, 17, 85, 212, 214
  unfolding 125
multiple
  comparisons 14, 187
  tests 189
multivariate analysis of variance *see* MANOVA
multivariate kurtosis *see* kurtosis
multivariate skewness *see* skewness

neural networks 16, 18, 103, 153
nonadditivity 59
nonlinear
  canonical analysis 210, 211
  distance analysis 214
  mapping 202
  methods 15, 17, 195
non-metric scaling 115, 124, 214
normality of data 79, 80, 83, 148, 168, 172
  directional 63
  joint 61
  marginal 61
null hypothesis 13, 53, 57, 82, 127, 161, 163, 166, 168, 169, 173, 190, 226, 228

object scores 208
optimisation 11
ordination 17, 105, 202
orthogonal
  axis 7
  polynomial 187
  projection 196, 215
outliers and outlier detection 8, 50, 148, 182, 229
OVERALS 210

path analysis 18
parameter 6, 7, 51, 151, 223
  dispersion 51
  location 51
partial correlation 22, 168
perceptron model 103

permutational distributions, tests 16, 173
Pillai trace 181, 184, 185, 189, 231
point estimate 13
polar nearest neighbour 96
population 6, 13
  principal components 80
prediction sum of squares 84
principal axes 80, 110
principal component 193, 206, 219
  analysis 9, 15, 50, 75, 86, 110, 196
    nonlinear 195, 206
    three-mode 85
  coefficients 76
  loadings 85, 211
  rotation 80
  scores 76, 139, 206
principal coordinate analysis 86, 109, 145
principal curves 196
principal inertia 132
probability model 13
probability plotting 52, 55, 57, 64
Procrustes
  analysis 80, 84, 134
    generalised 141
  rotation 135
  statistic 136, 139
projection 8, 9, 14, 44, 47, 64, 75, 92, 110
  criteria 92, 99
  pursuit 64, 85, 92
    density estimation 99
    regression 97
  stereographic 138
proximity 106
  matrix 106, 120
    asymmetric 125

quadratic
  approximation 215
  form 156
quadrature 155
quantification of categories 208

rank order proximities 116
reciprocal averaging 133
reduced rank approximation 87, 110
redundancy
  index 192
  variables 193
regression 13, 17, 21, 25, 76, 89, 111, 133, 182, 222, 226
  diagnostics 182
  isotonic 207
  nonparametric 16, 97
  partial 22
  polynomial 207
reification 9, 76
reflection
  of configurations 135, 141
repeated measures analysis 18, 39, 85, 168, 182, 187
residuals
  in linear model 177, 179, 227
  in metric scaling 114
  Pearsonian 131
risk function 149
robust estimates 148, 229
  of dispersion 66, 78
  of location 52, 66
  of scale 52, 66
robustness 27, 172, 233
  of classical scaling 111
rotation
  of configurations 135, 141
row profile 128, 132
Roy's largest root 54, 181, 185, 189, 231

sample 7
sampling distributions 17, 148, 156
SAS 112, 117, 122, 182
scaling 78
  dual 133
  individual difference 121
  metric (classical) 112, 138, 201, 214
  non-metric 115, 214
  three-way 121
  weighted classical 130
scatter diagrams 43, 46, 92
scatterplot smoother 197
scree plot 83, 111
selection of variables 82, 139, 189, 190
sensory data 120, 143
seriation 120
similarity 69, 105, 122
  matrix 106

simulated annealing 102
singular value decomposition 17, 76, 86, 87, 122, 132, 135, 200
size and shape 6, 10, 29, 77, 79, 137
skewness 58, 97, 173, 186
skew-symmetric matrix 125, 146
smoothing 95, 97, 197
spectral decomposition 109, 126
spectroscopic data 3, 181
sphericity test 83, 166
spline smoothing 16, 198
SPSS 86, 91, 182, 189, 190, 210, 228
standardisation 21, 70, 78
stars 46
steepest descent 100, 111
stepwise selection 191
stochastic optimisation 102
SSTRESS 112, 117, 215, 216
STRAIN 215, 216
STRESS 112, 116, 216
subspace 44
substitution sampling 154
sufficient statistics 65

Taylor series expansion 152, 153
test of
  dimensionality 233
  dispersions
    multi sample 171
    single sample 166
  equicorrelation 168
  isometry 79
  means
    multi sample 169
    single sample 163
    two sample 170, 221
  normality 55, 97
  sphericity 83, 166
test statistic 13, 172, 232
  see also Lawley-Hotelling trace, likelihood ratio, Pillai trace, T^2 statistic, Roy's largest root, Wilks' lambda
three-dimensional arrays 85
three-mode component analysis 85
three-way scaling 121
time series 6, 24, 39, 182
trace criterion 78, 92, 110, 181, 184, 185, 189
transformations 21, 30, 57, 59, 94, 105, 135, 138, 141, 203, 205, 215, 225
  Box-Cox 21, 60
translation
  of configurations 135, 141
trilinear model 122
trimming 66
T^2 statistic 54, 157, 164, 170, 186, 222
type one error 162, 188
type two error 162, 188

uniformly most powerful test 162
union-intersection tests 97, 164, 167, 168, 170, 181, 228

variables 1, 7, 18
  binary 1, 21, 32, 46, 178
  categorical 1, 70, 207
  dependent 177, 179
  dummy 178
  latent 15, 18
  nominal 209
  ordinal 209
  qualitative 10, 45
  quantitative 1, 10, 43, 45, 70, 177
variance matrix *see* covariance matrix
variance-covariance matrix *see* covariance matrix
varimax rotation 104

Wilks' lambda 54, 167, 170, 181, 184, 186, 189, 222, 231
within-group matrix 91